Communications
in Computer and Information Science   907

Commenced Publication in 2007
Founding and Former Series Editors:
Phoebe Chen, Alfredo Cuzzocrea, Xiaoyong Du, Orhun Kara, Ting Liu,
Dominik Ślęzak, and Xiaokang Yang

Editorial Board

More information about this series at http://www.springer.com/series/7899

Hongxiu Li · Ágústa Pálsdóttir
Roland Trill · Reima Suomi
Yevgeniya Amelina (Eds.)

Well-Being in the Information Society

Fighting Inequalities

7th International Conference, WIS 2018
Turku, Finland, August 27–29, 2018
Proceedings

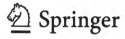
Springer

Editors
Hongxiu Li
Tampere University of Technology
Tampere
Finland

Reima Suomi
University of Turku
Turku
Finland

Ágústa Pálsdóttir
University of Iceland
Reykjavik
Iceland

Yevgeniya Amelina
Åbo Akademi University
Turku
Finland

Roland Trill
Fachhochschule Flensburg
Flensburg, Schleswig-Holstein
Germany

ISSN 1865-0929   ISSN 1865-0937 (electronic)
Communications in Computer and Information Science
ISBN 978-3-319-97930-4   ISBN 978-3-319-97931-1   (eBook)
https://doi.org/10.1007/978-3-319-97931-1

Library of Congress Control Number: 2018950433

This Springer imprint is published by the registered company Springer Nature Switzerland AG
The registered company address is: Gewerbestrasse 11, 6330 Cham, Switzerland

Preface

The present volume of the *Communications in Computer and Information Science* series includes revised versions of selected papers from the Well-Being in the Information Society (WIS 2018) conference, which took place in Turku in Finland, during August 27–29, 2018.

The WIS conference is a collaborative project of several universities, health institutes, and associations. It was organized by the University of Turku and the Baltic Region Healthy Cities Association – WHO Collaborating Centre for Healthy Cities and Urban Health in the Baltic Region, in co-operation with Åbo Akademi University, Tampere University of Technology, Turku University of Applied Sciences, and the Finnish National Institute for Health and Welfare.

The main theme of the conference this year was "Fighting inequalities." The outcomes of health and well-being are far from being equal for people, both across and within countries. To understand and address disparities in the health outcomes and in the distribution of health resources across population groups is not a new subject of concern. On the contrary, seeking ways to diminish, or preferably to eliminate, inequality in health and well-being across different groups has been a long-standing and ever-important challenge within the area of public health. The burden of inequality has a significant cost for both individuals and for society. Tackling it can therefore be seen as a fight for social justice and for better societies.

The focal point of the WIS conference has been from the beginning the use of information technology to promote equality in health and well-being. The subject has been approached from many different angles, with each participant bringing his or her point of view to it. Yet all of them have been working toward the same goal. That is, to address the question of how information technology can be used to remove the diverse barriers to good health and well-being that exist within society.

Information technology and the Internet have become a vital part of the daily lives of a great share of the population. This has in many respects brought about fundamental changes in the way that people work and conduct their private lives. For many, the adaption to these changes may be regarded as an achievement. This is the case for those who have been able to recognize the opportunities that technology may offer; who have had the capacity to embrace it and rise up to the challenge of taking it into their use. Others have not been as successful. It can even be said that information technology and digitalization have created negative effects for those groups in society who have been less fortunate at taking advantage of these new tools. The result is a digital divide that needs to be bridged if the aforementioned goal of using technology to bring about improvements that help in the fight for equality is to be achieved.

The WIS conference was now held for the seventh time. It started in 2006 and has since established itself as a biannual event. Throughout the years, we have had the pleasure of seeing the conference grow in maturity and strength, from taking its first steps in 2006, to this year reaching a stage in many ways similar to young adulthood.

A period in most people's lives characterized by interest and curiosity, brimming with questions touching upon the core of our existence, our purpose, and how we can attain the best quality of life. A period of daring and bold moves and uninhibited discussions, where unconventional opinions and looking outside the box are encouraged. And some of the questions that we ask, and the conclusions that we arrive at, may affect the directions that we take in life and how the future will unfold itself.

This is also how science must work. Science is about asking insightful questions that challenge the traditional way of thinking. It should also be about seeking answers that help to make advancements in the health and well-being of all groups within society. If progress is to be made, it is essential to be ready to look at things from new and innovative perspectives, and to have the courage to put forward unconventional viewpoints. To be ready to explore how other disciplines approach various matters, and to be willing to listen and learn from them. The WIS conference has allowed for the creation of a vibrant community of researchers and specialists that seek to do exactly this.

The success of the WIS conference can no doubt be in part attributed to its multidisciplinary nature. This has made it possible to bring together scientist and practitioners from several academic disciplines and professional specializations from around the world. The conference is a forum where participants meet and are given the opportunity to have thoughtful discussions about the gaps in information and knowledge of how disparities in health and well-being can be tackled. A forum where participants are given the possibility to share their current expertise and experiences and exchange their views on the latest developments within the field.

The WIS 2018 conference received a total of 42 submissions of which 45% were selected to be included in this volume through the review process. The selected papers reflect the diversity of the presentations, which were organized in two sessions.

The authors, who highlighted some important contributions to various areas of the conference theme, approached the matter in different ways. This includes papers on the advancement of digital competence and the use of information technology, by citizens in their everyday life, at the workplace, and to design new services. Others covered new and innovative ways to promote and manage human resources. A number of papers focused on how we can provide useful information and support to empower different groups within society, encouraging them to be involved in their own health, care, and well-being. In addition, papers considered the link between equality in health and well-being among different groups and the advancement of social justice and democracy.

A wide range of population groups were discussed in the papers. They covered citizens at all different age levels, from young children to elderly people. In addition, employees, managers, and professionals within the systems of health, welfare, and education, as well as those working in the business sector, were among the groups addressed.

Many people deserve thanks and acknowledgment for the hard work that they put into making this year's conference the success it has been. The event could not have taken place without the financial support of the Federation of Finnish Learned Societies, The Foundation for Economic Education, and Åbo Akademi University Foundation. We are deeply grateful to all for making our conference possible.

We would like to take this opportunity to give special thanks to the international keynote speakers, Isabel Ramos from the University of Minho in Portugal, whose lecture was titled "Augmented Collective Attention," Heikki Hiilamo from the University of Helsinki in Finland, who spoke about Debt as a "New Form of Inequality," Karen E. Fisher, from the University of Washington in United States, who gave a lecture about "Determinants of Information Poverty, Wealth, and Resilience in Refugee Camps: Effects of Gender, Place and Time," and Sascha Marschang from the European Public Health Alliance in Belgium, whose talk was entitled "Inclusive Digital Health in Europe: Opportunities and Gaps." All these keynote speakers come from different fields, each of them bringing their own unique experience and expertise. We feel both proud and privileged to have had the opportunity to host them at the conference.

Our thanks also go to the session chairs and all the authors and presenters of papers for their valuable contributions to the success of the conference and the publication of this volume. The papers all contribute to an understanding of the recent trends in research about how inequality can be fought.

Last but not least, our thanks go to the members of the Program Committee and external reviewers, who together with the program chairs invested their time generously in analyzing and assessing the papers to help ensure the quality of this publication.

It is our great pleasure and honor to present to the readers the outcome of the WIS 2018 conference. We hope that it will be an incentive to stimulate interest for further research about the fight against inequality in well-being.

July 2018

Reima Suomi
Ágústa Pálsdóttir
Roland Trill

Organization

WIS 2018 Organizing Committee

Reima Suomi (Conference Chair)	University of Turku, Finland
Hongxiu Li (Organizing Committee Chair)	Tampere University of Technology, Finland
Ágústa Pálsdóttir (Program Co-chair)	University of Iceland, Iceland
Roland Trill (Program Co-chair)	Flensburg University of Applied University, Germany
Jukka Kärkkäinen	The National Institute for Health and Welfare, Finland
Karolina Machiewicz	Baltic Region Healthy Cities Association, Finland
Marjut Putkinen	Turku University of Applied Sciences, Finland
Sanna Salanterä	University of Turku, Finland
Brita Somerkoski	University of Turku, Finland
Gunilla Widén	Åbo Akademi University, Finland

WIS 2018 Program Committee

Farhan Ahmed	Åbo Akademi University, Finland
Regis Cabral	FEPRO - Funding for European Projects, Sweden
Laurence Carmichael	The University of the West of England, UK
Wojceich Cellary	Poznan University of Economics, Poland
Preben Hansen	Stockholm University, Sweden
Sami Hyrynsalmi	Tampere University of Technology, Finalnd
Jonna Järveläinen	University of Turku, Finland
Ranjan Kini	Indiana University Northwest, USA
Stefan Klein	University of Münster, Germany
Peter Kokol	University of Maribor, Slovenia
Jani Koskinen	University of Turku, Finland
Winfried Lamersdorf	University of Hamburg, Germany
Hongxiu Li	University of Turku, Finland
Yong Liu	Aalto University School of Business, Finland
Thomas Mandl	University of Hildesheim, Germany
Hans Moen	University of Turku, Finland
Päivi Ovaskainen	University of Tuku, Finland
Agusta Palsdottir	University of Iceland, Iceland
Tero Päivärinta	Luleå University of Technology, Sweden
Niels Kristian Rasmussen	Ostfold County Council, Denmark
Kai Reimers	RWTH Aachen University, Germany
Alexander Ryjov	Moscow State University, Russia

Contents

E-health

Digital Society

Describing a Design Thinking Methodology to Develop Sustainable Physical Activity and Nutrition Interventions in Low Resourced Settings

Chrisna Botha-Ravyse[1,3](✉) [iD], Susan Crichton[2] [iD],
Sarah J. Moss[1] [iD], and Susanna M. Hanekom[3] [iD]

[1] Faculty of Health Sciences, Physical Activity,
Sport and Recreation Research Area, North-West University,
Potchefstroom 2531, SA, South Africa
chrisna.botha@nwu.ac.za
[2] Faculty of Education, University of British Columbia,
Kelowna V1V 1V7, Canada
[3] Center for Health Professions Education, North-West University,
Potchefstroom 2531, SA, South Africa

Abstract. The objective of the study is to describe how design thinking as a participatory process can be applied in determining how sustainable physical activity and nutrition interventions should be implemented in a low resourced community in South Africa. Physical inactivity is the 4th leading cause of mortality world-wide. Associated with inactivity, a high prevalence of obesity is reported. Evidence based research indicate that sustainable physical activity and nutrition interventions will reduce the burden of physical inactivity and obesity. Poverty, and its inherent lack of food security, further impacts the health of people living marginalized, increasingly urban lifestyles. The intent of the project is to change attitudes and behavior towards physical activity participation and nutrition choices. Design Thinking is typically implemented using a five-step process where the community is engaged with presenting the problem they experience, defining the problem, presenting solutions to the problem and finally developing a prototype in solving the problem they experience. The principle of the Design Thinking process is that the low resourced community holds part of the answer to the problem and has a desire to change their health. The proposed solutions, coming directly from the participants, are therefore considered viable. Once a desired prototype is developed and tested in the community, feasibility can be determined. The presence of these three factors, is expected to result in an innovation.

Keywords: Design thinking · Feasibility · Viability · Desirability
Innovation · Low-resourced communities · Physical activity · Nutrition

© Springer Nature Switzerland AG 2018
H. Li et al. (Eds.): WIS 2018, CCIS 907, pp. 3–13, 2018.
https://doi.org/10.1007/978-3-319-97931-1_1

1 Background

1.1 Introduction

More than five million premature deaths each year are caused by physical inactivity, making it one of the most significant contributors to the global burden of disease [1]. Research offers confirmation of the valuable effects of physical activity on psychological health and management of stress and burnout [2], but more importantly highlight the significance of physical activity in managing overall well-being, instead of just body weight [3]. Ding and Hu [4] conclude that encouraging physical activity and promoting a healthy diet are both equally essential to maintain a healthy body weight and diminish the risk of non-communicable Diseases (NCDs) and premature death. This paper aims to give a detailed representation of the methodology (grounded in the design thinking paradigm) we will implement in order to address physical inactivity and unhealthy eating in a low-resourced community in South Africa. We continue the first section with a brief sketch of the problem statement, followed by a concise listing of our aims and objectives in Sect. 2. In Sect. 3 we present design thinking and the theoretical framework in which we will carry out our future study, which flows into Sect. 4 where we offer a hypothetical application of our methodology. The last three sections of this paper are respectively dedicated to pitfalls, considerations and a succinct view of our future work in this study. Please be aware that this is not an empirical study, but rather a reflection and clarification of the methodology we are proposing for our future intervention activities.

1.2 Problem Statement

Physical inactivity and poor diet are associated with a wide range of non-communicable diseases (NCDs), which includes hypertension, stroke, coronary artery disease, type 2 diabetes mellitus, cancer and osteoporosis [5]. General physical inactivity results in the prevalence of a largely overweight population and this too is evident in South Africa, where obesity coexists with the less than sufficient levels of activity amongst the general population [6, 7]. Regular physical activity may also have other beneficial effects that provide protection against the development of NCDs, despite the already present primary risk factors [8]. The increased incidence of NCDs in South Africa accentuates the necessity to promote a healthy lifestyle through increased participation in physical activity and healthy eating habits [8]. It has been documented, however, that even though most people know that inactivity is a risk factor for heart disease, persons from low-resourced communities lack understanding on the execution, implementation, and management of physical activity [9]. This failure to change behavior is evidenced by the large number (57%) of South Africans that are treated with chronic prescription medication for conditions that are easily corrected through regular physical activity [10] and combined healthy eating [11].

Physical activity (PA), for obvious reasons, is featured in the World Health Organization's Global Action Plan for the Prevention and Control of NCDs 2013–2020 [12]. The plan informs public health policy and South-Africa has included this in their National Sport Plan of South Africa as one of the key performance areas [13]. Nearly one third of adults are inactive worldwide and there is an increased evidence-base on the associates and determinants of physical activity and effective interventions to increase PA [14]. There does however, remain a paucity in the evidence related to interventions in low and middle-income countries (LMICs). Multiple levels of impelling reasons are responsible for physical activity participation, or the lack thereof. These include individual, social, and environmental factors [6]. Individual factors such as (i) the need for confidence, (ii) motivation and time and (ii) environmental factors, including their physical neighborhood environments and safe accessibility to physical activity resources are all factors that individuals face and may hinder sustainable participation [15].

In one of our previous studies, a review focused specifically on physical activity implementation and healthy eating in South Africa [16], we concluded that research should focus on tactics that increase the knowledge of physical activity in the population and be linked with interventions to overcome barriers to activity. An advance toward being physically active should include education on how to be active with regards to duration, intensity, frequency and modalities of physical activity. Various physical activity programs have been implemented in South Africa, yet the level of physical activity in South African is at an average of 50% [12]. All previous interventions were based on solutions from the researchers with regards to increasing physical activity and implementing healthy nutrition. The aim of this paper is to describe the use of the Design Thinking process for developing sustainable PA and nutrition and to present the framework for how this study will be conducted. The Design Thinking process is based on the premise that communities know what they need, and the solution is also within them. The benefit of this approach in determining a sustainable physical activity and nutrition intervention is the fact that the community will form part of developing the solution and not just the researchers.

2 Research Objectives

The following objectives set for the study:

1. To describe the theoretical underpinning of design thinking;
2. To describe the Design Thinking process;
3. The design of a framework of Design Thinking in developing sustainable physical activity and nutrition interventions in low resourced communities.

3 The Process

3.1 The Theoretical Underpinning of Design Thinking

Collaborative design in software development is not a novel approach. One of the most used approaches, especially when it comes to software development for education purposes, McKenny's design cycle [17] is often used. However, although this and other similar approaches [18] include scope for context analysis and understanding the end user to help define the problem, they often neglect to explicitly direct researchers to actively engage the user community in defining the solution. Once again, creating a solution based on what researchers believe the users need, rather than a solution the user wants. This extends into the sustainability of research-designed interventions. That is, solutions which are wanted will be used, negating the novelty effect usage pattern of hypothesized interventions, described by high initial number of active users with a low retention rate going forward in time.

Design thinking on the other hand is a human-centered process honed at Stanford University's d.School [19]. This process is used in businesses, schools, organizations and numerous other settings to create change and foster innovation. Design thinking, as a process, encourages participants to develop a positive, proactive and optimistic stance toward addressing complex problems. Design thinking supports divergent, lateral thinking – thinking that promotes and encourages problem finding rather than quick, often short sighted, problem solving. Using design thinking, users come to realize it is possible "… to creatively attack the world's greatest problems and meet people's most urgent needs" [20].

Design thinking can be used to develop eight core abilities:

- Navigate ambiguity – ability to persist with the discomfort of not knowing
- Learn from others – ability to emphasize and embrace diversity
- Synthesize information – ability to make sense of information and find insight and opportunity
- Experiment rapidly – ability to quickly generate ideas in written, drawn or built forms
- Move between concrete and abstract – ability to move between needs, ideas, and define ideas
- Build and craft intentionally – ability to thoughtfully make or construct ideas into tangible, shareable forms
- Communicate deliberately – ability to form, capture and related stories, ideas, concepts, reflections and learnings to diverse audiences
- Design – ability to recognize a project as a design challenge and then decide on people, tools and techniques required to tackle it [19].

3.2   The Design Thinking Process

As described by d.School, Fig. 1 [19] illustrates the five steps of design thinking. These five distinct steps are Empathize, Define, Ideate, Prototype and Test. To determine the real problem a community experiences, an empathetic listener is needed to ask questions from the community to present the problem they are experiencing. The next step would be to clearly define the problem, as presented by the community. Through ideation, the community is then drawn into the process of supplying potential solutions to the problem they experience. The principle here, is that the answer to the problem lies within the person/people who have the problem. These steps are continuously repeated to make sure that correct information is obtained. Once a solution idea is formed, a prototype with regards to this solution can be developed. The community is then encouraged to further refine the prototype. This inclusive process of continuous refinement aims toward an iteratively improved prototype. Once a solution has been found, the testing of the prototype can be conducted.

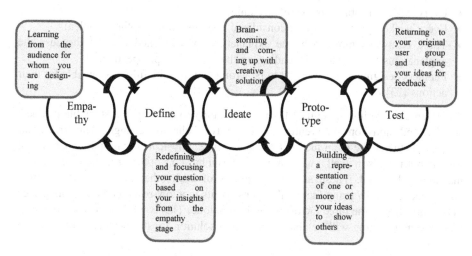

Fig. 1. The design thinking process (Adapted from: Stanford d.School)

Through the process of determining the problem based on the input of the community, we are in effect determining the desirable and desirability of exercise interventions and good nutrition within a low resourced community. Once this process is completed, it is important to understand the viability of the change that is about to take place. Therefore, the contribution of the community to the solution of the problem, makes the solution more acceptable with a high uptake and retention rate. When defining the problem and presenting with prototypes, the viability of the solutions is tested. The last step in the development of an innovation, is to conduct a larger-scale feasibility study with the uncovered prototype.

As a research methodology, design thinking can be found in the work of participatory design [21] and Collective Impact [22]. Both these approaches place the individuals being studied at the heart of the work and views them as participants in both the process and product. Both Participatory Design and Collective Impact include participants in all aspects of the research, from setting the research agenda and questions to determining metrics for evaluation and terms for data analysis.

Design thinking is well suited for research questions that are complex by nature and wicked. Wicked problems do not refer to mean problems, but rather to problems that seem impossible to solve – problems like many of the United Nations Sustainable Millennium Goals [23]. Ten characteristics of wicked problems include:

- There is no definitive formula for a wicked problem.
- Wicked problems have no stopping rule, as in there's no way to know your solution is final.
- Solutions to wicked problems are not true-or-false; they can only be good-or-bad.
- There is no immediate test of a solution to a wicked problem.

- Every solution to a wicked problem is a "one-shot operation"; because there is no opportunity to learn by trial-and-error, every attempt counts significantly.
- Wicked problems do not have a set number of potential solutions.
- Every wicked problem is essentially unique.
- Every wicked problem can be considered a symptom of another problem.
- There is always more than one explanation for a wicked problem because the explanations vary greatly depending on the individual perspective.
- Planners/designers have no right to be wrong and must be fully responsible for their actions [23].

When considering the aim of the research study to develop a sustainable physical activity and nutrition intervention will involve behavior change. This triangular interplay between the main factors behavior change, physical activity participation and healthy nutrition is in itself a wicked problem as it has no stopping rule and the solution may never be final. These are all symptoms of each other and an ever-changing environment with so many factors that participants in a low resourced community face this complexity of the three factors are indeed unique. This is why the researchers hope that Design Thinking will be able to provide a solution for this wicked problem.

4   Application of This Approach

The researchers identified the issues based on literature of developing and maintaining an active life style and improving nutrition amongst an identified low-income population in South Africa as wicked problems – problems without obvious and/or immediate solutions. The researchers recognized globally there have been numerous interventions "given" to low-income populations in the hope they would improve outcomes, change behaviors and address the risk of NCDs and premature death. A consistent finding of most of those interventions has been their inability to make sustained change [16].

As Einstein wisely noted, the definition of insanity is doing the same thing and expecting a different outcome. Keeping this in mind, the researchers turned to design thinking to create an iterative approach that focuses on problem finding, honoring participant voice, and ideation and iteration. The design thinking process allows researchers and participants to work together to create innovative ideas and possible interventions. The researchers suggest that it is through the ideation, prototyping and testing steps that Design Thinking comes into its own as a powerful, collaborative methodology, allowing participants to begin to make their thinking visible [24]. In a research context, prototyping can take the forms of storyboards of intervention steps or sketches of tools or resources [25].

As stated earlier, Design Thinking has five distinct steps. They do not need to be linear, and quite often, they are completed in a recursive way, moving from empathy to ideation to definition and re-definition to developing more empathy before prototyping promising ideas. To gain information with empathy, the researchers should identify (1) an initial set of open-ended questions (Fig. 1), and (2) identify the sectors of the population from which information should be gathered. Within the context of physical activity and nutrition, it is important to acknowledge that self-responsibility is a major factor in the development of sustainable interventions, therefore following the process with individuals from the community would be of importance. Other role players would be community health care workers that are employed by government to interact with the individuals in the community to ensure continuous interaction and health support.

To gain a clear understanding of what is happening in the community in question, field visits will be conducted. Table 1 gives a breakdown of how these principles will be applied in the community. In returning from the field visits, the researchers will begin to Define the challenges participants faced. This definition stage of the Design Thinking process encourages researchers to interrogate their assumptions based on the literature, their experiences and beliefs with the participants' comments and lived experiences from the participants. Based on the definition of the participant challenges, the researchers' can then begin the Ideation phase – the develop of potential solutions/interventions/ideas that might address the participant concerns. Ideas generated at this stage should be visualized by a medium that is both understandable and somewhat culturally sensitive to the community. For the low resource target community of this study, this would typically include storyboarding and graphical representations as opposed to online broadcasts that would be more suited to communities with a wider range of ICT possibilities. An example of this could be a frisbee with a visual plate model printed that will guide food selection and portion control but can also serve a plate. The storyboard and graphics would then be taken back to the community for their feedback, critique and ideation as well.

Table 1. A design thinking framework for low resourced communities

Design thinking steps	Application	Consolidation actions
Empathize	Interviews, focus groups and workshops to better understand the problem and desired solutions ***Initial target information from HCW:*** • Investigate working conditions and obtain possible improvements • Understand the perceived level of technology experience and competence ***Initial target information from community:*** • Current interaction with HCWs; • Understand their relationship with nutrition and physical activity • Determine their willingness to use mobile technology	Confirm findings with additional groups

(*continued*)

Table 1. (*continued*)

Design thinking steps	Application	Consolidation actions
Define	Synthesize all individual data gathering efforts into an inclusive and well-defined problem set *Hypothetical example:* Mobile solutions should be on simplified devices	Begin to develop initial ideas and confirm them with the participants
Ideate	Add detail to the ideas and relay them to the participants as workable solutions *Hypothetical example:* Application should be icon-driven as opposed to a textual interface	Work with participants to integrate participant ideation with researcher ideas
Prototype	• Before actual prototyping, develop comprehensive design principles to guide all further development • Commence storyboarding the solution content (be cognizant that **content** can be repurposed for multiple application modes) *Hypothetical example:* The logical order of icon selection starts with icon x, followed by icon y...	Take storyboards back to participants for their critique
Test	Allow participants to have a hands-on experience with the prototype *Hypothetical example:* Return to the field with a mock-up of the mobile application	Monitor participant engagement with prototype solution in the areas of: • Usage • Skill development; and • Behavior change Refine prototype as needed

5   Potential Pitfalls and Challenges and How to Overcome Them

Using Design Thinking as a methodology to gather data from low-resourced communities will most certainly not be without challenges and pitfalls. There are several factors that researchers will have to keep in mind. Firstly, language and culture might play a role and could influence the answers given by the participants. Making use of students that know the context well and speak the language of the people in the community will also help to eliminate some of the issues surrounding cultural differences. A fourth factor could be that researchers may be faced with distinct community groups who experience their environment differently, resulting in potentially conflicting data. The more traditional way to combat this is to ensure that you have a fully representative (and homogenous) community group. The risk however, is that you may encounter social structures where the more influential groups will drive the conversation and as a result, bias the data. With design thinking, researchers should rather keep different community groups apart and synthesize their data with background and context perceptions deeply considered. Physical problems such as hearing, whether by physiological or outside influencers, could influence the discussions. However, Design Thinking manages to curb communication interference in that the information the researchers thought the participants said should be sound boarded back to them before proceeding into the next phase. This will quickly determine any misinformed issues.

6 Considerations

Researchers are often influenced by external drivers into shaping a solution that fits greater international streams. For instance, one of the goals of the WHO is to make use of mobile technology to empower community members, especially those that cannot get to a clinic due to distance. As researchers we should identify where and how mobile technology could be incorporated into the current situation and provide this as a part of the scope definition when approaching the community. It is paramount though, in a Design Thinking approach, that community members are aware of this scope right from the outset. For example, this mobile approach could support the performance of health care workers. This can be attained by the distribution of clinical updates, learning materials, and reminders [26]. The use of mobile technologies may further enable health care providers to aid patients to improve their health in real time, empowering them to personalize their health care options and monitor their progress [27].

Having said all that it is important to remember that technology can be defined as the application of scientific knowledge for practical purposes, especially in industry [28]. This could mean that our idea of the technology our target community needs may differ from what they actually want. It might just be that a different type of technology could be more successful with them such a flyer or a booklet. Design Thinking does not tolerate the trivialization of community wants, but to remain sensitive to international drives, the best solution should incorporate both possibilities—a booklet augmented with a mobile platform perhaps.

We conclude that a Design Thinking Process is well-suited to tackling our wicked problem of decreasing the incidence of physical inactivity and poor nutritional habits in low-resourced communities. We foresee that Design Thinking is likely to bring alternative innovations and ideas to the table that are within the wants, rather than needs, of the community. Continued investigation of these innovations by means of a prototype will shape the outcome of the study through directing the very technologies being used to reach the outcomes of the study. Throughout the research journey, Design Thinking will continuously remind us that the best technology is the one most likely to bring forth a change in behavior. That is, the technology the community wants.

7 Future Work

This paper gives a theoretical background physical activity and nutrition intervention as a wicked problem. It describes the process of Design Thinking and presents the framework that will be used by the researchers to implement this process in their research. Report on the results gathered, the process of implementation and the prototyping that was created will be presented in future papers. Furthermore, once the prototype is accepted and approved by the community it will be developed to be a working application and then implemented and tested. The intervention will be followed for 1 year after the researchers are no longer involved to determine sustainability. Results on the success of the intervention will be reported.

References

1. Lee, I.M., Shiroma, E.J., Lobelo, F., Puska, P., Blair, S.N., Katzmarzyk, P.T.: Effect of physical inactivity on major non-communicable diseases worldwide: an analysis of burden of disease and life expectancy **380**, 219–229 (2012). https://doi.org/10.1016/s0140-6736(12)61031-9
2. Bradshaw, D., et al.: Provincial mortality in South Africa, 2000-priority-setting for now and a benchmark for the future **95**, 496–503 (2005)
3. Edwards, S.D., Ngcobo, H.S., Edwards, D.J., Palavar, K.: Exploring the relationship between physical activity, psychological well-being and physical self-perception in different exercise groups **27**, 75–90 (2005)
4. Ding, E.L., Hu, F.B.: Commentary: Relative importance of diet vs physical activity for health (2009). https://doi.org/10.1093/ije/dyp348
5. Reddy, S., et al.: Umthente Uhlaba Usamila-the 2nd South African national youth risk behaviour survey 2008 (2010)
6. Pratt, M., Perez, L.G., Goenka, S., Brownson, R.C., Bauman, A., Sarmiento, O.L., Hallal, P.C.: Can population levels of physical activity be increased? Global Evid. Experience **57**, 356–367 (2015). https://doi.org/10.1016/j.pcad.2014.09.002
7. De Vos, J.C.W., Du Toit, D., Coetzee, D.: The types and levels of physical activity and sedentary behaviour of Senior Phase learners in Potchefstroom **21**, 372–380 (2016). https://doi.org/10.1016/j.hsag.2016.06.005
8. Von Ruesten, A., Weikert, C., Fietze, I., Boeing, H.: Association of sleep duration with chronic diseases in the European Prospective Investigation into Cancer and Nutrition (EPIC)-Potsdam study **7**, e30972 (2012)
9. Moss, S.J., Lubbe, M.S.: The potential market demand for biokinetics in the private health care sector of South Africa **23**, 14–19 (2011)
10. Pedersen, B.K., Saltin, B.: Evidence for prescribing exercise as therapy in chronic disease **16**, 3–63 (2006)
11. Steyn, K., Fourie, J., Temple, N.: Chronic Diseases of Lifestyle in South Africa: 1995 – 2005. South African Medical Research Council, Cape Town (2006)
12. World Health Organization: Global action plan for the prevention and control of noncommunicable diseases 2013–2020, Report no. 9241506237 (2013)
13. DOSR: 'National Sport and Recreation Plan: National Sport and Recreation Plan', Department of Sport and Recreation (2016)

14. Bauman, A.E., Reis, R.S., Sallis, J.F., Wells, J.C., Loos, R.J., Martin, B.W., Lancet Physical Activity Series Working Group: Correlates of physical activity: why are some people physically active and others not? **380**, 258–271 (2012)
15. Mama, S.K., McCurdy, S.A., Evans, A.E., Thompson, D.I., Diamond, P.M., Lee, R.E.: Using community insight to understand physical activity adoption in overweight and obese African American and Hispanic women a qualitative study, **42**, 321–328 (2015)
16. Botha, C.R., Moss, S., Kolbe-Alexander, T.: "Be active!" revisiting the South African food-based dietary guideline for activity **26**, S18–S27 (2013)
17. McKenney, S., Nieeven, N., Van den Akker, J.: Educational design research. In: Van den Akker, J., Mckenney, S., Nieeven, N. (eds.) Design Research from a Curriculum Perspective, pp. 67–90. Routledge, Abingdon (2006)
18. Berthet, E.T., Barnaud, C., Girard, N., Labatut, J., Martin, G.: How to foster agroecological innovations? A comparison of participatory design methods, **59**, 280–301 (2016)
19. https://dschool.stanford.edu/resources/getting-started-with-design-thinking. Accessed 12 Feb 2018
20. Hatch, M.: The Maker Movement Manifesto: Rules for Innovation in the New World of Crafters, Hackers, and Tinkerers. McGraw Hill Professional, New York (2013)
21. Sharma, T., Mishra, P., Tiwari, R.: Designite-A Software Design Quality Assessment Tool, pp. 1–4. IEEE (2016)
22. Kania, J., Kramer, M.: Collective Impact. Stanford Social Innovation Review, New York (2011)
23. Weber, E.P., Khademian, A.M.: Wicked problems, knowledge challenges, and collaborative capacity builders in network settings **68**, 334–349 (2008)
24. Eisner, E.W.: The kind of schools we need: personal essays. ERIC (1998)
25. Buchenau, M., Suri, J.F.: Experience prototyping. In: Buchenau, M., Suri, J.F. (eds.) Book Experience Prototyping, pp. 424–433. ACM (2000)
26. Strachan, D.L., et al.: Interventions to improve motivation and retention of community health workers delivering integrated community case management (iCCM): stakeholder perceptions and priorities **87**, 111–119 (2012). https://doi.org/10.4269/ajtmh.2012.12-0030
27. Handel, M.J.: mHealth (Mobile Health)—Using Apps for Health and Wellness **7**, 256–261 (2011). http://dx.doi.org/10.1016/j.explore.2011.04.011
28. http://www.dictionary.com/. Accessed 28 Mar 2018

Behavioral Interventions from Trait Insights

Ulla Gain$^{(\boxtimes)}$, Mikko Koponen, and Virpi Hotti

School of Computing, University of Eastern Finland, 70211 Kuopio, Finland
{gain,virpi.hotti}@uef.fi, mikko@student.uef.fi

Abstract. Individuals have the stated and unstated beliefs and intentions. The theory of planned behavior is expressed by the mathematical function where beliefs have empirically derived coefficients. However, personality traits can help account for differences in beliefs. In this paper, we will find out how we can amplify behavioral interventions from text-based trait insights. Therefore, we research techniques (e.g., sentence and word embedding) behind text-based traits. Furthermore, we exemplify text-based traits by 52 personality characteristics (35 dimensions and facets of Big Five, 12 needs and five values) and 42 consumption preferences via API of the IBM Watson™ Personality Insights service. Finally, we discuss the possibilities of behavioral interventions based on the personality characteristics and consumption preferences (i.e., text-based differences and similarities between the individuals).

Keywords: Behavior · Belief · Intention · Insight · Personality trait

1 Introduction

Individual insights challenge our privacy. The GDPR (The General Data Protection Regulation) is setting the controllers and the processors to be responsible when they process the personal data "relating to an identified or identifiable individual" [1]. Personal data have been collected with and without consents of the humans that either identified or directly or indirectly identifiable natural persons (i.e., data subjects) [2]. For example, personal interests derived from tracking the use of internet web sites, personal or behavioral profile, and religious or philosophical beliefs can be used to identify the natural person [3]. Psychographics data (e.g., attitudes, interests, personality, and values) are used to fashion individually-targeted actions. For example, the Cambridge Analytica classified personalities according to the OCEAN scale (Openness, Conscientiousness, Extroversion, Agreeableness, and Neuroticism) and fashioned individually-targeted messages [4].

The intentions are the immediate determinants of behavior. It is possible to predict intentions the regressions of which are based on three independent determinants (i.e., attitude toward the behavior, subjective norm, and perceived behavioral control) of the intentions. The theory of planned behavior is expressed by the mathematical function $BI = a * AB + b * SN + c * PBC$ (where BI = behavioral intention, AB = attitude toward behavior, SN = social norm, PBC = perceived behavioral control, a, b and c = empirically derived weights/coefficients). The coefficients of the regressions are

© Springer Nature Switzerland AG 2018
H. Li et al. (Eds.): WIS 2018, CCIS 907, pp. 14–27, 2018.
https://doi.org/10.1007/978-3-319-97931-1_2

defined for the intentions of different kinds such as using cannabis, donating blood, buying stocks and engaging in leisure activities [5].

Background factors can help account for differences in beliefs. The background factors are divided into three groups. Personal factors are general attitudes, personality traits, values, emotions and intelligence. Social factors are age, gender, race, ethnicity, education, income and religion. Information factors are experience, knowledge and media exposure [5].

Behavioral interventions generally expose people to new information designed to change their behavioral, normative, and control beliefs. Hence, background factors (e.g., personality traits) can help account for differences in beliefs. For example, traits (e.g., helpfulness and independence) are dispositional explanations of behavior [5].

A composite application (e.g., mashups) can build by combining existing functions (e.g., APIs). For example, cognitive services or mashups of them [6] are used to manifest the behaviors and intents of the individuals. The manifested insights are algorithmically inferred from the raw data. For example, a speech or text can be extracted into tones and traits [7] the whole set of which forms a personal and behavioral profile with summarizing and manifesting preferences. There might be similarities between the traits of the individuals that are doing the same (or similar) things or are interested in the same (or similar) things.

In this paper, we figure out techniques that are behind text-based traits. Moreover, we produce text-based traits by the IBM Watson™ Personality Insights service [8]. We will clarify whether the traits insights of the IBM Watson™ Personality Insights service can be used in behavioral interventions. The IBM Watson™ Personality Insights service uses an open-vocabulary approach to infer personality characteristics (i.e., traits) from text input. The service deploys the word-embedding technique GloVe (Global Vectors for Word Representation) to attain the words of the input text into a vector representation (Sect. 2). Thereafter, the machine-learning algorithm calculates percentiles and raw scores of the personality characteristics from word-vector representations and consumptions preference scores from the personality characteristics (Sect. 3). Finally, we discuss whether behavioral interventions from text-based trait insights are reliable (Sect. 4).

2　From Text to Vectors

Raw text has to transform into a structured form. A bag-of-words is a sparse matrix where most of the elements are zero arises in real-world problems [9]. The bag-of-words is commonly followed by tf-idf (i.e., term frequency and inverse document frequency) weighted matrix weighting or we will produce the tf-idf weighted matrix from the text. When, we have the tf-idf weighted matrix we have to reduce dimensionality using separate methods (e.g., singular-value decomposition, SVD) or "we can feed the tf-idf weighted matrix directly into a neural net to perform dimensionality reduction" [10].

The dimensions of the matrixes have to reduce. Therefore, word or sentence embedding (Sect. 2.1) with several corpora of text [11] are used. The meaning of the word embedding is exemplified by the GloVe algorithm (Sect. 2.2).

2.1   Word and Sentence Embedding

Word or sentence embedding concerns natural language processing techniques via neural networks, or via matrix factorization. Dimensionality reduction techniques are applied to the datasets of co-occurrence statistics between words on a corpus of text.

Words are embedded in a continuous vector space where semantically similar words are embedded near to each other. The words that occur in the same contexts tend to share a similar semantic meaning. For example, the Turku NLP Group [12] has implemented the demo to illustrate the nearest words, the similarity of two words, and word analogy.

Word vectors are generated by algorithms. Each center word (cw) has surrounding words the symbol of which is sw (Fig. 1). The idea to convey the words of the sentence (i.e., text) into a matrix presentation is capture the embedded semantic and syntactic regularities from the sentence.

1)   The Finnish **capital** has warm **weather**

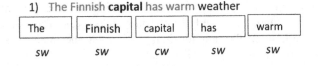

2)   The Finnish capital **has** warm weather

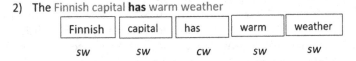

Fig. 1. Example sliding window size 5 from a word to a vector

Sentence embedding uses encoder-decoder models such as LSTM (long short-term memory) and CNN (convolutional neural network) to solve the sequence to sequence tasks [13] such as summarization [14]. Both supervised and unsupervised learning are applied [15].

2.2   Example of the GloVe Application

One of the most famous word embedding algorithm is GloVe [16]. It is used instead of word2vec [17], for example, in the IBM Watson™ Personality Insights service [18]. The Global Vectors for Word Representation (GloVe) the main function of which is to build co-occurrence function where the corpus is approved and co-occurrence values are calculated.

First, we created a vocabulary having 19 words (i.e., and, at, athlete, biathlon, compete, competition, distance, gun, guns, himself, human, interface, like, result, shooting, skiing, sometimes, sport, 50 km) from the statements as follows:

0. "gun interface skiing
1. human interface gun

2. sport interface human
3. biathlon interface sport
4. athlete interface biathlon
5. athlete sport competition at distance 50 km
6. athlete result distance 50 km
7. athlete like shooting and skiing
8. athlete like guns and skiing
9. Sometimes athlete compete competition
10. Sometimes athlete compete himself")

The vocabulary is tabulated tuples where each word has an index and number of occurrences. For example, the word 'gun' has the index zero and it occurs two times (0,2), the word 'interface' has the index one and it occurs five times (1,5), and the word 'skiing' has the index 2 and it occurs three times (2,3).

Second, the co-occurrences of the words are calculated [19]. The co-occurrences are tabulated triples where the first item is the index of the vocabulary word, the second item is the index of the context word, and the third item is the ratio of co-occurrence probability that the first item appears in the context of the second item. For example, the word 'gun' the index of which is zero concerns three triples (0,1,2.0), (0,2,0.5), (0,3,0.5) where the index one is the word 'interface', index two is the word 'skiing', and the index 3 is the word 'human'.

Third, the GloVe algorithm produces a co-occurrence matrix where the rows illustrate the vocabulary words and the columns illustrate the statements. For example, the statement "athlete sport competition at distance 50 km" the words of which are indexed as [4, 6–10] and the corresponding values for each word are calculated in the co-occurrence matrix (Table 1).

We will apply the model (i.e., the co-occurrence matrix), for example, for similarity evaluation. For example, there are 15 similarities (and, at, compete, competition, distance, gun, guns, human, interface, like, result, skiing, sport, sometimes, 50 km) of the statements in our example. In general, GloVe is very useful with natural language processing tasks such as demonstrating semantic and syntactic regularities. It can even find the correct words from outside of the ordinary vocabulary [19].

3 Example of Trait-Based Insights

First, we research techniques to get personality characteristics and consumption preferences via API of the IBM Watson™ Personality Insights service (Sect. 3.1). Second, we analyze trait insights (Sect. 3.2).

3.1 Traits via API of the IBM Watson™ Personality Insights Service

Web data are messy and it is time consuming to collect data from several channels by different APIs. Therefore, the Futusome service is used to make a data dump of web data. The data dump was created at 22.02.2018 11:15 UTC and it contains 53294 messages (Table 2) concern 'ampumahiihto' (biathlon) [20]. The data dump is the

Table 1. Example of the calculated values of the co-occurrence matrix

Vocabulary vs. statements	0	1	2	3	4	5	6	7	8	9
0 - gun										
1 - interface										
2 - skiing										
3 - human										
4 - sport						−0.0729962				
5 - biathlon										
6 - athlete						−0.318759				
7 - competition						0.17229				
8 - at						0.132553				
9 - distance						−0.529117				
10–50 km						−0.397189				
11 - result										
12 - like										
13 - shooting										
14 - and										
15 - guns										
16 - sometimes										
17 - compete										
18 - himself										

Excel file the fields of which are the author name, time stamp, channel type, message link, and message text.

The messages of each author are combined into 424-44168 words before the API call. Moreover, the retweets and duplicates of the forum posts are removed. Finally, there were 514 authors of the messages. It is possible to use the IBM Watson services in Python [21]. Therefore, Python is use to combine the messages, to call the IBM Personality Insights API [22], and to modify the API result by trait ids (Appendix A).

3.2 Percentiles and Scores

The IBM Watson™ Personality Insights service computes personality characteristics - five dimensions (i.e., Big Five or OCEAN) and 30 facets, 12 needs and five values. Big Five describes "how a person generally engages with the world", the needs describe what a person "hope to fulfill when [she] consider[s] a product or service", and the values (or beliefs) "convey what is the most important to [a person]" [18]. There are explanations for the high values of the needs and values. However, there are explanations both the high and low values of the dimensions and facets of the personality [23]. For example, if the cautiousness facet is 0.79 the explanation of which is that the individual is deliberate and she carefully thinks through decisions before making them [23]. There are percentiles and raw scores for the personality traits (i.e., dimensions and facets of Big Five, needs [24] and values [25]) – percentiles are normalized scores and raw scores are as the scores that based solely on the text [18]. It is observable that the

Table 2. Number of author per channel

Channel	Number of authors
blog_answer	161
blog_comment	136
blog_post	718
facebook_comment	2918
facebook_event	53
facebook_link	3082
facebook_photo	1356
facebook_post	111
facebook_status	674
facebook_video	299
forum_post	9916
googleplus_post	28
googleplus_post_comment	2
instagram_image	580
instagram_image_comment	102
news_comment	4496
twitter_retweet	4207
twitter_tweet	23935
youtube_video	34
youtube_video_comment	11

interpretations of the results differ a lot if we make the interpretation based on the percentiles or based on the raw scores (Appendix B).

IBM has identified 104 consumption preferences correlated with personality. IBM has selected 42 consumption preferences "for which personality-based classification performed at least 9 percent better than random classification" [18]. The consumptions preference scores (Appendix C) are derived from the personality characteristics (i.e., Big Five, needs and values) inferred from the input text [26]. There are eight categories having 42 preferences as follows [27]: 12 shopping preferences, 10 movie preferences, nine (9) music preferences, five (5) reading and learning preferences, three (3) health and activity preferences, one (1) entrepreneurship preference, one (1) environmental concern preference, and one (1) volunteering preference.

We realized that some personality characteristics correlate statistically significant with the consumption preferences. There are some minor differences in correlation coefficients when we compare correlations within the consumptions preferences versus the raw scores of the personality characteristics and the consumptions preferences versus the percentiles of the personality characteristics. However, we do not know how the words of the texts are mapped into the personality characteristics, as well we do not know how the personality characteristics affect the consumption preferences. Therefore, correlation calculations (Fig. 2) illustrate the relationships. The Person correlations are calculated by the rcorr function of the Hmisc (Harrell Miscellaneous) package [28].

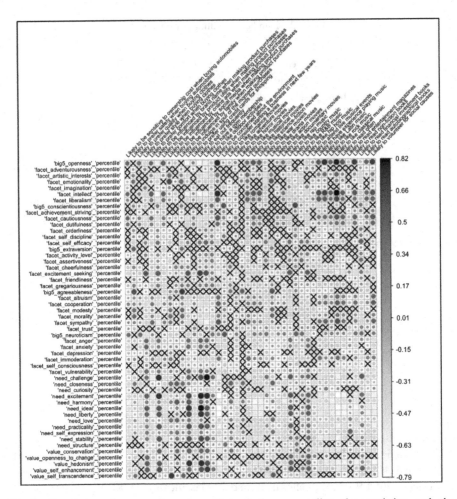

Fig. 2. Correlations between the percentiles of the personality characteristics and the consumption preferences, the cross is used when the statistical significance is <0.05

4 Discussion

The IBM Watson™ Personality Insights service computes personality characteristics - five dimensions and 30 facets of the Big Five, 12 needs and five values. We will explain the GloVe algorithm used in IBM Watson™ Personality Insights service. However, we did not know exactly how the values of the traits are calculated. However, the items of the International Personality Item Pool (IPIP) has been used [18]. There are many items (i.e., phrases or statements) used to describe people's behaviors. Answers (e.g., Very Inaccurate, Moderately Inaccurate, Neither Accurate, Nor Inaccurate, and Moderately Accurate) of the items (i.e., accuracies of the statements) affect negatively or positively to the results of the Big Five (i.e., dimensions and facets). For example, item-total correlations for the full sample have been calculated [29]. In general, the IPIP items are research-based relevant when people's behaviors are intervened. For example, the anger facet is related with the items "Get angry easily", "Get irritated easily", "Lose my temper", and "Am not easily annoyed" - the answers of the items "Get angry easily", "Get irritated easily", and "Lose my temper" have positive effects and the answers of the item "Am not easily annoyed" has a negative effect on the value of the anger facet [29].

Open and standardized measures in the pipelines from raw data to traceable results are required (Fig. 3). In general, when we assess the results of the calculations we have to understand the algorithms of APIs and how we interpret the results of the APIs.

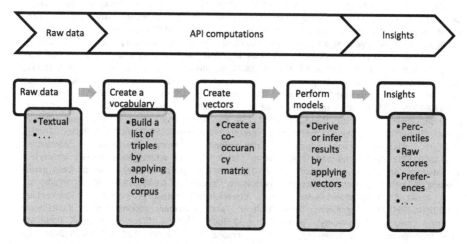

Fig. 3. Example of the pipeline

In many cases, the results of the APIs have to manipulate for further processing. Therefore, we have to have analytical, even statistical, tools for get interpretable and significant insights. Only some of the insights are derived straightforward way from the raw data. More and more, the insights are inferred by machine learning. For example, fitness trackers (e.g., BiAffect [30]) and other deep learning solutions based on Keras the examples of which give ideas of versatile uses. Keras [31] is the frontend that will use TensorFlow [32] as its tensor (i.e., an organized multidimensional array of numerical values [33]) manipulation library.

In future, we will build proof-of-concepts or solutions where the well-established corpora and IPIP items are used in word or sentence embedding. There seems to be semantic roles such as actions (e.g., avoid and believe) and objects (e.g., pressure and rule) in the IPIP items that can be related to certain personality characteristics which can be applied in word or sentence embedding. Furthermore, we will build the models where open source APIs and other building blocks (e.g., TPOT, the automatic machine learning tool [34]) are adapted within the artificially intelligent technologies such as Keras and TensorFlow.

Appendix A – Example of Big Five Traits and Facets of Them

[{'trait_id': 'big5_openness', 'name': **'Openness'**, 'category': 'personality', 'percentile': 0.9376988166491549, 'significant': True, 'children': [{'trait_id': 'facet_**adventurousness**', 'name': 'Adventurousness', 'category': 'personality', 'percentile': 0.6493499098483716, 'significant': True}, {'trait_id': 'facet_**artistic_interests**', 'name': 'Artistic interests', 'category': 'personality', 'percentile': 0.6158641904316721, 'significant': True}, {'trait_id': 'facet_**emotionality**', 'name': 'Emotionality', 'category': 'personality', 'percentile': 0.09685563208155124, 'significant': True}, {'trait_id': 'facet_**imagination**', 'name': 'Imagination', 'category': 'personality', 'percentile': 0.6558901273510154, 'significant': True}, {'trait_id': 'facet_**intellect**', 'name': 'Intellect', 'category': 'personality', 'percentile': 0.9894639896976287, 'significant': True}, {'trait_id': 'facet_**liberalism**', 'name': 'Authority-challenging', 'category': 'personality', 'percentile': 0.9603451147017372, 'significant': True}]}, {'trait_id': 'big5_conscientiousness', 'name': **'Conscientiousness'**, 'category': 'personality', 'percentile': 0.2023633519388825, 'significant': True, 'children': [{'trait_id': 'facet_**achievement_striving**', 'name': 'Achievement striving', 'category': 'personality', 'percentile': 0.3819686183228188, 'significant': True}, {'trait_id': 'facet_**cautiousness**', 'name': 'Cautiousness', 'category': 'personality', 'percentile': 0.6879031855220676, 'significant': True}, {'trait_id': 'facet_**dutifulness**', 'name': 'Dutifulness', 'category': 'personality', 'percentile': 0.48293181171869926, 'significant': True}, {'trait_id': 'facet_**orderliness**', 'name': 'Orderliness', 'category': 'personality', 'percentile': 0.44370659356923503, 'significant': True}, {'trait_id': 'facet_**self_discipline**', 'name': 'Self-discipline', 'category': 'personality', 'percentile': 0.3182111636651134, 'significant': True}, {'trait_id': 'facet_**self_efficacy**', 'name': 'Self-efficacy', 'category': 'personality', 'percentile': 0.7998622573834601, 'significant': True}]}, {'trait_id': 'big5_extraversion', 'name': **'Extraversion'**, 'category': 'personality', 'percentile': 0.32740091371308094, 'significant': True, 'children': [{'trait_id': 'facet_**activity_level**', 'name': 'Activity level', 'category': 'personality', 'percentile': 0.6317741938363013, 'significant': True}, {'trait_id': 'facet_**assertiveness**', 'name': 'Assertiveness', 'category': 'personality', 'percentile': 0.8306329369765959, 'significant': True}, {'trait_id': 'facet_**cheerfulness**', 'name': 'Cheerfulness', 'category': 'personality', 'percentile': 0.00807941409452484, 'significant': True}, {'trait_id': 'facet_**excitement_seeking**', 'name': 'Excitement-seeking', 'category': 'personality', 'percentile': 0.3802048384483194, 'significant': True}, {'trait_id': 'facet_**friendliness**', 'name': 'Outgoing', 'category': 'personality', 'percentile': 0.20476319548912464, 'significant': True}, {'trait_id': 'facet_**gregariousness**', 'name': 'Gregariousness', 'category': 'personality', 'percentile': 0.043608841680235544, 'significant': True}]}, {'trait_id': 'big5_agreeableness', 'name': **'Agreeableness'**, 'category': 'personality', 'percentile': 0.000139196908131467, 'significant': True, 'children': [{'trait_id': 'facet_**altruism**', 'name': 'Altruism', 'category': 'personality', 'percentile': 0.27667605621677194, 'significant': True}, {'trait_id': 'facet_**cooperation**', 'name': 'Cooperation', 'category': 'personality', 'percentile': 0.2588405142240412, 'significant': True}, {'trait_id': 'facet_**modesty**', 'name': 'Modesty', 'category': 'personality', 'percentile': 0.016171970864307328, 'significant': True}, {'trait_id': 'facet_**morality**', 'name': 'Uncompromising', 'category': 'personality', 'percentile': 0.04572387645340231, 'significant': True}, {'trait_id': 'facet_**sympathy**', 'name': 'Sympathy', 'category': 'personality', 'percentile': 0.4189960099898948, 'significant': True}, {'trait_id': 'facet_**trust**', 'name': 'Trust', 'category': 'personality', 'percentile': 0.7101433353200839, 'significant': True}]}, {'trait_id': 'big5_**neuroticism**', 'name': 'Emotional range', 'category': 'personality', 'percentile': 0.7190608517464266, 'significant': True, 'children': [{'trait_id': 'facet_**anger**', 'name': 'Fiery', 'category': 'personality', 'percentile': 0.6141639266814796, 'significant': True}, {'trait_id': 'facet_**anxiety**', 'name': 'Prone to worry', 'category': 'personality', 'percentile': 0.4031258151504815, 'significant': True}, {'trait_id': 'facet_**depression**', 'name': 'Melancholy', 'category': 'personality', 'percentile': 0.5512210695431201, 'significant': True}, {'trait_id': 'facet_**immoderation**', 'name': 'Immoderation', 'category': 'personality', 'percentile': 0.4743265563426596, 'significant': True}, {'trait_id': 'facet_**self_consciousness**', 'name': 'Self-consciousness', 'category': 'personality', 'percentile': 0.6938055709145589, 'significant': True}, {'trait_id': 'facet_**vulnerability**', 'name': 'Susceptible to stress', 'category': 'personality', 'percentile': 0.23619356766406913, 'significant': True}]}]]

Appendix B – Percentiles and Raw Scores for Personality Characteristics

Traits	MAX	MIN	RANGE	STDEV	>= 0,5	< 0,5
'big5_openness'_'percentile'	0,99999272	0,00019721	0,99979552	0,25239342	438	76
'big5_openness'_'raw_score'	0,88706392	0,63550973	0,25155419	0,03445183	514	0
'facet_adventurousness'_'percentile'	0,99369948	0,01115163	0,98254785	0,23450269	196	318
'facet_adventurousness'_'raw_score'	0,59354978	0,42354320	0,17000658	0,02647399	226	288
'facet_artistic_interests'_'percentile'	0,99945960	0,00094327	0,99851633	0,27172303	191	323
'facet_artistic_interests'_'raw_score'	0,83079255	0,50801079	0,32278176	0,04900104	514	0
'facet_emotionality'_'percentile'	0,94256578	0,00005502	0,94251076	0,20563892	56	458
'facet_emotionality'_'raw_score'	0,71247453	0,49052888	0,22194565	0,02909276	512	2
'facet_imagination'_'percentile'	0,99907260	0,00906165	0,99001095	0,22855610	244	270
'facet_imagination'_'raw_score'	0,88946019	0,61748317	0,27197703	0,03672788	514	0
'facet_intellect'_'percentile'	0,99997000	0,13810885	0,86186115	0,21534236	459	55
'facet_intellect'_'raw_score'	0,79298682	0,55684747	0,23613935	0,04899111	514	0
'facet_liberalism'_'percentile'	0,99996614	0,03811818	0,96184796	0,18044938	476	38
'facet_liberalism'_'raw_score'	0,71689733	0,42693163	0,28996570	0,04251613	496	18
'big5_conscientiousness'_'percentile'	0,93208986	0,01553764	0,91655222	0,19154162	133	381
'big5_conscientiousness'_'raw_score'	0,69761761	0,52748831	0,17012930	0,02707790	514	0
'facet_achievement_striving'_'percentile'	0,98021078	0,07244143	0,90776935	0,17754209	328	186
'facet_achievement_striving'_'raw_score'	0,79734461	0,61121356	0,18615105	0,02733258	514	0
'facet_cautiousness'_'percentile'	0,99891566	0,16685385	0,83206181	0,16985977	472	42
'facet_cautiousness'_'raw_score'	0,68602276	0,43145201	0,25457075	0,04347172	463	51
'facet_dutifulness'_'percentile'	0,98882544	0,00543148	0,98339396	0,21588716	424	90
'facet_dutifulness'_'raw_score'	0,71484403	0,59652344	0,11832059	0,01759053	514	0
'facet_orderliness'_'percentile'	0,91737009	0,00888474	0,90848535	0,17287961	70	444
'facet_orderliness'_'raw_score'	0,53960790	0,41651194	0,12309596	0,01794820	46	468
'facet_self_discipline'_'percentile'	0,87887458	0,00261368	0,87626091	0,16442561	112	402
'facet_self_discipline'_'raw_score'	0,62635834	0,43762067	0,18873766	0,02369677	503	11
'facet_self_efficacy'_'percentile'	0,99746356	0,01914470	0,97831886	0,20836749	433	81
'facet_self_efficacy'_'raw_score'	0,85165404	0,68024022	0,17141382	0,02447264	514	0
'big5_extraversion'_'percentile'	0,85316031	0,00021413	0,85294618	0,15698343	29	485
'big5_extraversion'_'raw_score'	0,59786466	0,39384086	0,20402380	0,03043173	230	284
'facet_activity_level'_'percentile'	0,99883398	0,05223746	0,94659652	0,19347593	422	92
'facet_activity_level'_'raw_score'	0,69615384	0,45730479	0,23884905	0,03561864	505	9
'facet_assertiveness'_'percentile'	0,99630464	0,00453865	0,99176598	0,18843876	423	91
'facet_assertiveness'_'raw_score'	0,77796798	0,51362774	0,26434024	0,03036737	514	0
facet_cheerfulness'_'percentile'	0,78121411	0,00028230	0,78093181	0,09913275	4	510
'facet_cheerfulness'_'raw_score'	0,64419029	0,50242397	0,14176633	0,02115610	514	0
'facet_excitement_seeking'_'percentile'	0,99599318	0,00626075	0,98973243	0,24644264	151	363
'facet_excitement_seeking'_'raw_score'	0,71602798	0,49772720	0,21830077	0,03404072	513	1
'facet_friendliness'_'percentile'	0,92948333	0,00148659	0,92799673	0,17329310	45	469
'facet_friendliness'_'raw_score'	0,63431531	0,41150170	0,22281362	0,03192251	379	135
'facet_gregariousness'_'percentile'	0,83189979	0,00055026	0,83134952	0,11622742	7	507
facet_gregariousness'_'raw_score'	0,50278498	0,28556612	0,21721886	0,03396248	1	513
'big5_agreeableness'_'percentile'	0,95605178	0,00000861	0,95604317	0,08182172	5	509
'big5_agreeableness'_'raw_score'	0,81004356	0,57132459	0,23871897	0,03129160	514	0
'facet_altruism'_'percentile'	0,98241031	0,01473785	0,96767246	0,22162725	233	281
'facet_altruism'_'raw_score'	0,77897969	0,62871642	0,15026327	0,02381936	514	0
'facet_cooperation'_'percentile'	0,99463106	0,00533903	0,98929203	0,23580043	288	226
'facet_cooperation'_'raw_score'	0,73308778	0,42557317	0,30751462	0,04535541	501	13
'facet_modesty'_'percentile'	0,98997596	0,00026704	0,98970892	0,22759168	105	409

Traits	MAX	MIN	RANGE	STDEV	>= 0,5	< 0,5
'facet_sympathy'_'percentile'	0,99945933	0,00381928	0,99564005	0,30182937	265	249
'facet_sympathy'_'raw_score'	0,78828240	0,56161583	0,22666657	0,04019655	514	0
'facet_trust'_'percentile'	0,99781079	0,07257401	0,92523678	0,17552606	476	38
'facet_trust'_'raw_score'	0,70319440	0,52578218	0,17741221	0,02874966	514	0
'big5_neuroticism'_'percentile'	0,98680995	0,00658912	0,98022083	0,18204013	418	96
'big5_neuroticism'_'raw_score'	0,59254319	0,32762498	0,26491822	0,03155862	180	334
'facet_anger'_'percentile'	0,99037872	0,00272110	0,98765761	0,25098703	152	362
'facet_anger'_'raw_score'	0,66372375	0,38370989	0,28001386	0,04558748	309	205
'facet_anxiety'_'percentile'	0,99639171	0,02271346	0,97367825	0,20679612	223	291
'facet_anxiety'_'raw_score'	0,77733565	0,45767138	0,31966427	0,04211487	507	7
'facet_depression'_'percentile'	0,99555493	0,10621226	0,88934267	0,16257691	398	116
'facet_depression'_'raw_score'	0,61414712	0,36946097	0,24468615	0,03105373	75	439
'facet_immoderation'_'percentile'	0,96704207	0,00253428	0,96450779	0,21574794	143	371
'facet_immoderation'_'raw_score'	0,57127299	0,39287410	0,17839889	0,02595308	146	368
'facet_self_consciousness'_'percentile'	0,99809895	0,07605338	0,92204557	0,17869400	466	48
'facet_self_consciousness'_'raw_score'	0,69900203	0,47135673	0,22764530	0,03359190	509	5
'facet_vulnerability'_'percentile'	0,97189714	0,07410908	0,89778806	0,20194751	184	330
'facet_vulnerability'_'raw_score'	0,58927446	0,37550465	0,21376981	0,03701366	75	439
'need_challenge'_'percentile'	0,92468369	0,00019484	0,92448886	0,25375082	161	353
'need_challenge'_'raw_score'	0,79624510	0,57270772	0,22353738	0,03954304	514	0
'need_closeness'_'percentile'	0,75439237	0,00078955	0,75360282	0,09073725	3	511
'need_closeness'_'raw_score'	0,82391566	0,65311115	0,17080451	0,02539221	514	0
'need_curiosity'_'percentile'	0,89598980	0,00077940	0,89521040	0,19778415	100	414
'need_curiosity'_'raw_score'	0,84978661	0,73338983	0,11639678	0,01691601	514	0
'need_excitement'_'percentile'	0,88776105	0,00075561	0,88700544	0,18802420	61	453
'need_excitement'_'raw_score'	0,78169551	0,43319445	0,34850106	0,05575661	504	10
'need_harmony'_'percentile'	0,84439695	0,00002536	0,84437160	0,10439782	9	505
'need_harmony'_'raw_score'	0,84422614	0,66933027	0,17489587	0,02732363	514	0
'need_ideal'_'percentile'	0,89183687	0,00056994	0,89126693	0,16862898	38	476
'need_ideal'_'raw_score'	0,74980865	0,53644105	0,21336760	0,03277839	514	0
'need_liberty'_'percentile'	0,68901309	0,00102373	0,68798935	0,10579846	5	509
'need_liberty'_'raw_score'	0,75498243	0,62100674	0,13397569	0,02178453	514	0
'need_love'_'percentile'	0,63373997	0,00008959	0,63365038	0,07737863	3	511
'need_love'_'raw_score'	0,78528577	0,58639983	0,19888594	0,03207787	514	0
'need_practicality'_'percentile'	0,99903799	0,00101467	0,99802332	0,19707437	47	467
'need_practicality'_'raw_score'	0,79478765	0,66110061	0,13368704	0,01723442	514	0
'need_self_expression'_'percentile'	0,59836123	0,00016548	0,59819575	0,08190370	3	511
'need_self_expression'_'raw_score'	0,68363269	0,55120559	0,13242711	0,02224307	514	0
'need_stability'_'percentile'	0,94827443	0,00015297	0,94812146	0,19595219	48	466
'need_stability'_'raw_score'	0,78630705	0,61947421	0,16683284	0,02571700	514	0
'need_structure'_'percentile'	0,95780887	0,00070619	0,95710268	0,20178786	109	405
'need_structure'_'raw_score'	0,74284251	0,60958235	0,13326016	0,01782846	514	0
'value_conservation'_'percentile'	0,88900241	0,00011655	0,88888586	0,12822282	9	505
'value_conservation'_'raw_score'	0,72046652	0,49965857	0,22080796	0,03394458	513	1
'value_openness_to_change'_'percentile'	0,86521953	0,03658561	0,82863393	0,17692143	163	351
'value_openness_to_change'_'raw_score'	0,82684265	0,71517560	0,11166705	0,01961785	514	0
'value_hedonism'_'percentile'	0,83739267	0,00621997	0,83117271	0,15964534	29	485
'value_hedonism'_'raw_score'	0,80105958	0,57847909	0,22258049	0,03754495	514	0
'value_self_enhancement'_'percentile'	0,98249652	0,00237073	0,98012580	0,27110894	213	301
'value_self_enhancement'_'raw_score'	0,79882592	0,58243124	0,21639468	0,03924734	514	0
'value_self_transcendence'_'percentile'	0,82490827	0,00005088	0,82485739	0,11985445	9	505
'value_self_transcendence'_'raw_score'	0,84817532	0,76965858	0,07851674	0,01099245	514	0

Appendix C – Consumption Preferences

Consumption preferences	1	0,5	0
Likely to like action movies	511	0	3
Likely to like adventure movies	509	0	5
Likely to prefer using credit cards for shopping	508	0	6
Likely to prefer quality when buying clothes	500	0	14
Likely to like documentary movies	500	0	14
Likely to attend live musical events	484	0	30
Likely to like rock music	483	13	18
Likely to like historical movies	481	0	33
Likely to like science-fiction movies	481	0	33
Likely to read non-fiction books	474	0	40
Likely to read autobiographical books	468	0	46
Likely to read often	462	0	52
Likely to like war movies	448	0	66
Likely to be sensitive to ownership cost when buying automobiles	444	52	18
Likely to prefer comfort when buying clothes	435	0	79
Likely to volunteer for social causes	422	0	92
Likely to have experience playing music	407	0	107
Likely to be concerned about the environment	375	118	21
Likely to like Latin music	373	44	97
Likely to be influenced by product utility when making product purchases	371	112	31
Likely to like classical music	365	113	36
Likely to read financial investment books	304	0	210
Likely to like outdoor activities	256	241	17
Likely to like musical movies	215	0	299
Likely to have a gym membership	194	0	320
Likely to be influenced by brand name when making product purchases	183	10	321
Likely to prefer style when buying clothes	174	0	340
Likely to like hip hop music	85	271	158
Likely to like rap music	78	359	77
Likely to eat out frequently	48	75	391
Likely to be influenced by online ads when making product purchases	47	0	467
Likely to like drama movies	44	0	470
Likely to prefer safety when buying automobiles	37	8	469
Likely to indulge in spur of the moment purchases	25	68	421
Likely to be influenced by family when making product purchases	23	0	491
Likely to like country music	9	271	234
Likely to like R&B music	9	451	54
Likely to be influenced by social media when making product purchases	8	0	506
Likely to read entertainment magazines	5	0	509
Likely to like romance movies	4	0	510
Likely to like horror movies	4	0	510
Likely to consider starting a business in next few years	3	308	203

References

1. The International Organization for Standardization: ISO 5127:2017(en) Information and documentation — Foundation and vocabulary (2017). https://www.iso.org/obp/ui#iso:std:iso:5127:ed-2:v1:en
2. The European Union: The European Parliament or the Council Regulation (EU) 2016/679 of the European Parliament and of the Council of 27 April 2016 on the protection of natural persons with regard to the processing of personal data and on the free movement of such data, and repealing Directive 95/46/EC (General Data Protection Regulation) (2016). https://eur-lex.europa.eu/legal-content/EN/TXT/HTML/?uri=CELEX:32016R0679&from=EN
3. The International Organization for Standardization, the International Electrotechnical Commission: ISO/IEC 29100:2011(en) Information technology — Security techniques — Privacy framework (2011). http://standards.iso.org/ittf/PubliclyAvailableStandards/index.html
4. Bruce, P.: The Real Facebook Controversy. Data Science Central (2018). https://www.datasciencecentral.com/profiles/blogs/the-real-facebook-controversy
5. Ajzen, I.: Attitudes, Personality and Behavior. Open University Press, Maidenhead (2005)
6. IBM: API mashup guide (2017). https://www-01.ibm.com/common/ssi/cgi-bin/ssialias?htmlfid=LBS03048USEN
7. Gain, U., Hotti, V.: Tones and traits - experiments of text-based extractions with cognitive services. Finnish J. eHealth eWelfare 9(2–3), 82–94 (2017). https://doi.org/10.23996/fjhw.61001
8. IBM: Getting started tutorial (2018). https://console.bluemix.net/docs/services/personality-insights/getting-started.html#gettingStarted
9. Davis, T.: Sparse matrix algorithms and software (2018). http://faculty.cse.tamu.edu/davis/research.html
10. Ingersoll, K.: An Intro to Natural Language Processing in Python: Framing Text Classification in Familiar Terms (2018). https://www.datasciencecentral.com/profiles/blogs/an-intro-to-natural-language-processing-in-python-framing-text
11. Wikipedia: List of text corpora (2018). https://en.wikipedia.org/wiki/List_of_text_corpora
12. Turku NLP Group: Models (2018). http://bionlp-www.utu.fi/wv_demo/
13. Zeng, W., Luo, W., Fidler, S., Urtasun, R.: Efficient Summarization with Read-Again and Copy Mechanism (2017). https://arxiv.org/abs/1611.03382
14. Google: Neural Machine Translation (seq2seq) Tutorial (2018). https://www.tensorflow.org/tutorials/seq2seq
15. Pagliardini, M., Gupta, P., Jaggi, M.: Unsupervised Learning of Sentence Embeddings using Compositional n-Gram Features (2017). https://arxiv.org/pdf/1703.02507.pdf
16. Pennington, J., Socher, R., Manning C.D.: GloVe: Global Vectors for Word Representation (2014). https://www.aclweb.org/anthology/D14-1162
17. Google: word2vec (2013). https://code.google.com/archive/p/word2vec/
18. IBM: The science behind the service (2018). https://console.bluemix.net/docs/services/personality-insights/science.html#science
19. Pennington, J., Socher, R., Manning, C.D.: GloVe: Global Vectors for Word Representation (2014). https://nlp.stanford.edu/projects/glove/
20. Futusome: Services (2017). https://www.futusome.com/en/services/
21. GitHub: watson-developer-cloud/python-sdk (2018). https://github.com/watson-developer-cloud/python-sdk/tree/develop/examples
22. IBM: Personality Insights – API reference (2017). https://www.ibm.com/watson/developercloud/personality-insights/api/v3/?python

23. IBM: Personality models (2018). https://console.bluemix.net/docs/services/personality-insights/models.html#models

24. IBM: Needs (2017c). https://console.bluemix.net/docs/services/personality-insights/needs.html#needs

25. IBM: Values (2017d). https://console.bluemix.net/docs/services/personality-insights/values.html#values

26. IBM: Interpreting the numeric results (2018). https://console.bluemix.net/docs/services/personality-insights/numeric.html#numeric

27. IBM: Consumption preferences (2018). https://console.bluemix.net/docs/services/personality-insights/preferences.html#preferences

28. The Comprehensive R Archive Network: Hmisc: Harrell Miscellaneous (2018). https://CRAN.R-project.org/package=Hmisc

29. Johnson, J.: Measuring thirty facets of the five factor model with a 120-item public domain inventory: development of the IPIP-NEO-120. J. Res. Pers. **51**, 78–89 (2014). https://doi.org/10.1016/j.jrp.2014.05.003

30. BiAffect: BiAffect (2017). http://www.biaffect.com/

31. Keras: The Python Deep Learning library (2018). https://keras.io/

32. TensorFlow: An open source machine learning framework for everyone (2019). https://www.tensorflow.org/

33. Wikipedia. Tensor (2018). https://en.wikipedia.org/wiki/Tensor

34. GitHub: EpistasisLab/tpot (2018). https://github.com/EpistasisLab/tpot

The Human Resources Debt in Software Business
Towards a Research Roadmap

Sonja M. Hyrynsalmi[1] ⓘ, Minna M. Rantanen[2] ⓘ, Johannes Holvitie[3] ⓘ,
Sami Hyrynsalmi[4(✉)] ⓘ, and Erkki Sutinen[3]

[1] University of Turku, Turku, Finland
smnyla@utu.fi
[2] Turku School of Economics, University of Turku, Turku, Finland
minna.m.rantanen@utu.fi
[3] Department of Future Technologies, University of Turku, Turku, Finland
{jjholv,erkki.sutinen}@utu.fi
[4] Pervasive Computing, Tampere University of Technology, Pori, Finland
sami.hyrynsalmi@tut.fi

Abstract. This conceptual-analytical paper presents and defines the concept of 'human resource debt' (i.e., HR debt). The presented concept draws from the software engineering field's recent work in the technical debt management, yet it departures from the existing conceptualizations by focusing on skills and competences of individual employees as well as emphasizing the need to manage the skill pool with conscious decisions. As with its paragons, this novel concept aims to help to understand, control and utilize better the phenomenon by using a simple metaphor. In addition, the metaphor, borrowed from the economics, also emphasizes the potential price that has to be paid back later. In the discussion, the ever-changing software industry is used as an example industrial domain; however, the concept should be generalizable to other fields. Finally, the paper lays foundations for future work and proposes initial actions needed for forming a proper research agenda.

Keywords: Human resource debt · Skills
Human resource management · Talent shortage · Technical debt

1 Introduction

There is no denying for the fact that our society is *digitalizating* at a fast pace. Yet, this is clearly only a part of continuum of series of industrial revolutions. These revolutions have shaped our society and industry through several distinct steps: steam power, mass production, and digitalization. Now, the humanity is entering to the era of full potential of artificial intelligence, robotization and nanotechnology—that is, the so-called fourth industrial revolution [1]. However, this time differences are, when compared to the past revolutions, the speed of change as well as the need for the new kinds of higher skills [2,3].

© Springer Nature Switzerland AG 2018
H. Li et al. (Eds.): WIS 2018, CCIS 907, pp. 28–41, 2018.
https://doi.org/10.1007/978-3-319-97931-1_3

In Finland, the software business is booming and software companies are more willing to grow than in years [4–6]. This has, not surprisingly, lead to a talent shortage of software professionals, the war for talents in the software industry, and to the different ways for software companies to cope with the problem [5,7,8].

However, Finland is only now waking up to the talent shortage in the software industry, and there are no fast actions planned by the government to ease the current situation [9]. This had leaded us to a situation where the companies themselves have to take an active role in both coping with the current situation (e.g., not taking too many projects without proper resources) as well as retraining existing staff for the new skills and competences needed.

This is a challenge that we have seen in our previous studies [6,10]: Companies can be reluctant to invest in retraining their existing workforce. As pointed out by several software business managers in a survey on the labour shortage [10], there are no guarantees that employees would not leave the company after expensive courses. Thus, naturally, this creates problems for both the companies as well as to the software professionals.

The aim of this paper is to use the experiences from the concept of 'technical debt', (a term widely used in the field and the literature of software engineering,) to better understand the aforementioned problem in the human resource management in the software companies. In the field of software engineering, technical debt is used to characterize possible future effects of, deliberately or indeliberately, using an non-exhaustive solution to a problem instead of the optimal one. The concept hence communicates to a software organization that a problem can be solved swiftly, but the intrinsics of the solution affect future delivery [11,12]. This also seems to be the case in the industry; for example, Klotins et al. [13] found that active start-ups have lower levels of perceived technical debt than closed or acquired start-ups.

In this paper, we present, initially define, and discuss about the novel concept of 'human resource debt'. With the human resource debt, we are referring to a situation where the companies are not taking care of retraining of their existing human resources, or they hire the most suitable candidates regardless of whether candidates meet all queried competences (due to labour shortage and high competition for workforce). Similarly than in monetary as well as in technical debt, hosting this sub-optimality can be expected to accrue additional costs—in a wider sense than only economic costs—in the future.

We focus on the human resource dept in software business by using a conceptual analysis [14]. In addition, we are also discussing a wider problem due to the nature of ICT: as ICT is a cross-cutting technology trough all industries, if HR debt is not managed well, it will cause a risk of slowing down of business and new innovations in most if not all fields of the industry. Further, we will discuss whether the software companies are taking human resource debt consciously. We go through the best practices of software companies' ways to tackle the technical debt. In addition, we will discuss and propose a formation of a roadmap for future work for this new opening.

Finally, the remaining of this paper is organized as follow. Section 2 reviews extant literature on human resource management in the software industry, whereas Sect. 3 presents an overview on the recent work on management of technical debt. In Sect. 4, we will discuss on the concept of 'human resource debt'. Finally, Sect. 5 summarizes the key arguments of this study and lays some building blocks for the future roadmap.

2   Human Resource Management and the Software Industry

What is Human Resource Management (HRM) depends on the perspective that one takes. First, HRM can be defined as a generic activity that takes place whenever one person controls and coordinates the labor of another person in the production of a good or service. From this broad perspective, HRM can be seen as labour management, which has history as long as human civilization [15]. Personnel management and HRM has also a long history from the start from industrial revolutions but in the academic it gained real visibility starting from the 1980s [16].

HRM can also be more specifically defined as the management or administrative function in business, government, and nonprofit organizations that is responsible for handling employment, or personnel, issues. From this perspective HRM, is seen as an activity, that is often handled by a department of its own, often labeled as Human Resources (HR). Thus, this perspective is all about the practices of HR, such as the employee selection, compensation, training and other labour related matters [15]. In environments where HRM has evolved, HRM professionals and departments have also developed their skills in order to ensure the best possible result [17].

In the beginning of the new millennium, the field of HRM research adopted also a third definition with even more specialized meaning. From this perspective, HRM is a new and improved philosophy and approach to manage people in organizations. The traditional system of managing people is embodied in personnel management and industrial relations. From this perspective HRM, is a management philosophy that highlights a participative form of management, in which employees are seen as human assets instead of commodities and the employment as a positive-sum game instead of a zero-sum game [15]. HRM is also seen as a much longer development chain where much of previous choices and strategies will affect the downstream results [18].

Thus, it is not a surprise that HRM has been tackling the challenges of revolutions of technology and change of skills set and competences. Organizations of all sizes are moving toward more knowledge-based business and employees are expected to continuously learn and update their knowledge and skills. HRM is now days seen as a major competitive advantage which cannot be directly copied to the other companies [17].

There are also differences how HRM is managed in small and big enterprises. The extant research has shown that small companies do not give formal training to their employees as professionally as larger companies do [19, 20]. Furthermore, it has been even pointed out that HRM is one of the most crucial stumbling blocks at new or small enterprises—even among high-technology firms, which usually invest more in the human resources than other kinds of small businesses. That is not a surprise as small and new companies are often investing more in productization and business growth and HRM will become important a lot later [21].

There are two main reasons identified why small enterprises do not focus enough to HRM, included training of the existing staff. Firstly, the management does not recognize the benefits of proper HRM or HRM blueprints. Secondly, the management in small and new companies is well aware of the benefits on training; however, they still see the costs of training and competence building of employees too high [20, 22]. In addition, training of the staff is also seen more as a formal kind of an action at the small and new entrepreneurs. Therefore, staff members' personal development stays shadowed in the bigger picture. This is especially typical to small and medium size companies which employees are already lower educated [18].

The software industry is widely recognized as a highly knowledge-based field of economy and most of the enterprises in the field of software industry are mainly small and niche market ventures although there are also really big players in the industry. In the software industry, companies can produce large information system products with small teams and companies main resources are knowledge and communications rather than natural resources or physical labour [23]. Still, despite the size of software companies, enterprises of software industry manage to be relatively well represented in different workplace happiness and well-being competitions such as 'Great Place to Work'[1] among others.

3   Technical Debt and Its Management

Technical debt is a concept which was initial coined by Cunningham [24]. This definition has been expanded later in for example [11, 25, 26]. The reader is encouraged to revise the last definition especially; as it represents the consensus in the field.

The concept of technical debt explains that all software constructs carry sub-optimal solutions. These can be deliberate—cutting corners to release earlier—or indeliberate—inexhaustive understanding of requirements or lacking knowledge about applicable practices. Nevertheless, the solutions deliver required functionality and as such the release is acceptable. The problem—the technical debt—realizes when development is continued on top of these solutions: the sub-optimalities need to be either resolved or added solutions must conform to the sub-optimality. As a result, the implementing organization is less effective in delivering functionality as debt resolving reserves a part of the resources.

Technical debt management is a support function of software development. Technical debt management can be divided into three main phases: identification,

---

[1] http://www.greatplacetowork.net/.

estimation, and decision making. Identification needs to capture and document single sub-optimal solutions into manageable technical debt items (TDI). The TDIs form a technical debt list (TDL) which is an exhaustive description of all technical debt residing in a system-under-development. Every TDI should at least describe wherein the technical debt resides (i.e. what are the affected implementation components), how severe the debt is (i.e. how far from the considered optimal the current solutions is), and how potent the item (i.e. how probable it is that the sub-optimality will affect the implementation of other solutions; the debt propagates to affect the referring solutions) [27].

The second phase, the technical debt estimation consists from updating and extrapolating the TDL. Updating consists from revising afore described potency and severity characteristics for all TDI in the TDL. If the TDL is not kept current, there is a high chance that items are re-identified or decision making is done on stale information. Further, TDI may interact with one another causing items to merge or split; changing their overall potency or severity drastically. Automated ways to carry out the updating exist, but as they generally base on rule-matching, they can not directly update a subjectively produced TDIs [28,29]. Instead, the combination of both automatic and manual updating is encouraged to retain both updating efficiency and information quality [27,30].

Extrapolating the estimation consists from considering a given development horizon and delivering an estimate on the effects of technical debt for it. For example, if the horizon consists from developing only the component A and the TDL does not describe technical debt for it, it can be stated that as long as development is constrained to A with no outside references, the effects of technical debt are non-existent. Assuming the TDL exhaustively captures all technical debt.

The decision making phase consists from ensuring that, first, technical debt related information is readily available when relevant decisions are made during software development and, secondly, about inputting the extrapolation estimates in a consumable form to support decision making. The existence of a TDL is an important premise here as it both ensures that technical debt is documented and thus noted as a project steering artifact and it enables comparing the technical debt items directly to backlog items (i.e. functional deliverables). There are different approaches to facilitate technical debt decision making [31], but at the core, the exercise is about cost-benefit optimization.

As was referred in the previous paragraph, the cost of technical debt can be associated to components and probability of propagation. When this is combined with information about the estimated excess cost of implementing a backlog item on top of sub-optimal, existing, components the cost-benefit question is fully formed: for component X and for the duration of N iterations, is the cost of resolving technical debt in X higher than paying the interest for N iterations? If the answer is yes, then it is more reasonable to pick only backlog items and implement them whilst making adaptations on top of the sub-optimalities. If the answer is no, then the technical debt should be resolved in full prior to implementing any backlog items [32].

4   Human Resource Debt and Its Management

4.1   Motivation and Approach

In the case of software industry, it is notable that the latest form of HRM started to emerged in the 1980s [15] and it has a lot of similarities with the socio-technical design, that gained interest in organizational information systems (ISs) development in previous decades. For example, one of the cornerstones of socio-technical design is that in order to create an optimally working system it is required that people who are actually doing the work are heard and the quality of work life is assured when developing new technical systems [33, 34].

At the time, companies had problems to recruit new employees as well as to keep existing ones. Socio-technical approach was seen as a solution for this problem. It was strongly believed that by improving the quality of work life and guaranteeing meaningful tasks for employees by increasing the communication between managers, employees and developers of technical systems these problems could be minimized. In other words, employee participation to the decision making about their work was seen as a key to make the company appeal and be a good place to work. This could also be seen in the quality of the end-product and thus, better quality of work life can be also a competitive advantage [34, 35].

Changed atmosphere in the case of organizational culture and competition in the 1980s were not favourable for socio-technical approach, but it still left its mark to the development of ISs [36–38]. Thus, the general paradigm shift towards the appreciation of people in work affected the software industry from two different fronts.

In addition, the software industry is currently in a situation where companies in the field have problems in finding and keeping skilled employees. On the one hand, the problem is that the companies do not have the resources or knowledge to offer less-skilled employees enough training to become skilled. On the other hand, people who are skilled are also eager to change the employee for better benefits or attractiveness of an other company, which does not motivate software companies to invest in the training of the employees [6, 10]. This clearly is a HRM problem and it is effecting specially to the small and middle size software companies and their growth potential. That is, there would be a market need for a useful conceptualization and decision support mechanisms.

In this paper, we follow the conceptual-analytical research approach as defined in Järvinen's classification [39]. According to Järvinen [14], the conceptual-analytical approach can be characterized with two main sub-approaches. In the first, the work starts from hypotheses or assumptions that are used to derive a model or a framework. In the second sub-approach, previous empirical studies are analyzed and their results generalized towards to a model, framework or a theory. Our approach follows mainly the former while it is heavily influenced by the extant empirical work in the field of the software industry.

4.2   Towards a Model

For this study, we draw from the metaphor of 'technical debt' and its management to define the concept of 'human resource debt'. The objective of the papers is propose the model, lay some building blocks for the future inquiries and require a formation of a research agenda. The conceptual-analytical approach of this paper starts from empirical observations that helped us to formulate the assumptions.

In our previous studies [6,8,10], it was noted that some software businesses were often bypassing training and development of their software development personnel. The reasons varied. For example, an individual respondent, as reported in [10], points out that *"There is a specific problem on the software side that the competence is largely outdated in five years. Employers generally can not afford or are not willing to retrain people to today's tools and requirements because it is considered a society's task."* Furthermore, it was revealed that companies might not want to invest in an expensive training as there is a risk that an employee could change the employer shortly after [10].

These lead us to the observation: Some companies are struggling with managing the development of their employees' skills and competences—e.g., their human resources—in the software industry. Furthermore, the second observation is that several companies have frequently pointed out that they are lacking time which affects to various functionalities of the company [6,8]. That is, they might not even have time for retraining and advance the skills and competencies in their company. However, as the companies often seek to grow, it has to be acknowledged that personnel development might be an issue that can be addressed later in the company as other issues at a hand might be more important.

Thus, we start with an assumption, which draws from the technical debt and its management, that a company can consciously take a 'skill loan' for being able to meet the short-term objectives whereas those decisions might have harmful implications in the long-term and setting the loan might be expensive later. This is similar than in the technical debt—by conscious decision, the developers might improve, e.g., time-to-market by accepting a lower production quality.

Thus, we initially define the HR debt as *conscious decisions and actions not to invest in, e.g., skill and competence developments, training and lowering recruitment standards in order to achieve various short-term benefits while being aware that in a long-term period, these can cause remarkable drawbacks.* Respectively, the 'HR debt management' concept refers to management of HR debts in various ways.

There are a few remarks in the definition that should be noted. Firstly, it should be acknowledged that the most of the companies who are not investing in the skill and competence development are currently doing this likely without conscious decisions. That is, due to, e.g., lack of time or proper HRM, companies have adopted this kind of a way of working. Yet, it should not be considered as a HR debt. To properly gain advantage from HR debt, decisions – including benefits and drawbacks—should be clearly analyzed.

Secondly, the benefits gained or drawbacks endured from HR debt do not need to be monetarily. While in the technical debt management, the economic consequences are often emphasized. Yet, in the HRM, the implications do not need to be only directly monetarily, but they can be related to, e.g., well-being and work satisfaction. Naturally, these can be indirectly linked back to the economic consequences.

Third, a clear difference between a loan and a technical debt is that one can rarely decide not to pay the loan and its interest back. Whereas technical debt items can be discarded (e.g. technical debt is rejected when the product is removed from the use) or tolerated (e.g. products that are used but not updated anymore) without significant consequences. HR debt, however, relates more on a loan than on technical debt. That is, one cannot avoid the consequences of the HR debt.

4.3 Comparison with Other Concepts

It is worthwhile to note differences between the HR debt and the concept of 'social debt' by Tamburri et al. [40]. The social debt is defined as *"a cumulative and increasing cost in the current state of things, connected to invisible and negative effects within a development community. These effects might need some digging in order to be found since they are connected to undesirable, often implicit characteristics in the organizational and social structure emerging in development communities. These characteristics produce an additional cost, e.g., increase the time needed for development"* [41].

Our points of departure are the following. First, the work by Tamburri et al. [41] emphasize the interactions inside the software development community and problems caused by it. As the opposite point of view, the HR debt focuses on individuals, their skills and competences. Second, the social debt approach focuses still on the implications touching on the different areas of software engineering, such as architecture and development processes. The HR debt focuses more on a company and management level areas.

Furthermore, there are inherited links between the two concepts. For example, Tamburri et al. [41] point out that the social debt might cause instances of technical debt. As an example, they describe a case where a socio-technical decision to change the programming language caused waste by unnecessary implementations. Similarly, also the HR debt can cause technical debt—not having a well-qualified developer can cause that, e.g., the solutions are not top-notch. However, this yet expands the limits of the technical debt and its management— according to overall views of 'technical debt', the debt instances, or at least their management, should be based on conscious decisions. This, however, might not be the case in either of the examples presented.

In addition, there are several different aspects of technical debt; for instance, Tom et al. [42] use four dimensions: code debt, documentation debt, architecture debt, environmental debt, and testing debt. Whereas HR debt might have relations to the most of these dimensions, there are no clear connections between those.

5   Conclusion, Discussions and Future Work

To the best of the authors' knowledge, this is among the first academic papers to open the discussion on the human resource debt and its management. This study presented our arguments for the need of and an initial definition of the concept. This conceptual-analytical paper aims to lay the base for further work and pinpoint some fruitful research areas. Therefore, we are briefly discussing the promising research avenues. The following list does not aim to cover all necessary aspects; instead, it is hoped to inspire academics with various backgrounds to take a look on the HR debt.

Implications of HR Debt Management. The basic assumption is built on the premises that not investigating in the skill development of employees, a company achieves benefits in a short-term period (c.f. money received in a loan). However, the detriments of this decision are appearing the long-term period (c.f. interests of a loan).

Therefore, the fundamental question in the HR debt concept is whether there are real implications caused by conscious decision and management of HR debt or not. Furthermore, it should be studied would a company achieve greater good by taking HR debt and managing it properly than in other ways. For example, a company could decide to take HR debt by recruiting a less-skilled workforce in order to be able to deliver a product or a service quicker to the market—even while its architecture, technical quality or feature lists would suffer from using non-competent developers.

Monetary Aspects of HR Debt Management. As with the most definitions of the technical debt, the money is often—but not always—present also in the HR debt concept. While the possible lack of economic aspects was noted in the proposed definition of the concept, still the different monetary aspects should be analyzed. Also when we are talking about HR debt in software industry, we have to remember that ICT skills and competences are also a cross-cutting factor through industries. If a human resource debt in software business is consciously treated with negligence and not taken care of, the consequences and the financial damages can be major.

Dimensions of HR Debt. In the field of technical debt management, different dimensions or aspects of technical debt has been identified [42]. Whether HR debt approach is found useful, a fruitful research would be to study and identify are there more nuances or sub-types of HR debt. For example, would there be differences been different skills and competence areas, or should HR debt be divided according to technical and other kinds of competences. In addition, there might be differences in the HR debt regarding of having a deep understanding on certain technologies versus having a wide-ranging understanding about several different technology families.

Modelling and Analyzing HR Debt. An important aspect for understanding and following the HR debt is to have ability to model, identify and keep track on the made HR debt decision. That is, the HR debt decisions might be crucial for the future development of a company and therefore these should be properly documented. In addition, documenting different instances also would help to analyze the HR debt more.

In the field of the technical debt management, different tools have been proposed for capturing (e.g. [30]) and documenting (e.g. [43]) technical debt in software engineering projects. Similar development could be useful also for the HR debt management, yet keeping in mind that there are remarkable differences between the abstraction levels and nuances of these two concepts. For instance, it is likely that there are remarkable number of technical debt issues whereas the number of HR debt instances are likely few. However, a more formal model for documenting and keeping a track of the instances would be useful for the overall HR debt management.

HR Debt Management and the Software Industry. It should be noted that recruitment is always a greater risk for small enterprises than it is for big companies. Small companies have to be always one step ahead and they have to be more aware about conscious HR debt. Because of the growing talent shortage in the field on software industry and ongoing significant technical revolution, the employee engagement is growing more and more important. Software companies are usually small but have managed to shine in employee satisfaction competitions. In the near future, maintaining small software businesses depend largely on how well they succeed to manage HR debt in their company.

One interesting future work possibility could be to research how HR debt was handled in the early 2000 s' when there was huge demand for software professionals, mostly influenced by Nokia's success in the mobile phone industry, and how that HR debt is still seen at the field on Finnish software industry. Are those Nokia engineers still unattractive in the eyes of recruiters and is it because they came to the industry with no training at the time of the last IT-bubble and their skills were not developed during their career?

HR Debt Awareness and Higher Education. Nonetheless, even though HR debt is a good tool for taking over the management of skills and competences in companies, the awareness about HR debt should be present every day and through employees career. The software industry is well-known by its nature that employees are excepted to train themselves by new skills through their career. Lifelong learning should not be only the burden of an employee and companies should give the tools and possibilities for the employees to train themselves properly. Because software industry is a knowledge-intensive industry, the higher education institutions have to reinvent themselves if they want to be also enabling the lifelong learning of software professionals and in that way enable the well-being of software industry. The higher education institutions need more agile methods to offering education and they are also ones whose responsibility should be to raise the awareness of HR debt.

Ethical Aspects of the HR Debt Management. Whenever people, their personal development—or lack of it as in the HR debt—and its management are intertwined, ethical questions are prevalent. While in the domain of the technical debt management, the implications are mainly focusing on artifacts such as the program code or documentations. In the case of the HR debt management, different implications touches individual employees.

Therefore, moral philosophical aspects of conscious HR debt management should be discussed and overall rules for an ethically justified conduct should be laid. For example, treating people only as a resource might contradict with classic Kantian ethics that one should not treat people *'just as a means to an end'*, instead people should always be treated *'also as ends in themselves'*. That is, gambling with employees as well as with their individual skills and competences, in the sake of the HR debt management, might subjugate them just as the means, not as the ends. Thus, while the HR debt management might be a promising tool for boosting, e.g., the short-term growth of the company, the recent development of the HR management towards more ethical justifiable should also be acknowledged.

The aforementioned research avenues certainly are not all fruitful directions inside the HR debt domain. Nevertheless, this study is among the first opening the discussion on this metaphor and concept. In this study, we have identified different research issues that would help to better understand and characterize the HR debt. However, more work is needed in order to create a proper research agenda for advancing this domain.

References

1. Schwab, K.: The fourth industrial revolution. Foreign Affairs (2018). https://www.foreignaffairs.com/articles/2015-12-12/fourth-industrial-revolution. Accessed 23 Jan 2018
2. OECD: New Markets and New Jobs. No. 255 in OECD Digital Economy Papers. OECD Publishing (2016). https://doi.org/10.1787/5jlwt496h37l-en
3. World Economic Forum: The Future of Jobs: Employment, Skills and Workforce Strategy for Fourth Industrial Revolution. Global Challenge Insight Report, World Economic Forum, Geneva, Switzerland (2016)
4. Luoma, E., Rönkkö, M., Tahvanainen, S.: Ohjelmistoyrityskartoitus 2017. (Finnish software industry survey 2017) (2017). http://www.softwareindustrysurvey.fi/wp-content/uploads/2017/10/Oskari2017-vfinal.pdf. Accessed 23 Jan 2018
5. Tieto- ja viestintätekniikan ammattilaiset TIVIA ry: Ohjelmisto-osaaminen Suomen talouskasvun ja uudistumisen jarruna - vuonna 2020 Suomesta puuttuu 15 000 ohjelmistoammattilaista (2017). http://www.tivia.fi/lehdistotiedote/ohjelmisto-osaaminen-suomen-talouskasvun-ja-uudistumisen-jarruna. Press release
6. Hyrynsalmi, S.M., Rantanen, M.M., Hyrynsalmi, S.: Do we have what is needed to change everything? A survey of Finnish software businesses on labour shortage and its potential impacts. In: Proceedings of 13th IFIP TC9 Human Choice and Computers Conference: "This Changes Everything", pp. 1–12 (2018)

7. Metsä-Tokila, T.: Kasvun mahdollistajat - ohjelmistoala ja tekninen konsultointi. Tech. rep., Työ- ja elinkeinoministeriö TEM, Helsinki (2017). http://www.eva.fi/wp-content/uploads/2018/04/eva_analyysi_no_62.pdf

8. Hyrynsalmi, S.M., Rantanen, M.M., Hyrynsalmi, S.: The war for talents in software business: how Finnish software companies are perceiving and coping with the labour shortage? (2018, manuscript in review)

9. Ahopelto, T.: Nollaksi vai ykköseksi. Eva analyysi no 62, Elinkeinoelämän valtuuskunta EVA, Helsinki (2018). http://www.eva.fi/wp-content/uploads/2018/04/eva_analyysi_no_62.pdf

10. Hyrynsalmi, S.M., Rantanen, M.M., Hyrynsalmi, S.: The war of talents in software business: polarisation of the software labour force? In: Proceedings of 7th Wellbeing in the Information Society: Fighting Inequalities, pp. 1–12 (2018)

11. Avgeriou, P., Kruchten, P., Ozkaya, I., Seaman, C.: Managing technical debt in software engineering (dagstuhl seminar 16162). In: Dagstuhl Reports, vol. 6, no. 4, pp. 110–138 (2016). https://doi.org/10.4230/DagRep.6.4.110

12. Holvitie, J.: Technical debt in software development – examining premises and overcoming implementation for efficient management. Ph.D. thesis, University of Turku, Turku, Finland (2017)

13. Klotins, E., et al.: Exploration of technical debt in start-ups. In: ICSE-SEIP 2018: 40th International Conference on Software Engineering: Software Engineering in Practice Track, p. 10. ACM, New York (2018). https://doi.org/10.1145/3183519.3183539

14. Järvinen, P.: On a variety of research output types. Series of Publications D - Net Publications D-2004-6, Department of Computer Sciences, University of Tampere, Tampere, Finland (2004)

15. Kaufman, B.E.: Early Human Resource Management: Issues and Themes, pp. 1–35. Cornell University Press, Ithaca (2008)

16. Legge, K.: What is Human Resource Management?. Macmillan Press Ltd., Hampshire (1995)

17. Burke, R.J., Ng, E.: The changing nature of work and organizations: implications for human resource management. Hum. Res. Manag. Rev. 16(2), 86–94 (2006). https://doi.org/10.1016/j.hrmr.2006.03.006. The New World of Work and Organizations

18. Cardon, M.S., Stevens, C.E.: Managing human resources in small organizations: what do we know? Hum. Res. Manag. Rev. 14(3), 295–323 (2004). https://doi.org/10.1016/j.hrmr.2004.06.001

19. Brown, C., Hamilton, J.T., Hamilton, J., Medoff, J.L.: Employers Large and Small. Harvard University Press, Cambridge (1990)

20. Storey, D.J., Westhead, P.: Management training in small firms - a case of market failure. Hum. Res. Manag. J. 7, 61–71 (1997). https://doi.org/10.1111/j.1748-8583.1997.tb00282.x

21. Baron, J., Hannan, M.: Organizational blueprints for success in high-tech start-ups: lessons from the Stanford project on emerging companies. Calif. Manag. Rev. 44(3), 8–36 (2002). https://doi.org/10.2307/41166130

22. Storey, D.J.: Exploring the link, among small firms, between management training and firm performance: a comparison between the UK and other OCED countries. Int. J. Hum. Res. Manag. 15(1), 112–130 (2004). https://doi.org/10.1080/0958519032000157375

23. Nowak, M.J., Grantham, C.E.: The virtual incubator: managing human capital in the software industry. Res. Policy **29**(2), 125–134 (2000). https://doi.org/10.1016/S0048-7333(99)00054-2

24. Cunningham, W.: The wycash portfolio management system. ACM SIGPLAN OOPS Messenger **4**(2), 29–30 (1993)

25. McConnell, S.: Managing technical debt, pp. 1–14. Construx Software Builders Inc. (2008)

26. Kruchten, P., Nord, R.L., Ozkaya, I.: Technical debt: from metaphor to theory and practice. IEEE Softw. **29**(6), 18–21 (2012)

27. Seaman, C., Guo, Y.: Measuring and monitoring technical debt. In: Advances in Computers, vol. 82, pp. 25–46. Elsevier (2011)

28. Letouzey, J.L.: The SQALE method for evaluating technical debt. In: Proceedings of the Third International Workshop on Managing Technical Debt, pp. 31–36. IEEE Press (2012)

29. Fontana, F.A., Pigazzini, I., Roveda, R., Tamburri, D., Zanoni, M., Di Nitto, E.: Arcan: a tool for architectural smells detection. In: 2017 IEEE International Conference on Software Architecture Workshops (ICSAW), pp. 282–285. IEEE (2017)

30. Holvitie, J., Leppänen, V.: Debtflag: technical debt management with a development environment integrated tool. In: 2013 4th International Workshop on Managing Technical Debt (MTD), pp. 20–27 (2013). https://doi.org/10.1109/MTD.2013.6608674

31. Seaman, C., et al.: Using technical debt data in decision making: potential decision approaches. In: Proceedings of the Third International Workshop on Managing Technical Debt, pp. 45–48. IEEE Press (2012)

32. Zazworka, N., Seaman, C., Shull, F.: Prioritizing design debt investment opportunities. In: Proceedings of the 2nd Workshop on Managing Technical Debt, pp. 39–42. ACM (2011)

33. Cherns, A.: The principles of socio-technical design. Hum. Relat. **29**(8), 783–792 (1976)

34. Enid, M.: The story of socio - technical design: reflections on its successes, failures and potential. Inf. Syst. J. **16**(4), 317–342 (2016). https://doi.org/10.1111/j.1365-2575.2006.00221.x

35. Mumford, E.: Technology and freedom: a socio-technical approach. In: Coakes, E., Willis, D., Lloyd-Jones, R. (eds.) The New SosioTech. CSCW, pp. 29–38. Springer, Heidelberg (2000). https://doi.org/10.1007/978-1-4471-0411-7_3

36. Bødker, S., Grønbæk, K., Kyng, M.: Cooperative design: techniques and experiences from Scandinavian scene, pp. 157–175. Lawrence Erlbaum Associates Inc., New Jersey (1993)

37. Hirschheim, R., Klein, H.K.: A glorious and not-so-short history of the information systems field. J. Assoc. Inf. Syst. **13**, 188–235 (2012)

38. Petter, S., DeLone, W., McLean, E.R.: The past, present, and future of "is success". J. Assoc. Inf. Syst. **13**, 341–362 (2012)

39. Järvinen, P.: Research questions guiding selection of an appropriate research method. Series of Publications D - Net Publications D-2004-5, Department of Computer Sciences, University of Tampere, Tampere, Finland (2004)

40. Tamburri, D.A., Kruchten, P., Lago, P., van Vliet, H.: What is social debt in software engineering? In: 2013 6th International Workshop on Cooperative and Human Aspects of Software Engineering (CHASE), pp. 93–96 (2013). https://doi.org/10.1109/CHASE.2013.6614739

41. Tamburri, D.A., Kruchten, P., Lago, P., van Vliet, H.: Social debt in software engineering: insights from industry. J. Internet Serv. Appl. **6**(1), 10 (2015). https://doi.org/10.1186/s13174-015-0024-6
42. Tom, E., Aurum, A., Vidgen, R.: An exploration of technical debt. J. Syst. Softw. **86**(6), 1498–1516 (2013). https://doi.org/10.1016/j.jss.2012.12.052
43. Guo, Y., et al.: Tracking technical debt – an exploratory case study. In: 2011 27th IEEE International Conference on Software Maintenance (ICSM), pp. 528–531 (2011). https://doi.org/10.1109/ICSM.2011.6080824

The War of Talents in Software Business
Polarisation of the Software Labour Force?

Sonja M. Hyrynsalmi[1] (iD), Minna M. Rantanen[2] (iD), and Sami Hyrynsalmi[3](✉) (iD)

[1] University of Turku, Turku, Finland
smnyla@utu.fi
[2] Turku School of Economics, University of Turku, Turku, Finland
minna.m.rantanen@utu.fi
[3] Pervasive Computing, Tampere University of Technology, Pori, Finland
sami.hyrynsalmi@tut.fi

Abstract. The modern business world is undergoing digitalisation in fast pace and, therefore, more jobs are born in the field of information and communication technology (ICT). Only in Finland, one of the leading countries in digitalisation, there is an estimated need for 7,000–15,000 software professionals while the demand for skilled labour is growing every year. The skill set required from professionals is also changing and different skills are needed in the future. ICT companies are facing problems of finding highly skilled professionals to ensure their rapid growth and new innovations. At the same time, when companies are fighting for the talents, there are ICT professionals unemployed. Offered and requested skills are not meeting in the ICT industry, which can lead to bigger problems in the eyes of workers and companies. This study focuses on the skill polarisation between software professionals at the war of talents by using data collected with a survey (n = 90) to software businesses. The results reveal some signs of ongoing skill polarisation in the field and its possible impacts are discussed.

Keywords: Software business · Skill · Competence
Skill polarisation · War for talents

1 Introduction

As pointed out already by an ancient Greek philosopher Heraclitus, over two millenia ago, *"everything changes and nothing stands still"*. This old wisdom, that the only constant is the change itself, remains true even for the modern day working life. Both the job titles and the duties of a single job are constantly evolving. However, changes in the work life are a part of a bigger picture. It is widely deemed that we are now living on a new technological era or a start of the fourth industrial revolution [1]. Currently, the digitalised world is affecting every aspect of our lives and it is expected to create new possibilities from machine learning, robotics, nanotechnology as well as from artificial intelligence [1,2].

© Springer Nature Switzerland AG 2018
H. Li et al. (Eds.): WIS 2018, CCIS 907, pp. 42–52, 2018.
https://doi.org/10.1007/978-3-319-97931-1_4

Even the work itself is digitalisating and demands for skills and competencies of new kinds are arising as an impact of new technologies and innovations [3].

Every industrial revolution has affected the labour market and there are no reasons to estimate that this revolution would be an exception. New work duties will be born and old ones will fade out as an impact of automatisation and digitisation. Therefore, new skills are vital in both old and new occupations. In addition, it has been discussed that this revolution will most likely affect differently to the women and men as well as people from different age groups [4]. Right now only 17% of the almost 8 million ICT specialists are women. It is said that because of currently unequal share of caring and house works, women will have less time to invest in training and life-long learning, which is crucial in the fast changing ICT sector and jobs. Still, attracting more women to ICT sector is estimated to lead to economic growth, with more jobs and increased GDP [5].

However, there is a problem at our hands right now: Where to find people, with those new skills, to be the changemakers? For example, in Finland, one of the leading countries in digitalisation and innovations [6], the estimated need for software professionals during 2017–2018 varies from 7,000 to 15,000—in addition, the need is estimated to grow yearly by 3,800 person [7–9]. Authors of this study have already researched how software companies are perceiving the labour shortage and investigated that there is an ongoing *war for talents* between software companies in Finland [10,11].

This paper turns the perspective around and studies the polarisation of labour force in the software industry. In this study, we are addressing whether there is a *war of talents* between the software professionals and how the employers are perceiving this phenomenon. That is, we study the signs of skill polarisation inside the workforce in the software industry. In this study, by 'skill polarisation' we are referring to a development process where those capable with modern technologies are fought for, whereas those skilled with other technologies, such as obsolete frameworks, are passed over. This study departs from the previous studies on the labour polarisation by focusing on the internal structure of a single industrial field and specifically on the skill polarisation.

To answer the research objective, we use the responses of the survey for the top managers of Finnish software companies regarding the labour shortage in the industry. We are interested to see if there really is an on-going war of talents between software professionals and why and how software industry see the situation. We present a qualitative thematic analysis to the open-ended responses (n = 90) given by the managers. The results show that highly talented software professionals seem to be able to choose the company they work for, and the respondents are perceiving that largest companies are able to provide the best benefits as well as a high wage. Yet, also the opposite seems to be true. Often, it is mentioned that there are applicants that are skilled with obsolete technologies.

It is worthwhile to note that software business is widely considered as an industrial field of highly skilled labour. As the work is seen as an important part of modern people's identity and life, an ongoing polarisation in a high-skill field might endanger the well-being of employees in the information society.

That is, the polarisation process might produce a group of highly educated and experienced ICT employees who are unable to find work, which in the end will affect the well-being of the individuals of this group. To fight against this trap of skills, actions are needed from the governmental, academic as well as from the private stakeholders.

The rest of this paper is structured as follows. First, the background is presented in Sect. 2 and it is followed by a description of the empirical data acquisition process in Sect. 3. Section 4 presents the results and the impacts of this study are discussed in Sect. 5. Lastly, Sect. 6 concludes the study.

2   Background

Every industrial revolution has affected our society vastly. New kind of business opportunities, jobs and demands for new skills had arisen first from the mechanisation of industry, then from the mass production, after that from the automation and robotics in industry and now from the digitisation and smart solutions. Every industrial revolution has affected the jobs, erased old occupations and gave birth to new ones. However, the differentiating issue this time is the speed of changes, and that is causing more problems than excepted from the learnings of the past revolutions [12,13].

A high-skilled worker usually has a degree from a college, technical school or university. Previous research has shown that demands for high-skilled labour has grown every decade hand in hand with every industrial revolution [14]. It has been studied that nowadays an employee possess greater variety in the skills and competencies compared, for example, with a worker at the 1970s [15]. The software business is not the only industrial field which needs ICT professionals who can code, make applications or analyse data. This revolution, at the latest, will make it clear that ICT is, nowadays, everywhere—and the need for skilled ICT workers is everywhere. Today's software professional is not only a technical expert, he also posses new kinds of 'soft skills', such as self-direction, information-processing, problem-solving and communication [16].

The need for the skilled workforce has already lead some of the researchers to talk about a global 'war for talents' which refers to employers' competition for employees [17,18]. For example, World Economic Forum has stated that there are already now difficulties in order to recruit talents for some job families, such as data analyst, database and network professionals, and electrotechnology engineers [4]. World Economic Forum is also forecasting that open vacancies for ICT specialists in a large scale are going to be harder to fill in the near future [4].

European Commission's study has estimated that by 2020 there will be 756,000 unfilled vacancies for ICT professionals in the whole economy [19]. It is also estimated that in the next decades there is going to be growing demand especially for more advanced digital skills compared with the low-skill ICT labour [20]. In developed countries, the ageing of the population has also its effect on the situation. More talented workers are retiring than there are new ones entering to the job markets [21]. Therefore, it is not a surprise, that software professionals are nowadays said to be one of the most hunted occupations [22].

In addition, those high-skilled experts, including software professionals, are in the sight of every growth-seeking country who wants to ensure a high level of know-how in their country. A large number of countries, among the leading immigration countries (e.g. USA, Canada and Australia), are polishing their talent attraction management strategies and political moves for talent migration. For instance, Sweden and the Netherlands have tax discounts for highly educated workers, Germany and France have launched 'scientific visa' and 'green cards' to attract high-skilled workers from the countries not belonging European Economic Area (EEA) [23,24]. All of these actions have been done to prevent major problems in each country's economics and abilities to produce innovations, which have been seen to be in problems if the right kind of work force would be missing.

Thus, the lack of right skills and competencies is a global problem and its effect are already visible in some countries. Finland, for instance, is evidently facing a severe labour shortage in the ICT industry. The need for software professionals is already now varying from 7,000 to 15,000 and the estimated need for new workers in the industry is growing 3,800 per year. However, a fundamental problem is that only around 1,100 students graduate from the field of computer science and technology yearly [7–9]. Therefore, Finnish software companies are forced to work overtime and limit their growth expectations [7,11].

There are signs that Finland might be losing its potential for being one of the leading countries in digitalisation. Also, this can be the case with other top countries, most of them from the Nordics [25]. In global rankings, Finland has also lost its place in top 5 innovative countries[1]. It cannot be stated that that is because of the labour shortage in the software industry; however, it may have been among the one of the reasons as the ICT industry is fuelling innovations in other industrial fields with its solutions. In addition, Finland does not have a change to lose in this competition because already now the ICT industry is the second largest industrial field in the country, after the paper and pulp industry, and it covers 11.4% of Finnish national export yearly [26].

Next, we move our discussion to the polarisation of job markets. This is a useful research area to explain and understand the development in the software industry. The concept of *'job polarisation'* refers to a recent development of job markets towards two end-points: well-paid high-skill jobs, and low paid least-skill jobs [27]. At the same time, jobs belonging to a middle of this spectrum are disappearing. This kind of development has been reported already in the 1980s in the U.S. [28] and from early on, the technological change has been accounted as one of the reasons [29]. The development has since steadily continued in the U.S. [30,31] and the similar phenomenon has also been observed in Europe [32]. However, as discussed by Goos and Manning [27], this development is not only a result of skill-biased technological change; also, the level of routine manual and routine cognitive jobs have been decreasing [33].

---

[1] World Economic Forum. "South Korea and Sweden are the most innovative countries in the world". https://www.weforum.org/agenda/2018/02/south-korea-and-sweden-are-the-most-innovative-countries-in-the-world/. Accessed April 10, 2018.

While the majority of the previous studies have focused on nation-wide analyses, there are also analyses focusing on, e.g., the sub-national level [34,35]. However, in this paper, we focus on development inside a single industrial field instead of general population. Yet, the extant literature of job polarisation might help to explain and understand the potential consequences of polarisation inside an industrial field. In our case, we focus on the 'skill polarisation' which refers to the development of two end-point categories for employees: those who are highly skilled in relevant modern technologies, and those who are skilled yet in, e.g., obsolete technologies.

3   Research Process

The empirical material for this inquiry is collected via an electronic survey [36] sent to the members of the Finnish Software Industry & Entrepreneurs Association (*Ohjelmistoyrittäjät ry*). The association represents software entrepreneurs in Finland and it has over 600 members, including software companies, their managers as well as the field's central influencers. The questionnaire was sent by the association by the request of Helsingin Sanomat[2] at the beginning of the fall 2017.

The questionnaire consisted of two parts. In the first part, a company's vision for the forthcoming growth and requirement of more labour was asked. In the second part, open-ended questions regarding the labour shortage's impact on the company was presented. Overall, 160 answers were gathered, thus, indicating that approximately one-fourth of the members responded to the questionnaire.

This study continues the work done previously by us in [10,11]. In [10], we studied how the Finnish software businesses perceive the labour shortage in the field of ICT with a quantitative analysis. We showed that there are signs of the labour shortage influencing on the growth and innovations in the field. In [11], we used a qualitative analysis to identify the reasons and consequences of the labour shortage.

During the analyses of the data, it was noted that frequently appearing theme in the open-ended answers is the division between the high- and less-skilled labour. This division motivates this study and this paper departs from the previous ones by focusing on the '*war of talents*' instead of the '*war for talents*'.

To study this divide between high- and less-skilled labour, we use a qualitative analysis of the open-ended answers. We focused on the subset of answers discussing or emphasising this skill divide. The overall analysis follows the basic steps of the thematic analysis [37]. Two researchers, who are familiar with the dataset, identified the answers belonging to our subset. In the meetings of the authors, the subset was went through and overall themes related to phenomenon

---

[2] Kempas, K. "Koodareita haetaan yhä useammin ulkomailta, koska Suomessa ei riitä osaajia – jotkut yritykset haluavat olla 'sataprosenttisesti suomalaisia'". Helsingin Sanomat, October 5th, 2017.

at hand was identified. As the results of the meeting, the themes were selected and agreed between all authors.

All respondents were numbered, from #1 to #90, and in the direct quotations, we are identifying different respondents with the unique identifier. All answers were given in Finnish and the presented quotations were translated by the authors. Finally, as all answers are treated confidentially, we have removed such details that could help to identify a company.

4 Results

In the responses of the top level managers, a clear division between 'high-skilled' software professionals and 'less-skilled' software professionals. Among those respondents, who have not perceived the labour shortage, a commonly given explanation was that there is abundance of offering in the less-skilled software professionals whereas it is hard to find the highly skilled professionals. For example, respondents reported that:

- *"There are enough basic-level programmers, but not necessarily enough skilled and able to understand modern platforms."* (ID #50);
- *"There seems still to be some experts on the market. Especially in the resource rental market, there seems to be over-supply and low prices. [...] highly skilled labour is hard to recruit, even tough there is workforce available."* (ID #83); and
- *"There are some basic-level experts* [available in the job market] *but experienced professionals are under the rock."* (ID #48).

Highly skilled professionals were characterised by, on one hand, the know-how on modern technologies, tools and frameworks. On the other hand, experience was often mentioned. Several times the respondents mentioned that they have been forced to recruit people under the set pre-requirements to be able even to fill the position. For example, a respondent points out that it is *"[h]ard to find normal-level programmers, but so far I have found only when I have been ready to make compromises on the knowledge and experience"* (ID #30).

However, it is a worth noting that experience alone is not all as there is a mismatch of skills offered and requested. For a simple example, please consider the following. Due to the boom of Nokia's phones in the early 2000s, there are lots of those skilled with, e.g., Symbian operating system whereas the companies are nowadays looking for Android and iOS professionals. Also new technological paradigm changes, such as cloud computing and robotic process automation, have emerged in the last few years and the experience of the previous generation's tools, processes and frameworks is no more as valuable as it used to be.

As a consequence of the labour shortage and especially on the lack of high-skilled professionals, several respondents report that salaries of the high-skilled professionals have been started to grow over the limits. Therefore, several respondents pointed out that small or medium-sized companies cannot anymore compete of experts with salaries. On the positive side, when the competition with salaries is not seen as productive, the companies have turned their focus on work well-being issues. As pointed out by a respondent, *"[r]ecruiting, especially finding more experienced developers, is difficult. On the other hand, competition from the experts forces us to pay attention to management and to the fact that the workplace also has enough to provide for the employees. When these things are fine, it will ultimately affect the whole company's result. This also makes software firms leaders in the Finnish employers' scene"* (ID #25).

On the negative side, companies were divided whether to invest into retraining and competence building of less-skilled employees or not. As characterised by one respondent that *"[t]here is a specific problem on the software side that the competence is largely outdated in five years. Employers generally can not afford or are not willing to retrain people to today's tools and requirements because it is considered a society's task"* (ID #61). Furthermore, it was pointed out in a few responses that it is possible that an employee changes the company after an expensive training. However, there were also those respondents emphasising that competence building is something that employers should support and pay. For instance, a respondent reported that *"the [Inter]net offers quite a lot of self-study material in the form of different courses. Our firm invest and pay these for employees"* (ID #70).

In addition, it was also pointed out in single answers that the employers are often seeking for 'unicorns', extremely skilled and yet cheap employees. Finally, several respondents pointed out that the experts are active to change jobs and compete employers against each others. As discussed by a respondent *"The salary demand of available workers is beginning to rise unrealistically high. Too often a motivation for people who exchange jobs often is just raising wages, which is a strong signal that a person should not be hired—he will also easily switch to the next company"* (ID #14). Similar kinds of observations were reported also by other respondent, who stated that *"It is important to pay attention to the employee's well-being at work because otherwise the experts will go away. Wage growth is also significantly higher than the national average, almost 10 % per year"* (ID #64). However, as pointed out also in this answer, the positive consequence is that the companies are forced to focus on the well-being in the work in order to keep the high-skilled experts.

5   Discussion

We recapitulate our study's key findings in the following three observations:

- While there is an overall labour shortage in the software industry, there seems to be a constant supply for less-skilled software professionals whereas high-skilled professional are highly sought for.
- High-skilled professionals are characterised, not only by experience but also by competencies on—or ability to learn—modern technologies.
- High-skilled professionals compete employers against each others for raising wages. Also, they easily change employers which is a reason why some of the firms are not interested to invest into the training and competence building.

Altogether, these hints on the possible polarisation of the labour inside the software industry. However, due to the overall labour shortage, also less-skilled are, at least now, able to get jobs. Nevertheless, the miss-match of skills and jobs is creating a market for skilled. During the war for talents, skilled workers can bid between employees and at the same time less-skilled professionals have to take what is offered—even if it is a job where overtime work is done because of the lack of resources and labour shortage. Those less-skilled workers will find themselves at the skill trap—to success in the field of ICT they should master new technologies and skills but they do not get enough support and retraining from their present employees because of time and resource limits. Thus, the war of talents can lead to situation where the skill and competence development of some of the ICT professionals slows down. This could lead to seizing of development level of the ICT professionals' skills and competencies in general, which is not ideal.

Meanwhile, companies are looking for affordable yet highly skilled people with competence in specific technologies. In the survey, it became clear that these people are rare and hard to find. It could be stated, that in the war of talents these people are like *unicorns*—mythical creatures that simply do not exist. Highly skilled people seem to know that they are the ones that everybody needs and wants, which raises their expectations about the compensation as well as other benefits. However, it has also become apparent that monetary compensation is not enough—also the quality of the workplace is an important factor affecting the desirability of the workplace. Companies working in the ICT field have become known for breaking the model of traditional workplace by focusing on comfort and bringing pleasure to offices.

Creating playgrounds for adults is not all that these companies are doing. Perhaps a more sustainable approach is taken by companies that offer training and competence building as part of the employment. However, as multiple respondents stated, training requires a lot of resources, which companies are already short of because of the labour shortage. It was hinted that training could also be a waste if workers choose to leave the company, which often is the case with high-skilled workers. On one hand, training the employees could help to prevent polarisation by narrowing the gap between less- and high-skilled workers.

On the other hand, this phenomenon could also put the companies in unequal positions, since bigger companies are more likely to be able to invest in the salaries and training of their employees as well as to well-being and activities in the workplace. Smaller companies often lack the extensive resources of time and money. Furthermore, the responses from smaller firms emphasise chronic hurry, which might imply less time is left for competence building of employees. However, smaller companies do have the advantage of lower hierarchies, which could mean that they are able to react to the desires of their employees faster than bigger companies. Since changes require resources, there is a limit to which they can be acted upon especially in the small companies. Thus, competition for high-skilled personnel could lead to increasing inequality between companies.

The field of ICT is drastically fast-phased in its development. Development of old and new technologies requires a lot of skills, competencies as well as company resources. Vacuum of skilled employees has created a suitable ground for the war of talents, which could lead to a decrease of the overall skill and competence level. War of talents does not particularly encourage skilled people to update their skill sets and competencies—especially when training is seen as something that binds the limited resources of a company. This could lead to a situation where today's skillful and competent people are tomorrow's outdated relics.

If the polarisation becomes reality, it could result in a situation where the field has only a little true knowledge and a lot of people with none to mediocre skills and competencies. This could lead to increasing the turn-over of employees, decreasing job satisfaction and raising levels of unemployment. The war of talents might become a war of shooting stars, a war between people at the peak of their skills and competencies, but who are not able to up-date their skills.

Consequences of this phenomenon can be really harmful to the whole industry of IT. However, to understand the war of talents and its impacts on the IT, we should research it further. It would be beneficial to conduct empirical investigations amongst the employees in the field of IT. How do they see and feel the war of talents? Do they have the resources to develop their skills and competencies? Do they feel that they can be the winners in this war? In other words, how is the war of talents affecting the well-being of the professionals in the field of ICT?

Finally, this study is naturally limited by its method and focus on a single Nordic country. As it is known, often people, who are the most interested in the phenomenon under study, answer to the questionnaire and this can, therefore, create a bias to the responses. Furthermore, Finland's software industry has its own characteristics (e.g., the implications of the post-Nokia era) which makes direct generalisation to other economies hard. Nevertheless, this study opens interesting avenues for future inquiries.

6   Conclusions

This paper studied the polarisation employees inside the software industry. Based on an analysis of a survey, we found that there are signs of divergence to those highly skilled and fought for the experts of modern technologies and to those less-skilled experts (i.e., the war of talents). This is a noteworthy observation as the software industry and the ICT field are widely considered as a high-skill industry. This kind of development can lead to significant inequalities in the well-being in the work in future information societies.

Acknowledgements. The authors wish to thanks Managing Director *Rasmus Roiha* and Finnish Software Industry & Entrepreneurs Association for sharing the dataset used in this study.

References

1. Schwab, K.: The fourth industrial revolution. Foreign Affairs, January 2018. https://www.foreignaffairs.com/articles/2015-12-12/fourth-industrial-revolution. Accessed 23 Jan 2018
2. Hermann, M., Pentek, T., Otto, B.: Design principles for industrie 4.0 scenarios. In: 2016 49th Hawaii International Conference on System Sciences (HICSS), pp. 3928–3937 (2016). https://doi.org/10.1109/HICSS.2016.488
3. OECD: New markets and new jobs. In: OECD Digital Economy Papers, No. 255. OECD Publishing (2016). https://doi.org/10.1787/5jlwt496h37l-en
4. World Economic Forum: The future of jobs: employment, skills and workforce strategy for fourth industrial revolution. Global Challenge Insight report, World Economic Forum, Geneva, Switzerland (2016)
5. European Institute for Gender Equality (EIGE): Women and men in ICT: a chance for better work-life balance (2018). http://eurogender.eige.europa.eu/system/files/events-files/women_and_men_in_ict_presentation.pdf. Accessed 8 Apr 2018
6. Digibarometri 2016: Helsinki, Finland (2016). http://teknologiateollisuus.fi/sites/default/files/file_attachments/digibarometri-2016.pdf
7. Luoma, E., Rönkkö, M., Tahvanainen, S.: Ohjelmistoyrityskartoitus 2017 (Finnish software industry survey 2017) (2017). http://www.softwareindustrysurvey.fi/wp-content/uploads/2017/10/Oskari2017-vfinal.pdf. Accessed 23 Jan 2018
8. Tieto- ja viestinttekniikan ammattilaiset TIVIA ry: Ohjelmisto-osaaminen Suomen talouskasvun ja uudistumisen jarruna - vuonna 2020 Suomesta puuttuu 15 000 ohjelmistoammattilaista (2017, press release). http://www.tivia.fi/lehdistotiedote/ohjelmisto-osaaminen-suomen-talouskasvun-ja-uudistumisen-jarruna
9. Naumanen, M., et al.: Tekbaro 2017. Tekniikan akateemiset TEK, Helsinki (2017)
10. Hyrynsalmi, S.M., Rantanen, M.M., Hyrynsalmi, S.: The war for talents in software business: how Finnish software companies are perceiving and coping with the labour shortage? (2018, manuscript in review)
11. Hyrynsalmi, S.M., Rantanen, M.M., Hyrynsalmi, S.: Do we have what is needed to change everything? A survey of Finnish software businesses on labour shortage and its potential impacts. In: Proceedings of 13th IFIP TC9 Human Choice and Computers Conference: "This Changes Everything", pp. 1–12 (2018)
12. Katz, L.F., Margo, R.A.: Technical change and the relative demand for skilled labor: the United States in historical perspective. Working Paper 18752, National Bureau of Economic Research, February 2013. https://doi.org/10.3386/w18752
13. Frey, C.B., Osborne, M.A.: The future of employment: how susceptible are jobs to computerisation? Technol. Forecast. Soc. Change **114**, 254–280 (2017). https://doi.org/10.1016/j.techfore.2016.08.019
14. Falk, M., Biagi, F.: Relative demand for highly skilled workers and use of different ICT technologies. Appl. Econ. **49**(9), 903–914 (2017). https://doi.org/10.1080/00036846.2016.1208357
15. Becker, S.O., Muendler, M.A.: Trade and tasks: an exploration over three decades in Germany. Econ. Policy **30**(84), 589–641 (2015). https://doi.org/10.1093/epolic/eiv014
16. Spiezia, V.: Jobs and Skills in the Digital Economy. OECD Observer (2016)
17. Chambers, E.G., Foulon, M., Handfield-Jones, H., Hankin, S.M., Michaels, E.G.I.: The war for talent. McKinsey Q. **1**(3), 44–57 (1998)
18. Beechler, S., Woodward, I.C.: The global 'war for talent'. J. Int. Manag. **15**(3), 273–285 (2009). https://doi.org/10.1016/j.intman.2009.01.002. The Emerging CEO Agenda in Multinational Companies

19. European Commission: The Digital Single Market - State of Play. European Union (2017). https://doi.org/10.2759/746724
20. Berger, T., Frey, C.B.: Digitalization, jobs and convergence in Europe: strategies for closing the skills gap. Technical report, University of Oxford (2016)
21. Mahroum, S.: Europe and the immigration of highly skilled labour. Int. Migr. **39**(5), 27–43 (2001). https://doi.org/10.1111/1468-2435.00170
22. Lehner, F., Sundby, M.W.: ICT skills and competencies for SMEs: results from a structured literature analysis on the individual level. In: Harteis, C. (ed.) The Impact of Digitalization in the Workplace. PPL, vol. 21, pp. 55–69. Springer, Cham (2018). https://doi.org/10.1007/978-3-319-63257-5_5
23. Chaloff, J., Lematre, G.: Managing highly-skilled labour migration - a comparative analysis of migration policies and challenges in OECD countries. OECD Social, Employment and Migration Working Papers, No. 79 (2009). https://doi.org/10.1787/225505346577
24. Bauer, T.K., Kunze, A.: The demand for high-skilled workers and immigration policy. IZA Discussion Paper No. 999, RWI: Discussion Papers No. 11 (2004)
25. Chakravorti, B., Bhalla, A., Chaturvedi, R.S.: 60 Countries' Digital Competitiveness, Indexed. Harvard Business Review, Watertown (2017)
26. Haaparanta, P., et al.: 100 vuotta pientä avotaloutta - Suomen ulkomaankaupan kehitys, merkitys ja näkymät. Technical report, Valtioneuvoston selvitys- tutkimustoiminta (2017)
27. Goos, M., Manning, A.: Lousy and lovely jobs: the rising polarization of work in Britain. Rev. Econ. Stat. **89**(1), 118–133 (2007). https://doi.org/10.1162/rest.89.1.118
28. Bluestone, B., Harrison, B.: The growth of low-wage employment: 1963–86. Am. Econ. Rev. **78**(2), 124–128 (1988)
29. Bluestone, B.: The Polarization of American Society: Victims, Suspects, and Mysteries to Unravel. Twentieth Century Fund Press, New York (1995)
30. Autor, D.H., Katz, L.F., Kearney, M.S.: The polarization of the U.S. labor market. Am. Econ. Rev. **96**(2), 189–194 (2006)
31. Autor, D.: The Polarization of Job Opportunities in the U.S. Labor Market: Implications for Employment and Earnings. The Brookings Institution, Washington, D.C. (2010)
32. Goos, M., Manning, A., Salomons, A.: Explaining job polarization: routine-biased technological change and offshoring. Am. Econ. Rev. **104**(8), 2509–2526 (2014)
33. Autor, D.H., Levy, F., Murnane, R.J.: The skill content of recent technological change: an empirical exploration. Q. J. Econ. **118**(4), 1279–1333 (2003)
34. Abel, J.R., Deitz, R.: Job polarization and rising inequality in the nation and the New York-northern New Jersey region. Curr. Issues Econ. Finan. **18**(7), 1–7 (2012)
35. Terzidis, N., van Maarseveen, R., Ortega-Argilés, R.: Employment polarization in local labour markets: the dutch case. Technical report 358, CPB Netherlands Bureau for Economic Policy Analysis (2017)
36. Dillman, D.A.: Mail and Internet Surveys: The Tailored Design Method. Wiley, New York (2007)
37. Braun, V., Clarke, V.: Using thematic analysis in psychology. Qual. Res. Psychol. **3**, 77–101 (2006). http://eprints.uwe.ac.uk/11735

Unworthy Guardians: Nappula Child Welfare Information System

Jouko Kiesiläinen[1], Minna M. Rantanen[2(✉)], Olli I. Heimo[2],
and Kai K. Kimppa[2]

[1] Hyvinvointipalvelut Arjessa Oy, Hakakatu 12, 20540 Turku, Finland
jouko.kiesilainen@arjessa.fi
[2] Department of Management and Entrepreneurship,
Turku School of Economics, University of Turku, 20014 Turku, Finland
{minna.m.rantanen,olli.heimo,kai.kimppa}@utu.fi

Abstract. In this paper we examine a Finnish child protective service software Nappula. We point out some of the problems with the system in relation to the information stored and used. It shares some of the problems which are prevalent in patient information systems without exactly being one. Some of these problems include, but are not limited to privacy problems and a lack of possibility of correcting data in certain situations, amongst other ethical issues. We point out that the system has issues which cannot be justified in accordance to what the values of child protective services, social services, and the society are.

Keywords: Child protective services · Social services · Information systems
Ethics

1 Introduction

In this paper we are focusing on ethical challenges of the Finnish social welfare platform Nappula. It is used to document and report on the welfare of children. Child welfare in Finland has been in the centre of public discussion and its practices have been looked into closely. In 2012 the Ministry of Social Affairs and Health researched the state of Finnish child welfare's practices. In the report it was stated that: "The four most important bases for child welfare's controls are good practices, accountability, transparency and effectiveness." [1, p. 62]. As a part of transparency is good reporting and most children's homes this means daily reporting to the database. Nappula is currently the main database of its kind in Finland. Nappula is a product of a privately-owned company called Fastroi [2].

One section of Finnish child welfare is preventive work, done in schools, national day care centres and child health centres. Its main purpose is to prevent possible social risks. Another section provides open services that are available for those families who already are customers of social welfare services. In this situation social welfare strives to help families and their children in their own home. It is important to note that a child can be taken in custody if social care has evidence to show that the child's development or health is in jeopardy [3, 4].

H. Li et al. (Eds.): WIS 2018, CCIS 907, pp. 53–63, 2018.
https://doi.org/10.1007/978-3-319-97931-1_5

According to the Finnish national institute of health and welfare's statistics, children's custody rates have grown dramatically. When in 1993 there was 9000 children and youngsters living outside of their homes, in the end of year 2015 same number was over 18 000 doubling the numbers in just over 20 years. From these 18 000 children and youngster nearly 10 000 were taken to custody. Approximately half of the children in care at the end of 2014 were placed to children's homes. The rest of the children were placed to foster families [5].

What is recorded in the system varies between organizations. Especially what is recorded, and in particular, what is left unrecognized and thus unreported varies between departments and individuals within organisations. The interests of the child may remain in the shadow of the interests of the organisation and the public system – the same one which is at least partially removed from the guardian's supervision in the interest of the child – is unable to protect the interests of the child. In addition, written text about the guardians may not be appropriate or fair. Also the use of euphemisms and code words may occur in the system culture, and the supervising body cannot follow them.

2   What Is Nappula? – Documentation in Finnish Child Welfare

In Finnish child welfare, documentation and reporting is regulated by law. Documenting is one way to control and keep decision making transparent in child welfare. Careful documentation is important for a child and his family as well as the employee's legal security. A child's legal protection requires accurate and up-to-date documentation. Improving child and family involvement, making visions more visible and getting a child's voice heard are named as the key goals of the documentation. Describing the customer's life history and life situation increases the employee's understanding. Documentation of child welfare goals is relevant to the child and his or her parents [4].

The purpose of documentation is also to keep information, to inform colleagues and to make work and thinking visible. Documentation supports a systematic work and customer process and highlights the expertise of a social worker or other child protection worker (e.g. an educator). It improves the continuity and structuring of work. Documenting increases the sense of job control and provides the necessary knowledge base for the development of client work [4].

The law on access to information is governed by the Act on the Openness of Government Activities 11 §. The contents of the authority's document shall be provided orally or by means of a document to be read by the authority, reproduced or listened to, or provided by a copy or a printout. Information on the public content of a document must be provided as requested, unless the compliance with the request for a large number of documents or the difficulty of copying the document or any other comparable reason causes unreasonable disadvantage to official activity [6: 11 §, 16 §].

This demand has created a need for different kinds of documentation databases. In the field of child welfare there are different kinds of databases available, most of them are owned by private companies. One of the most popular databases in Finland is

Nappula, which is largely used in the private sector, like in children's homes and Non-Governmental Organizations (NGOs).

Privately produced and upkept Nappula database offers a large range of possibilities to store information about a child who lives in a children's home or is otherwise in contact with social services. The information can be viewed by a child's social worker and certain workers in the children's home. Even though it is provided by law which workers can see child's documents [7], it depends on the children's home, how well the spirit of the law is fulfilled. Even though National Supervisory Authority for Welfare and Health tries to follow children's homes actions, also in documentation, it doesn't do it without heavy reasons or evidence [8]. So in theory, it is possible that even workers who do not work with a child can observe the child's information.

The information Nappula includes is wide: from day to day reports, through yearly compilations, to medications and parents' contact information. In brief, it contains all information about a child. Usually the reports also include children home's workers' remarks on the child's parents and the child's behaviour. Reports have significant power: they are used as a base for social workers' decisions [4: 26 §, 33 §, 9].

Children and their parents have a right to read the reports and demand corrections when needed according to National Institute for Health and Welfare's recommendation, sharing documents via e-mail is a risk [10] and that's why documents are given usually in printed form via mail. This is problematic: Nappula reports can be updated within 24 h, but these updates cannot be seen in printed versions that are given to parents.

3 Nappula in Practice

In Nappula the system's user rights can be defined by the child protection organization itself. Employees generally have fewer rights than employers, social workers or middle management. It is up to the organization who will see the child's information. What is recorded in the system varies between organizations. Especially what is recorded, and in particular, what is left unrecognized and thus unreported varies between departments and individuals within organisations.

In the system there are management tools and a so-called "message booklet" that can be used to exchange information between employees of the department. This exchange of information is informal and does not appear in the official reports of the child – or in reporting on the child's parents. In other words, this information is limited to a select number of staff, and therefore does not formally exist but may end up to a person who decides on a child's supporting actions. From every child there is a file with picture, reason for custody, the child's educator or foster family, daily reports made by child protection workers, whether a child is in the child protection department or not and whether child has any restrictions given by social workers (for example, restriction to go outside).

When opening a client profile file, there is very comprehensive information about the child (Fig. 1). The middle bar shows the name, identity code, county that child has come from, service contract with the county's social service, educators, child's parents and their contact details. The blue text can contain for example school information, social worker information and a free field that can contain any information. From the grey top bar you can find among other things medication information, care and education plans, restrictions, file bank and seasonal summaries. When writing a report, a written report can be sorted by type, such as schooling, health and other similar issues.

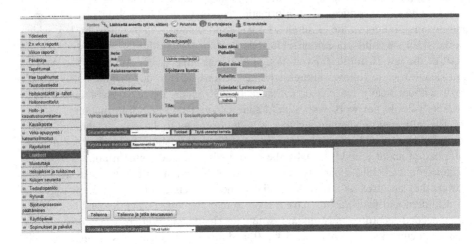

Fig. 1. Client profile in Nappula.

As one can notice, the Nappula software can contain plenty of information about child. While the rights of different employees are often restricted within a company or organization, access to rights is not actively monitored by an outside authority. This allows various abuses and possibly even actions that are against the law. Ultimately, the privacy of the child is not secured. This is in clear contradiction with the good practice described by Finnish National Institute for Health and Welfare (THL): Child protection should be legally and ethically justified, and therefore the existence of written evidence becomes significant. Documenting is demanding because the authors and the documenters have a lot of power and responsibility [4].

One of the challenges of the software is that a child's parents do not have direct access to all information, but can only receive them by asking separately from a social worker. In practice, this means printed documents that do not show for example corrections or other subsequent changes that have been made to reports. Some of the information exchange also does not appear in printed documents: for example, in the "message booklet" information can be exchanged and it does not appear in the official documents. This is a risk for the parent's and child's legal protection: employees can cover their activities, exchange unauthenticated information (e.g. through the "message booklet") and influence the child's process strongly.

Although the Nappula system has been created for reporting on the child, in practice, the child's parents are also the subject of information processing. According to good reporting practices, documentation must include all relevant information about the child [4]. This means that parents will inevitably be subject to evaluation. This is problematic because parents have very poor possibilities to influence what information is shared about them. This gives great power to the educators, social workers and other staff that work with the children to decide how they describe the children's or the parent's behaviour. This issue has now been raised, but nothing has been done to it [4]. Liability for a public act does not reach all those who make reports, as all child welfare workers are not public servants.

Usually a child protection worker has 24 h to correct the text. This also depends on the access rights, and some employees can fix the reports later. However, there is a possibility that the reports are not corrected, but the correction requests are subsequently recorded in addition to that text. In practice parent's disputed, and possibly wrongly reported, information stays in documents. These postings may affect later decision-making, for example in cases which deal with parents' abuse of alcohol. If the employee has registered a suspicion of excessive use of alcohol and the parents' correction is later recorded, the final decision will be interpreted by the decision making social worker. Therefore the problem of correcting reports is visible both at technical and social level. Also the interests of the child may remain in the shadow of the interests of the organisation and the public system – the same one which is at least partially removed from the guardian's supervision in the interest of the child – is unable to protect the interests of the child. On the other hand a social worker who has 70 to 100 "clients" simply cannot follow all the reports and their quality [11, p. 24].

The Nappula system has similar problems as the Finnish Wilma system [12, 13]. The target of the system does not know what is written about them in the system. However, on top of this, it seems to have overlapping qualities with eHealth systems containing data both about possible medications and treatments. Moreover, it is a system which has information that can be used against those who are the subjects of the information without the possibility for them to defend themselves, have knowledge of what is written about them and thus have no chance to correct the information if it is incorrect. Yet again the system data is monitored by the government officials but they do not have enough time (as pointed above) to check and correct all of the inputted data. The point is that the data is stored by the system provider to media owned and controlled by them, and this increases the chances of possible misuse of the data by the system provider and its employees.

4 Nappula and Patient Information Systems

Nappula is an information system used in child welfare which is a part of social services. Social services are in close relation to healthcare. In Finland there is also an active attempt to digitalise all public services – including social services and public healthcare [14]. This reform is built around the National Service Path, which is also a key feature in the official Social Service and Health Care (SOTE) reform, which is a wider reform of social and healthcare services. Digitalisation of public services attempts to make once collected citizen information available for all governmental institutions through the National Service Path [15]. Thus, these reforms will bring social services and healthcare even closer to each other and could make changing information between them easier.

Currently both healthcare information systems and child welfare systems are working mainly under the same laws of handling private information [see e.g. 7], but there are also some more specific laws that apply to patient and healthcare providers [see e.g. 6, 16–18]. However, there are some major differences in the interpretations of these laws that affect the way these information systems are designed and used. Patient information systems (PISs) are used to handle patient information which contains data about patients' health and other information that is needed in healthcare to treat patients [19].

Handling patient information in mainly in electronic form in and between healthcare institutions has required a lot of work around structures and regulations. In healthcare patient information is seen as one of the core instruments in successful healthcare delivery. Thus, there has been a lot of effort in making it as unambiguous as possible by using predetermined structures instead of natural language. Although natural and free text is still used to clarify structured entries, in PISs the information is mainly structured [20]. In other words, patient information is a collection of predetermined pieces of information instead of long texts.

Besides the way of making the entries there are also a lot of regulations about how patient information should be handled in healthcare. For instance, in healthcare the one who makes the entry to the PIS is the one that is responsible of correctness of the entry and the maker of the entry should always be visible also to the patient that the information is about. The patient has a right to check the information written about them and also the right to apply for correcting the information if it is incorrect. If the information is corrected, new corrected information is added to the system next to the incorrect one [19]. Thus, the information once entered in the PISs is not ever removed by any one.

Patient information should be accessed only in cases when a member of healthcare staff is treating a patient. However, to access the information there should always be consent from the patient. In most cases getting into treatment is considered consenting to accessing the information within the organisation, but transferring patient information between organisations should always be the patient's choice. To prevent forbidden access each patient information system should contain a log system that collects data about persons accessing the information. Information about the persons accessing the data is not available to patients, since it is information about healthcare professionals [19, 21].

In contradiction, Nappula contains mainly natural language instead of structured information [22]. This makes the marking more vulnerable to misinterpretations than for example structured information handled in PISs. However, it must be noted that the information in healthcare is in many cases more data driven than in child welfare. But, it must also be noted that in healthcare the practitioners using more free language have structures and rules how to make the entries to provide the necessary and correct information to their colleagues and patients [23]. In child welfare there seems to be no such structures, since each person favours their own way of making the entries [22].

Another big difference between healthcare and child welfare seems to be the responsibility about the correctness of the inserted information. In healthcare, each person making the entries is responsible, whereas in child welfare the responsible party is not the one entering the information, but rather the superior of that person [19].

What comes to the right to check the information, it must be noticed that in case of PISs this applies only to one's own information. In case of a minor for instance, patient information can be visible to guardians or other legal representatives, unless the child forbids it. However, patient information can contain also information about the patient's family members and since that information is not about the patient, this information is not available to the patient [19]. In case of child welfare systems such as Nappula, the information is often about a child – a minor that is then considered to be the client. However, Nappula contains vast amount of information for example about family members and it is possible that this information is not available to the guardians [23]. Thus, Nappula can contain more information that cannot be checked.

This creates a dilemma: the child's representatives such as guardians should see the information collected about the children (and about them), but legally neither the child nor the guardians have the right. Information can be denied from the children or their representatives based on that the information is about somebody else, whereas guardians can be denied the access to that information because it is a part of child's personal information and not theirs.

Thus, people are not able to see what is written about them in these records. Since they cannot see what is written, they cannot check whether the information is correct. If the information in Nappula is incorrect, how people are supposed to know about it and how they can correct it? This together with the lack of responsibility when making entries creates an even greater problem, since there is a possibility to write arbitrary entries that are then considered to be correct without inspection and that incorrect information can be acted upon.

5 Nappula and Values

According to Leavitt [24] and Nurminen and Forsman [25] the change in technological solutions make a change also in work. Therefore IS creation and use has consequences for its users, the organisation, for other organisations, and for the targets of the system. These targets experience impact in their lives as the IS is used. When designing ISs, it is noteworthy to consider that decision in design that changes the system also changes the effects of the system on those who it is used upon [26, p. 5]. The goals of the designer are required to be good and the consequences proper (see e.g. [27–30]). Values (albeit not necessarily ethical values) are always designed into a system [28, pp. 35–39]. An information system without a purpose is not worthy of designing or producing. Purpose brings forth the values. The values in design might differ from the values of the users of the system, for example, the values connected to an IT designer's work differ from the values connected to a medical practitioners' work [29, 30] (see also [31, 32]).

Values and attitudes highlight the things that the people in the organisation as a collective see important. These are affected by and affect the norms, which are official and unofficial rules that the people act upon within the organisation. Norms can be laws as well as unofficial codes of conduct [33]. Healthcare has been strongly affected by the norms above; laws and rules that have shaped the ways of working considerably. Healthcare strongly relies on hierarchies, principles and rules, which can be seen as a result of strict discipline and order which have been used in unifying the actions [34].

Despite the strict rules and norms also human values have a particular role in healthcare. In Finland, ethical codes frame the values that guide the daily actions in healthcare. These codes highlight the value of human life, respect for self-determination, protection of human life and promotion of health [35]. Besides general ethical codes, doctors for example have their own professional ethical code that determines goals of the task as well as ethical liabilities of a doctor [36]. These codes have their roots in medical ethics, which is based on the four principles of autonomy, beneficence, non-maleficence and justice [31]. Rules and laws concerning the handling of the patient information in PISs at least should reflect the values of healthcare. For example they typically aim to support the autonomy and justice through the right of the target, the patient to see and correct the entries made in a PIS.

Hence Nappula is very similar to PISs and should inherit both the values of healthcare and child protection. As mentioned earlier, the four most important bases for child welfare's controls are "good practices, accountability, transparency and effectiveness." [1, p. 62]. In Nappula the documents can be changed afterwards. Therefore they can also be changed to justify actions made after the document was first written even though the original document does not contain any justification for these actions – to avert the accountability and consequences for the misdemeanours of the child protection. Hence the accountability from the aforementioned actions can be seen as lacking.

Transparency seems also be missing for there can be forms which are not available to those who they handle and cannot be accessed by any other than the childcare workers. When the parent is both in the role of "the representative for the child" and "the subject", the system does not give a transparent view for the child nor their representatives. Whereas transparency requires the possibility to see what actions are undertaken and why, these secret documents blur the vision of the process.

Finnish National Institute for Health and Welfare [37] state that the good practices of child protection are (1) the dignity and fundamental rights of the customers, (2) the benefit of the child, (3) interaction, (4) the quality of the work of the professional staff and (5) responsible decisions and operating culture. As shown above, the fundamental rights do not concern the Nappula system where the information is not being transparent. It is hard to defend oneself or one's children when some of the information one is being accused of is kept secret. Also the quality of work and the responsible decisions can be questioned because of the possibility in the system to change the documents.

That does not mean that the quality of work is bad or that there are no responsible workers, the problem is that the system itself does not promote these kinds of practices. If the Nappula system would promote these values, those responsible should not be able to change the documents afterwards. Therefore it seems that at least some of the good practices are not implemented into the system.

Thus it seems that all these three have been sacrificed to the altar of efficiency – mostly in economical viewpoint. Therefore it can be argued that the Nappula system mainly represents the efficiency of child care without inheriting other values from the requirement list given by the Ministry of Social Affairs and Health.

6 Conclusions

The aforementioned dilemma is not a small one. Whereas the guardians are not users of the information system but rather targets of the use as well as their children are. The only one guarding the correctness of the information is the same person writing it. Compared to the medical records there therefore cannot be a checking system to verify the information and thus it can lead to misinformation or even disinformation if the one adding the information is malicious about the targets of the use spreading within the system. This can lead to numerous problems.

One of the problems is the integrity of data. While a normal procedure in healthcare is that the patients check the information written about them, the information cannot be changed (after 24 h) thus leaving the possibility for misinformation to be written to the system – and to stay there. Moreover, the information is not always available for the guardian, and in this case the misinformation stays in the system even when it could have been corrected within 24 h.

As mentioned before, unauthorised use of data is possible with the system and thus the privacy of the children and their parents, the targets of the use is at stake. The system should be redesigned to meet proper privacy standards.

As discussed in Sect. 5, the system should support the values of the organisation but in this case it does not seem to fulfil that demand. On the contrary Nappula seems to have changed the values of the organisation with its structure thus affecting the values of the whole organisation. As the system is designed to suspect both the child and the parent as possible "criminals" who require child protective services, the information flow is more like one from mental institution rather than health care: the patients are not trusted and must be treated even against their will. The inherent value of the organisation – to protect the child – is built to serve the work process of the social worker and the organisation, not the value of the organisation changing the organisational value of protect the child to the value of suspect the parent and the child.

One of the major drawbacks with Nappula is that it is not procured and tailored to meet the needs of the office but merely "bought" from the producer and thus it is lacking various components and finesses required from the information system for the child social services. It serves the social services not only as the best but as the most used system, other, less used systems being very similar – which might explain the overlooking of the aforementioned serious flaws. Hence it seems that either Nappula should be largely redesigned or replaced by a system that is tailored not only to the needs of child protective services as a government office but especially to the values of the child protective services as an entity.

References

1. Kananoja, A., Lavikainen, M., Oranen, M.: Toimiva lastensuojelu – selvitysryhmän loppuraportti [Working child welfare]. Sosiaali- ja terveysministeriön raportteja ja muistioita 2013:19. Sosiaali- ja terveysministeriö, Helsinki (2013)
2. Fastroi: Fastroi Webpage (2018). https://fastroi.fi/en/. Accessed 9 Mar 2018
3. Heino, T., Oranen, M.: Lastensuojelun asiakkaiden koulunkäynti – erityistäkö? [Schooling of clients of child welfare – special?]. In: Jahnukainen, M. (ed.) Lasten erityishuolto ja -opetus Suomessa, 13 edn, pp. 217–248. Vastapaino, Tampere (2012)
4. Finnish National Institute of Health and Welfare (THL): Lastensuojelun käsikirja [Child welfare handbook] (2016). https://www.thl.fi/en/web/lastensuojelun-kasikirja. Accessed 9 Apr 2018
5. Kuoppala, T., Säkkinen, S.: Lastensuojelu 2014 [Child protection 2014] Finnish National institute of health and welfare (THL) (2015)

6. Laki viranomaisten toiminnan julkisuudesta 621/1999 Oikeusministeriö. Edita Publishing Oy. https://www.finlex.fi/fi/laki/ajantasa/1999/19990621

7. Henkilötietolaki 22.4.1999/523 Oikeusministeriö. Edita Publishing Oy. http://www.finlex.fi/fi/laki/ajantasa/1999/19990523

8. Laki yksityisistä sosiaalipalveluista 922/2011 Oikeusministeriö. Edita Publishing Oy. https://www.finlex.fi/fi/laki/alkup/2011/20110922#Lidp450368240

9. Lastensuojelulaki 417/2007 Oikeusministeriö. Edita Publishing Oy. https://www.finlex.fi/fi/laki/ajantasa/2007/20070417#P52

10. Laaksonen, M., et al.: Asiakastyön dokumentointi sosiaalihuollossa [Documenting client work in social welfare]. Opastusta asiakastiedon käyttöön ja kirjaamiseen Raportti 54/2011 Finnish National institute of health and welfare (THL), Helsinki (2011)

11. Valvira: Valtakunnallinen lastensuojelun henkilöstöselvitys. Selvityksiä 1:2014. Valvira (Sosiaali- ja terveysalan lupa- ja valvontaministeriö), Helsinki (2014)

12. Heimo, O.I., Rantanen, M., Kimppa, K.K.: Wilma ruined my life how an educational system became the criminal record for the adolescents. Comput. Soc. Spec. Issue Ethicomp. 45(3), 138–146 (2015)

13. Heimo, O.I., Rantanen, M.M., Kimppa, K.K.: Three views to a school information system: Wilma from a sociotechnical perspective. In: HCC13: This Changes Everything, IFIP TC9 Human Choice and Computers Conference, in Poznan, Poland, September 2018 (2018, in print)

14. Ministry of Finance (2017): Digitalisoidaan julkiset palvelut [Digitalization of public services]. http://vm.fi/digitalisoidaan-julkiset-palvelut. Accessed 11 Dec 2017

15. Ministry of Social Affairs and Health, Ministry of Finance (2017): Digitalisaatio – Sote- ja maakuntauudistus [Digitalization – social, healthcare and regional reform]. Ministry of Social Affairs and Health and Ministry of Finance (STM and VM). http://alueuudistus.fi/soteuudistus/digitalisaatio. Accessed 28 Dec 2017

16. Laki potilaan asemasta ja oikeuksista 785/1992 Oikeusministeriö. Edita Publishing Oy. http://www.finlex.fi/fi/laki/ajantasa/1992/19920785?search%5Btype%5D=pika&search%5Bpika%5D=Laki%20potilaan%20asemasta%20ja%20oikeuksista

17. Terveydenhuoltolaki 30.12.2010/1326 Oikeusministeriö. Edita Publishing Oy. http://www.finlex.fi/fi/laki/ajantasa/2010/20101326?search%5Btype%5D=pika&search%5Bpika%5D=terveydenhuoltolaki

18. Laki terveydenhuollon ammattihenkilöistä 559/1994 Oikeusministeriö. Edita Publishing Oy. https://www.finlex.fi/fi/laki/ajantasa/1994/19940559

19. Ministry of Social Affairs and Health: Potilasasiakirjojen laatiminen ja käsittely - Opas terveydenhuollolle [Preparation and handling of patient information – guidebook for healthcare]. Sosiaali- ja terveysministeriön julkaisuja 2012:4. Ministry of Social Affairs and Health (Finland). Juvenes Print – Tampereen Yliopistopaino Oy, Tampere (2012)

20. Virkkunen, H., Mäkelä-Bengs, P., Vuokko, R.: Terveydenhuollon rakenteisen kirjaamisen opas, Osa I, Keskeisten kertomusrakenteiden kirjaaminen sähköiseen potilaskertomukseen [Guidebook for structured recording in healthcare. Part 1, Recording of central structures of narrative in electronical patient information system]. National Institute of Health and Welfare, Helsinki: Juvenes Print – Suomen Yliopistopaino Oy (2015)

21. Vuokko, R., Suhonen, J., Porrasmaa, J.: Sairaanhoitopiirin yhteisen potilastietorekisterin ja KanTa-suostumustenhallinnan toiminnallisuuksien määrittely – Potilaan informointi, suostumus ja kiellot. [Defining functionalities of hospital districts shared patient information record and consent management of Kanta – patient informent, consent and prohibitions]. Terveyden ja hyvinvoinnin laitoksen raportti 63/2012. National Institute for Health and Welfare, Helsinki (2012)

22. Vierula, T.: Lastensuojelun asiakirjat vanhempien näkökulmasta [Examining Child Welfare Documents from a Parental Perspective]. Doctoral thesis, Tampere University. Suomen Yliopistopaino Oy – Juvenes Print, Tampere (2017)
23. Data Protection Ombudsman: Sosiaalihuollon asiakastietojen käsittelystä - päivitetty 7.9.2016 [About handling of social services' client information – updated 7 Sept 2016] (2016). http://www.tietosuoja.fi/material/attachments/tietosuojavaltuutettu/tietosuojavaltuute tuntoimisto/oppaat/sS7Y8nd6n/TSV_LOGO_ARVOT_20110222162112.pdf
24. Leavitt, H.J.: Applying organizational change in industry: structural, technological and humanistic approaches. In: March, J. (ed.) Handbook of Organizations. Rand McNally, Chicago (1965)
25. Nurminen, M.I., Forsman, U.: Reversed quality life cycle model. Paper presented at the human factors in organizational design and management-IV: development, introduction and use of new technology - challenges for human organization and human resource development in a changing world, Stockholm, Sweden, 29 May–2 June 1994 (1994)
26. Johnson, D.G.: Computer Ethics. Prentice Hall, Upper Saddle River (2001)
27. Moor, J.H.: Just consequentialism and computing. Ethics Inf. Technol. 1, 65–69 (1999)
28. Tavani, H.T.: Ethics & Technology: Ethical Issues in an Age of Information and Communication Technology, 2nd edn. Wiley, Hoboken (2007)
29. Heimo, O.I., Kimppa, K.K. Nurminen, M.I.: Ethics and the Inseparability Postulate. In: ETHIComp 2014, Pierre & Marie Curie University, Paris, France, 25–27 July 2014 (2014)
30. Heimo, O.I.: Icarus, or the idea toward efficient, economical, and ethical acquirement of critical governmental information systems. Ph.D. thesis manuscript, Turku School of Economics, University of Turku (2018 – in review)
31. Gillon, R.: Medical ethics: four principles plus attention to scope. BJM 309(118), 184–188 (1994)
32. Koskinen, J.S., Heimo, O.I., Kimppa, K.K.: A viewpoint for more ethical approach in healthcare information system development and procurement: the four principles. In: Eriksson-Backa, K., Luoma, A., Krook, E. (eds.) WIS 2012. CCIS, vol. 313, pp. 1–9. Springer, Heidelberg (2012). https://doi.org/10.1007/978-3-642-32850-3_1
33. Valta, M.: Sähköisen potilastietojärjestelmän sosiotekninen käyttöönotto: seitsemän vuoden seurantatutkimus odotuksista omaksumiseen [The sociotechnical implementation of an electronic patient record. A seven-year follow-up study from expectations to adoption]. Doctoral thesis, University of Eastern Finland (2013)
34. Wrede, S.: Suomalainen terveydenhuolto: jännitteitä ja murroksia [Finnish Health care system: tensions and revolutions]. In: Kangas, I., Karvonen, S., Lillrank, A. (eds.) Terveyssosiologian suuntauksia [Directions in Health Sociology], pp. 189–205. Gaudeamus Kirja, Helsinki (2000)
35. National Advisory Board of Social Welfare and Health Care Ethics ETENE: Ethical Grounds for the Social and Health Care Field. ETENE-publications 34. National Advisory Board of Social Welfare and Health Care Ethics ETENE, Ministry of Social Affairs and Health (2012)
36. The Finnish Medical Association: Code of Medical Ethics (2014). https://www.laakariliitto. fi/en/ethics/. Accessed 04 Mar 2018
37. Finnish National Institute of Health and Welfare (THL): Lastensuojelun laatusuositus [Quality proposal for child protection]. Sosiaali- ja terveysministeriön julkaisuja 2014:4, Helsinki (2014)

Social in Virtual – Viewpoints into the Development of Online Rehabilitation

Sirppa Kinos[1(✉)] and Laura Jussila[2]

[1] Turku University of Applied Sciences,
Joukahaisenkatu 3, 20720 Turku, Finland
sirppa.kinos@turkuamk.fi
[2] Finnish Parkinson Association, Suvilinnantie 2, 20900 Turku, Finland

Abstract. The emphasis of this article is in examining the phenomena "social in virtual" and related key concepts (social rehabilitation, social support, interaction), in light of previous research. Key viewpoints include the special characteristics of technology-mediated interaction, the building of trust in interaction, the activities of an instructor and peer support. Virtualization and digitalization are world-changing megatrends. Rehabilitation, along with many healthcare services, is at least partially transitioning to a virtual environment. This brings rehabilitation and adaption training into the person's home, which saves time and expense. Online adaptation training course experiences obtained from the Verkkosova project of the Finnish Parkinson Association are discussed briefly to introduce a real-life element to the phenomena. It can be concluded that face-to-face interaction is not a mandatory requirement in peer support. When planning and guiding online rehabilitation group, it is important to recognize the special characteristics of technology-mediated interaction and acknowledge the group processes as well as the informational, emotional and behavioural aspects affecting the creation of trust. The use of two instructors is recommended. However, communications technology and networks, along with IT skills of citizens should improve, in order to take full advantage of new prospects which online rehabilitation creates.

Keywords: Rehabilitation · Online interaction · E-health

1 Introduction

Virtualization and digitalization are world-changing megatrends. Digitalization refers to the integration of digital technology with everyday life by means of digitization, in other words, by changing image, sound, signals or documents into bits and bytes. Virtualization plays a key role in this. The term 'virtual' (as well as the term 'web') often refers to communications taking place online. The Internet of Things and the Internet of Everything bring together people, processes, things and objects, thus connecting consumers, society, services and industry. This is one of the reasons why digitalization is a key project for Sipilä's government in Finland. Digitalization enables scalability, meaning that one product can be duplicated into a limitless number of products with nearly the same costs. The goal is to develop both the efficiency and the user-centred nature of services. Principles concerning the digitalization of services will be created for all public services (Sitra Megatrends 2016; Juhanko and Jurvansuu 2015, p. 5, pp. 18–19; Finland, a land of solutions. Strategic Programme of Prime Minister Juha Sipilä's Government 29 May 2015).

The development of the information society has changed our ways of understanding the world and our concept of community. Rehabilitation and adaptation training is at least partially transitioning to a virtual environment. Even though the benefits of scalability cannot be utilized in full, other advantages can be seen in virtualization. This brings rehabilitation and adaption training into the individual's home. It is a safe and comfortable environment for rehabilitation and the guidance of rehabilitation and supports the transition of new habits learned in rehabilitation to everyday life. The Internet also helps overcome geographical obstacles without travel and other costs (Ahtiainen and Auranne 2007; Kolehmainen et al. 2012).

Use of ICT in support of health and health-related fields (eHealth) is indeed cost-effective method in health-care services, health surveillance and health education. It is increasingly popular worldwide: more than half of WHO Member States have an eHealth strategy. For the present, online group rehabilitation has only had minor piloting, compared with piloting of individual rehabilitation like therapies (especially physiotherapy, psychotherapy and speech therapy). The terminology of the sector has not been established: some of the terms used include distance rehabilitation, online rehabilitation, telerehabilitation and virtual rehabilitation. In this article, the term online rehabilitation is applied (Global diffusion of eHealth: making universal health coverage achievable 2016, pp. 5–6; Salminen et al. 2016, p. 17; Eichenberg et al. 2013; Keck and Doarn 2014; www.Mielenterveystalo.fi; Heikkinen 2011; Oksa 2012; Kinos et al. 2014, p. 4; Karppi 2011, p. 15).

2 Adaptation Training as Part of Social Rehabilitation

Rehabilitation is a systematic, multidisciplinary activity intended to help the customers fulfil their life projects and maintain control of their lives in situations where their opportunities for social survival and integration are threatened or weakened. Becoming disabled or being diagnosed with a chronic disease is a challenge to both the person themselves and their loved ones. Uncertainty, fear and the feeling of losing control of one's life are natural consequences of having an illness or a disability create changes in various aspects of life. Adaptation training may provide support in such a situation (Järvikoski and Härkäpää 1995, 2004).

Research findings in many countries prove that long-term peer group activities support adaptation to a new challenging situation in life. Those group activities may carry a name psychoeducation, self-efficacy education or psychosocial rehabilitation, for instance. An adaptation training course is a Finnish rehabilitation innovation with goals directed at the core of social rehabilitation. As a section of rehabilitation, social rehabilitation has been quite vague in terms of content. It refers to operations intended to support the social capacity of the person. According to Järvikoski and Härkäpää (2004, 2014), social capacity includes managing one's everyday chores, interactive relationships and the roles required by one's environment. Good social capacity means strong inclusion and relationships in the community (Linsey et al. 2016; Cook et al. 2016; Alburquerque et al. 2016; Järvikoski and Härkäpää 2004, 2014).

In Finland, The Social Welfare Act (1301/2014) describes social rehabilitation as part of social services. According to the act, social rehabilitation refers to enhanced support provided by means of social work and social guidance to increase social capacity, prevent social exclusion and promote inclusion. Social rehabilitation includes assessing social capacity and need for rehabilitation, training on managing everyday chores and control of one's life, group activities and support for social, interactive relationships.

Adaptation training is a process in which an ill or disabled person builds a new relationship with themselves and their environment. The purpose of the training is to support the person in understanding the significance of illness or disability from the perspective of identity and good everyday life. Rehabilitation experts and a peer group provide support in the process (Järvikoski and Härkäpää 2004, 2014; Vilkkumaa 2014).

3   Group Activities Enable Social and Peer Support

Adaptation training is conducted as a group activity, either in short periods in a rehabilitation unit or as regular group meetings in outpatient rehabilitation. The group aspect enables social support to have an impact. The key factors are the realization of a sense of community and the trust in the support and strength of the group. Social support may refer to mental and physical support and comfort received from other people. Kumpusalo lists five forms of social support: material, functional (e.g. a favour), informative, emotional and mental (e.g. a shared ideology, belief or philosophy). Social support has been observed to have a considerable impact on health, including the prevention and treatment of depression. Peer support, in turn, refers to social support provided by a person with experiences in the challenge in question (e.g. an illness or disability) and shares some characteristics with the supported person. Peer support providers empathy and experiential knowledge. It also helps normalize one's experiences and get over the feeling of shame. Peer support is assumed to possess some qualities not provided by other forms of social support. However, very little is known about the mechanisms through which the impacts of peer support are conveyed (Streng 2014; Keski-Luopa 2014; Hiilamo and Tuuli-Henriksson 2012; pp. 210–211; Kumpusalo 1991, p. 14; Laimio and Karnell 2010, pp. 18–19; Vilkkumaa 2014).

From the perspective of social rehabilitation and adaptation training, one of the key questions is the creation of an online environment enabling the type of interaction that allows peer support to be conveyed. As a trend, online rehabilitation is on the rise also in Finland and supported by Kela (the Finnish national insurance institution). According to Kela's rehabilitation standard, online rehabilitation can be used to, for example, implement the contents of rehabilitation as well as communications and exercises between periods of rehabilitation (Vilkkumaa 2014; Approved Kela standards of outpatient and institutional rehabilitation enacted in 2016).

4   Comparisons Between Face-to-Face and Technology-Mediated Interaction

Online interaction is one form of technology-mediated interaction. According to Sivunen, technology-mediated interaction refers to the interaction between two or more people by means of some form of communications technology. Various forms of communications technology differ according to, for example, whether the interaction is synchronous (real-time) or asynchronous, in other words, whether the tool creates a delay in the interaction. They also differ in terms of their interactive properties, i.e. whether the parties of the communication have equal opportunities to communicate. Some tools enable the participants to hear and/or see each other. In the other hand, interaction may be simply textual. The anonymity, or whether the sender and recipient of the message can identify each other, also varies according to the tool. Some tools are primarily designed for communications between two parties and others for sending messages from one person to several people (Sivunen 2007, pp. 30–31).

Different tools of communication require different interaction and communication skills. Technology-mediated interaction has been studied both in Finland and abroad since the 1990s. Many studies have shown that it differs from face-to-face communication. According to the results of an Aalto University research group led by Professor Lauri Nummenmaa, no digital channel of interaction matches face-to-face interaction in terms of diversity. This particularly applies in terms of emotions, the intimacy of social relationships and the meaningful network and, through these, mental and somatic health. Figure 1 presents the level of interactive diversity in various tools of communication compared to face-to-face interaction (Currell et al. 2010; Suvivuo et al. 2013; Kinos et al. 2014; Nummenmaa 2015; Nummenmaa 2010, pp. 142–145).

Emotions play a vital role in regulating human behaviour. Our emotions affect our abilities of observation and thinking, such as the functions of long-term memory, the direction of attention and decision-making processes. The face and its expressions are the most important tool of non-verbal communication between humans. On the other hand, we can use our bodies in a number of ways to express emotions, for instance by stepping closer or further away or by using various positions and motions. The primary purpose of expressing emotions is social communication, and sharing one's emotions promotes interaction between individuals. Spoken language is the most important channel of communication. In addition to the content and meaning of words, it utilizes the acoustic properties of voice (for example pitch, emphasis, rhythm and various signals, such as crying or laughter). These acoustic properties of voice influence the emotional response triggered by the spoken message in its listener. Few tools of communication enable non-verbal communications (Nummenmaa 2010, 30, pp. 79–84).

For the present, even the most diverse communications technology does not enable physical touch, which is one of the reasons why technology-mediated interaction cannot match face-to-face interaction in terms of expressing emotions or the intimacy of social relationships. Touch is an important channel for communicating emotions and creating social relationship. It is also a key tool in the professional practices of the rehabilitation sector (including physiotherapy and occupational therapy) (Suvilehto et al. 2015; Nummenmaa 2015; Karppi 2011, p. 17).

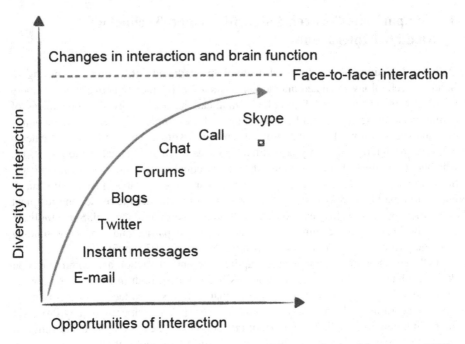

Fig. 1. Diversity of interaction when using various tools of communication (Nummenmaa 2015).

On the other hand, words can also touch. In his final book, author Lundán (2006, p. 178) describes this as follows:

"A person trying, as accurately as possible, to verbally describe to another person what they feel and what is real to them is, in my opinion, the highest form of communication. Even through words, we can come close enough to each other to sense each others' hopes, fears, beliefs, love. When words become sensations that is literature."

Even when using synchronous tools of communication transmitting the image and audio in real time, the interaction may still remain thinner, more distant, emotionless and less comprehensive than face-to-face interaction. The process described by Lundán, the transformation of words into sensations, requires a skilful writer. Skills are also required for the development of a sense of community in technology-mediated interaction, compensating, wherever possible, for the limitations introduced by tools of communication in the interaction and, on the other hand, utilizing their advantages. However, we know that the Internet with its communities and discussion groups is an important part of social life for many people. They use it to create friendships and develop intimacy in a diverse, creative manner by, for example, using text. It also pays to remember that an open connection for dialogue and positive social interaction as such may already enable important processes that harmonize one's emotional life (Marila and Ylinen 2002, p. 28, 33, 56; Nummenmaa 2010, p. 203).

5   Advantages of Various Tools of Communication from the Perspective of Interaction

According to Sivunen's research, technology-mediated interaction may also be more functional in terms of social characteristics than face-to-face interaction. It forms mental images as much as face-to-face interaction but those images are based on different processes. Using only text instead of, for example, image and sound, the person can put more effort into editing the text. If the communications are not time-sensitive but rely on, for example, e-mail or a blog, the time limits of communication are reduced. In addition, all the modern tools of communication enable interaction regardless of physical location. This is a clear advantage in rehabilitation and adaptation training where the traditional, institutional methods result in considerable travel and accommodation costs and compensation for loss of income (Sivunen 2007, p. 33).

The question of the advantages and disadvantages of various tools of communication is not quite simple. Various tools can be used to both increase and decrease the social distance of the parties. For example, e-mail is used for sending both personal, emotional messages and bad news with the purpose of avoiding an immediate response from the recipient. Even though technology-mediated interaction is often assessed to be more superficial, some studies show that people are more likely to ask each other personal questions and talk about themselves in a less general and superficial manner in technology-mediated interaction than face to face (Mäkiniemi et al. 2011, p. 8; Sivunen 2007, p. 168–170).

In face-to-face interaction, the topics discussed remain more confidential due to the fact that they have not been stored anywhere but, on the other hand, they are also more fleeting, emphasizes Sivunen (2007, p. 88, 200). The discussions do not necessarily result in documented materials one can review later. Many tools of communication, such as discussion forums, enable the messages to be stored. Storage is a key feature, especially from the perspective of exercise-oriented interaction.

On the Internet, the certain anonymity, social distance and small number of clues given to the parties of interaction concerning each other may encourage participation. Even though the possibility of misunderstandings may be greater than in face-to-face interaction, it may be easier to process unpleasant and difficult things online without the fear of losing face. Online, it is also easier to withdraw from interaction of one's own accord than in face-to-face interaction. In addition, it is easier to leave various tasks undone (Mäkiniemi et al. 2011, pp. 8–9; Sivunen 2007, p. 38, 88, 118; Marila and Ylinen 2002, p. 33).

When using both an audio and video connection (e.g. Skype or video conference), misunderstandings in interaction are not as likely as when interacting by means of mere text, for example. Video and audio make it easier to form a mental image of another person. Sensing and conveying moods is also easier when the meanings are also carried by gestures and facial expressions. On the other hand, online meetings enabling real-time audio and video connection may also entail technical issues more frequently. Even a slight delay in the audio may interfere with the interaction (Suvivuo et al. 2013, p. 245; Kinos et al. 2014, pp. 7–8; Sivunen 2007, pp. 156–171).

Interaction and the activities of a group online are also a matter of technology. According to Sivunen, the tool of communication must be chosen based on what best suits the intended use. A functional IT infrastructure is vitally important. Technical issues weaken the experiences of presence and contact and may draw the attention away from the actual topic. They also increase the negative assessments of technology-mediated interaction. In fact, functional technology and sufficient IT skills of the participants are a basic requirement for all interaction taking place online (Sivunen 2007, pp. 156–171; Osman 2011, p. 3; Juhanko and Jurvansuu 2015, p. 19).

6 Trust as a Prerequisite for Peer Support

A group can be defined as consisting of three or more people with a shared goal and rules for their activity. Groups may be continuous and long term. They are formed in interaction. The size of the group is one of the influencing factors. The members of the group are determined by having an individual and the members of the group define themselves as part of the group and thereby becoming attached to it (Mäkiniemi et al. 2011, p. 11; Marila and Ylinen 2002, p. 28; Sivunen 2007, p. 45).

The key element in grouping and attaching oneself to a group is trust. Trust is the prerequisite for the creation of team spirit and cohesion in a group, thus enabling experiences of peer support. This takes time. The constancy of the group is also important to enable its members to get to know each other and develop shared methods. Constancy also plays a role in attaching oneself to the group and having the motivation to work with the group (Marila and Ylinen 2002, pp. 10–16; Sivunen 2007, p. 85) (Fig. 2).

In the creation process of trust, the first factor to be observed is the rational, informed level. It means assessing the reliability of other members and the advantages and disadvantages to be gained from interaction. The second observable factor in the creation of trust is the affective, in other words, emotional level. This refers to the emotions of concern, liking and caring about another person, for example. A third factor, a behavioural level related to demeanour and action, can also be identified. These three levels are interconnected and may form a circle. Trust is built through thinking and emotions and becomes visible through behaviour. Behaviour, in turn, may create more trust in the group members. On the other hand, distrust may create a circle or reducing trust (Marila and Ylinen 2002, pp. 10–16, 40–42; Isoherranen 2012, pp. 54–57; Sivunen 2007, p. 176).

A group in which the members are efficiently attached and feel thorough belonging and trust is able to offer close-knit and supportive interaction, in other words, peer support. It includes the opportunity to talk about oneself and one's experiences, engage in social presence and reduce one's feelings of insecurity. On the other hand, the experience of being a member of a group also has to do with how well the group member feels the other members participate in the activities and belong in the group. If the assessments concerning the other group members are weak, this may weaken the person's own sense of being a member of the group. The opportunity of experiencing peer support is increased by a sense of similarity, a "common denominator", as well as experiences shared between the group members. It is also increased by shared

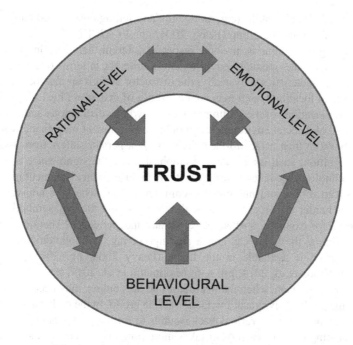

Fig. 2. The creation process of trust: circle of trust

meanings and stories created in discussions and developing the culture of the group. A sense of community can be created with surprisingly few words, often utilizing factors such as humour (Isoherranen 2012, pp. 38–40; Marila and Ylinen 2002, p. 82; Sivunen 2007, pp. 176–189).

According to Marila and Ylinen, it is easier for a group to get to know each other and maintain trust when interacting face-to-face. Relational communication, i.e. communication connected to interactive relationships, is considered more difficult in technology-mediated communications. The same applies to expressing presence, interest and activeness. Sometimes, it is possible to meet both face-to-face and by technology-mediated means. In those situations, the timing of meeting face-to-face is crucial as technology-mediated interaction is most frequent before and directly after meeting face-to-face. If meeting face-to-face is not possible, particular attention must be paid to getting to know each other, creating trust and grouping. This is a vital task of the group's instructor (Marila and Ylinen 2002, p. 31; Sivunen 2007, pp. 91–92).

7   Activities of the Instructor of an Online Group

The instructor of an online group plays a particularly crucial role in all the stages of the group's development. The instructor guides the group processes that, according to Peavy, are interaction, agreeing on work methods, decision-making and settling issues and conflicts. In this task, the instructor needs a variety of skills, such as reaction skills (e.g. listening), interactive skills (e.g. motivating and setting boundaries) and functional skills such as observing the group (Peavy 2004, pp. 30–32; Kim 2000, pp. 174–184).

Directing a group online is, in some respects, different than directing a group that meets face-to-face. The operating environment is different in terms of physical, social and symbolic characteristics. Physically, the instructor and group members are all in a different physical location which may create a sense of distance. Physical touch is also prevented. The locations of the group members may have distractions and noise. From the perspective of a social environment, an online environment may enable withdrawal and passivity more than a face-to-face situation. If a person suffers from issues with speech or cognition, such issues may be emphasized as the significance of speech is higher in technology-mediated interaction than in face-to-face interaction. It is also more difficult to follow and interpret the communications when the non-verbal communication is harder to perceive, even with a video connection. A symbolic environment includes, for example, a sense of safety and independence. Therefore, in online adaptation training, the home can create an empowering, symbolic environment if an undisturbed space is available in the home (Peavy 2004, pp. 30–32; Kim 2000, pp. 174–184; Kinos et al. 2014, pp. 4–6; Mäkiniemi et al. 2011, pp. 11–14).

According to Sivunen, when the instructor operates online, they need to pay special attention to the goals, activity and interaction of the group. In the early stages, their task is to encourage people from various backgrounds to form a group, act together and be motivated. Getting to know each other takes more time than in face-to-face interaction. The instructor promotes it with a number of grouping tasks, using a sufficient amount of time for them. When the group is taking its first steps, it is important to make an agreement on confidentiality and secrecy. After getting to know each other, the instructor guides the group's discussion on the goals of the group activity and makes them more tangible. The instructor also supports continuous motivation and awareness of the goals in the group throughout the process. Mäkiniemi, Ahola and Peltonen emphasize the sense of social presence created by the instructor by, for example, following the discussion and posing additional questions. The instructor also activates the participants to interact by encouraging them and serving as an example. The instructor personally expresses their emotions and moods, thus creating an atmosphere for socio-emotional discussion. With various exercises, the instructor supports the mutual interaction of the group members by, for example, asking them to comment on a message sent by another member (Sivunen 2007, pp. 121–122; Mäkiniemi et al. 2011, p. 14).

Support is also needed in the use of communications technology and tools. The instructor learns to use them and, if necessary, arranges external support for group members. The instructor organizes online meetings and guides the discussion. If the video and audio connection is real-time, the instructor gives the group members a chance to talk one at a time to avoid members interrupting each other. This is conducted by talking as directing speech through eye contact or gestures is not possible. The instructor ensures that even the quietest participants are given the chance to express their views in the group, possibly by setting limits to the most active participants (Osman 2011, pp. 2–3; Kinos et al. 2014, pp. 5–6; Suvivuo et al. 2013, pp. 241, 244).

It is important to observe that the creation of trust in the group requires both exercise-oriented and emotional communications from the instructor. The instructor may promote confidentiality by showing commitment, enthusiasm and optimism. They observe the atmosphere in the group and the interaction between the members, help settle conflicts and support the activities of the group with their own interventions (Sivunen 2007, pp. 121–125).

8 Implementation of Adaptation Training Courses Online and Feedback from Participants

Adaptation training was developed in online environment in the Verkkosova project (2015–2017), funded by Finland's Slot Machine Association, the Finnish Parkinson Association and Turku University of Applied Sciences (https://www.parkinson.fi/hankkeet). The four courses had a total of 28 participants. The participants were required to have basic skills in the use of computers and the Internet. They were also required to have access to a computer or tablet, an Internet connection, webcam and a headset. The participants were asked to provide feedback in an electronic questionnaire at the end of the course and in an electronic questionnaire and telephone interview six months after the end of the course (Tenhunen et al. 2016). The purpose of the feedback was to obtain information on reaching the goals of the adaptation training and, particularly, whether the goals of conveying peer support were realized. Another topic of interest was whether the opportunity for a physical encounter was significant in terms of grouping (cf. Heikkinen 2011).

Each course lasted eight weeks. Two of the courses started with a shared weekend meet. Two of the courses did not include any physical encounters. At the beginning of the course, an IT expert provided personal guidance in the use of the hardware and software. The weekly online meetings through the Skype or OpenTokRTC applications lasted from 90 min to two hours. There were seven (in addition to the weekend meet) or eight (no weekend meet) of such meetings altogether.

The contents and themes of the course were similar to those on institutional adaptation training courses (e.g. Kela/rehabilitation and adaptation training courses). Traditionally, adaptation training is a multiprofessional activity in which information and expertise on medicine, physiotherapy, psychology, treatment and social work is utilized to support the participants. On the online course, each meeting had a specific theme. The participants were given exercises related to the themes between the meetings (see Table 1), which is unusual in adaptation training courses organised face-to-face. As in all adaptation training, the objective of online training is to support the participant in adjusting to living with a chronic disease. The adaptation process is promoted by the peer support and information received during the course. For this reason, the stages of the adaptation process or crisis are taken into account in the structure of the course. An instructor thoroughly acquainted with the special characteristics and challenges of online guidance work was always present during online meetings. In addition to the instructor, the meetings were joined by an expert of the theme discussed. The requirements of guiding a group in an online meeting are challenging, which is why the presence of two experts was justified (Saari 2012; Hiivola et al. 2016; Heikelä-Välimäki 2016).

Table 1. Themes and instructors of online meetings

Theme of the meeting	Instructors
1. Start of course and getting to know each other	Course instructor and IT expert
2. Falling ill	Course instructor and peer
3. Mood and adaptation	Course instructor and psychologist
4. Parkinson's disease and its characteristics	Course instructor and neurologist
5. Social security and welfare	Course instructor and social worker
6. Physical exercise as part of self-care	Course instructor and physiotherapist
7. Nutrition and sexuality	Course instructor, dietitian and sex therapist
8. End of course and association activities	Course instructor and representative of the Finnish Parkinson Association

Means to enable peer support were planned for each theme. As mutual interaction may lead to development of trust and trust enables sharing and hence peer support, the opportunities for interaction (provided by both the online meetings and the exercises carried out between the meetings) were utilized. In the online meetings the participants shared with the group what they learned from the exercises. They were encouraged to discuss online (by Skype or OpenTokRTC) outside those meetings, as most of the participants also did. During the online meetings, the grouping of the participants was supported with various introductory exercises and by sharing experiences and feelings. Professionals helped the participants to structure the new information.

The feedback provided by the participants conveys quite a positive image of the online adaptation training. The personal goals of the participants were in line with the general goals of adaptation training. The goals included receiving peer support, information about the illness, advice for everyday issues and support for psychological well-being. Most of the participants had reached their goals to a high or very high degree. There was correlation between the activity of the participant and the experience of having their own well-being improved by taking part in the online group. Most of the participants felt that they received a high or very high amount of peer support. Based on the feedback, the group with no weekend meet scheduled at the beginning of the course felt it easiest to form a group and received the most peer support. There were quite many technical issues. For example, the headphones and microphone were incompatible or the Internet connection was too weak. The support of an IT expert was required throughout the course. On the other hand, many participants felt that their IT skills improved considerably. After six months, most of the participants still kept in touch with the other participants (via Skype, for instance) and felt that the peer support provided by the online course still had an impact on their everyday life. Most of the participants also reported that they did not receive peer support elsewhere (Kaisko and Kanerva 2016, pp. 15–16; Eriksson and Lantela 2016, p. 21; Tenhunen et al. 2016, pp. 37–38, 28; Di Mariano and Valmunen 2016, pp. 20–21; Arvola 2016; Kinos 2017).

9   In Conclusion

It is possible to experience peer support even in a group that does not meet face to face. Face-to-face interaction is not a mandatory requirement in peer support. This conclusion is supported by many informal online groups. A large number of groups and communities are only active online and their participants report receiving peer support. These groups are often created spontaneously around some common denominator. When such groups interact in a manner that creates trust, interaction providing social support in its various forms is possible. However, many people are excluded from groups due to the spontaneity and unpredictability of the activity.

Target-oriented and systematic rehabilitation and adaptation training activities cannot leave grouping, the creation of trust and, thus, the opportunities of peer support up to chance. By recognizing the special characteristics of technology-mediated interaction, various tools can be used creatively, utilizing their best features. By acknowledging the group processes and the informational, emotional and behavioural aspects affecting the creation of trust, the development of the group can be influenced. Thorough planning of the online course is, therefore, important, using the goals supporting the participants' adaptation process as a starting point. The know-how of the instructor is also vitally important. The instructor must learn about the special characteristics of guiding an online group and the means to tackle its challenges. One of the key challenges is that technology-mediated interaction can easily be more vague, distant and unemotional than face-to-face interaction. This requires the instructor to invest in getting to know each other, becoming a group and creating and maintaining trust. The use of two instructors provides exceptionally good opportunities for observing the activities of the group in practice, supporting its mutual interaction and motivate and activate individual participants to join in. This creates excellent opportunities for peer support.

However, online activities are not the best option for everyone. Illnesses and disabilities, for example, can make such activities difficult. Diseases affecting the motor system, such as Parkinson's disease, can cause difficulty in controlling one's movements and result in slowness of movement, rigidity and shaking. Parkinson's disease may also weaken facial expressions and monotonize speech. These symptoms may hinder online interaction. Advanced Parkinson's disease may also create cognitive issues (Marttila et al. 2000).

It can also be stated that communications technology, Internet connections and software have yet to reach a level required to fully support online interaction intended to create trust and, therefore, develop peer support. Disconnected devices result in disconnected interaction processes. In addition, the IT skills of the citizens need to be generally improved to make online group activities and peer support available to all.

References

Sitran Megatrendit (2016). http://www.slideshare.net/SitraFund/sitran-megatrendit-2016. Accessed 05 May 2018

Juhanko, J., Jurvansuu, M. (toim.): Suomalainen teollinen Internet – haasteesta mahdollisuudeksi. Elinkeinoelämän tutkimuslaitos. Raportit nro 42 (2015). https://www.etla.fi/wp-content/uploads/ETLA-Raportit-Reports-42.pdf. Accessed 05 May 2017

Ratkaisujen Suomi: Pääministeri Juha Sipilän hallituksen strateginen ohjelma (2015)

Ahtiainen, M., Auranne, K.: Hyvinvointiteknologian määrittely ja yleisesittely. In: Suhonen, L., Siikanen, Y. (toim.) Hyvinvointiteknologia sosiaali- ja terveysalalla – hyöty vai haitta? Lahden ammattikorkeakoulun julkaisu. Sarja C (2007)

Kolehmainen, P., Ikonen, J., Turunen, J.: Työikäisten liikuntaneuvonta etäohjauksen keinoin. Opinnäytetyö. Mikkelin ammattikorkeakoulu (2012)

Global Diffusion of eHealth: Making universal health coverage achievable. Report of the third global survey on eHealth. World Health Organization Geneva (2016)

Salminen, A.L., Heiskanen, T., Hiekkala, S., Naamanka, J., Stenberg, J.H., Vuononvirta, T.: Etäkuntoutuksen ja siihen läheisesti liittyvien termien määrittelyä. In: Salminen, A.L., Hiekkala, S., Stenberg, J.H. (toim.) Etäkuntoutus, Kela Helsinki (2016)

Eichenberg, C., Wolters, C., Brahler, E.: The internet as a mental health advisor in Germany Results of a national survey. PLoS ONE 8(11), e79206 (2013)

Keck, C.S., Doarn, C.R.: Telehealth technology applications in speech-language pathology. Telemed. e-Health 20(7), 653–659 (2014)

https://www.mielenterveystalo.fi. Accessed 03 Jan 2018

Heikkinen, M.: Small, closed virtual communities. Case: power and support from the net rehabilitation courses for people with multiple sclerosis. University of Tampere (2011)

Oksa, M.: Verkon käyttö kuntoutuksessa on tätä päivää. Opinnäytetyö. Satakunnan ammattikorkeakoulu (2012)

Kinos, S., Asteljoki, S., Suvivuo, P.: Special features of counselling work carried out through interactive TV. In: Saranto, K., Castrén, M., Kuusela, T., Hyrynsalmi, S., Ojala, S. (eds.) Safe and Secure Cities. Communications in Computer and Information Science 450. WIS proceedings (2014)

Karppi, M.: Interaktiivinen etäkuntoutus ikääntyneen toipilasajan tukena. Pro gradu –tutkielma. Tampereen yliopisto (2011)

Järvikoski, A., Härkäpää, K.: Mitä kuntoutus on? In: Suikkanen, A., Härkäpää, K., Järvikoski, A., ym. (toim.) Kuntoutuksen ulottuvuudet. WSOY Porvoo (1995)

Järvikoski, A., Härkäpää, K.: Kuntoutuksen perusteet. WSOY Helsinki (2004)

Linsey, K., Fauser, M., Ossig, C., Hermann, A., Storch, A.: Feasibility and effectiveness of a low-threshold psychoeducative group-intervention for depression in Parkinson's disease. In: MDS Congress Germany (2016). https://www.mdscongress.org/Congress-2016.htm. Accessed 20 Jan 2018

Cook, D., McRae, C., Kumar, R.: Impact of self-efficacy education on physical and psychosocial functioning in newly-diagnosed Parkinson patients. In: MDS Congress Germany (2016). https://www.mdscongress.org/Congress-2016.htm. Accessed 20 Jan 2018

Alburquerque, D., Rojas, N., Tapia, S., Reyes, P., Silva, C., Chana-Cuevas, P.: Program evaluation empowerment of people with Huntington's disease (HD) and their families: using goal attainment scaling (GAS). In: MDS Congress Germany (2016). https://www.mdscongress.org/Congress-2016.htm. Accessed 20 Jan 2018

Järvikoski, A., Härkäpää, K.: Teoreettisia näkökulmia psykososiaaliseen sopeutumiseen ja sopeutumisvalmennukseen. In: Streng, H. (toim.) Sopeutumisvalmennus. Suomalaisen kuntoutuksen oivallus. RAY Helsinki (2014)

Social Welfare Act 1301/2014

Vilkkumaa, I.: Ihminen suhteessa ympäristöönsä. In: Streng, H. (toim.) Sopeutumisvalmennus. Suomalaisen kuntoutuksen oivallus. RAY Helsinki (2014)

Kela/kuntoutus- ja sopeutumisvalmennuskurssit. http://www.kela.fi/kuntoutus-ja-sopeutumisval mennuskurssit. Accessed 01 Oct 2017

Streng, H. (toim.): Sopeutumisvalmennus. Suomalaisen kuntoutuksen oivallus. RAY Helsinki (2014)

Keski-Luopa, L.: Sopeutumisvalmennus postmodernissa yhteiskunnassa. In: Streng, H. (toim.) Sopeutumisvalmennus. Suomalaisen kuntoutuksen oivallus. RAY Helsinki (2014)

Hiillamo, H., Tuulio-Heriksson, A.: Terapiaa, lääkkeitä ja toisia ihmisiä. Sosiaalisen tuen merkitys masennuksesta toipumisessa. Sosiaalilääketieteellinen aikakauslehti 49, 209–219 (2012)

Kumpusalo, E.: Sosiaalinen tuki, huolenpito ja terveys. Sosiaali- ja terveyshallinnon raportteja 28. Valtion painatuskeskus Helsinki (1991)

Laimio, A., Karnell, S.: Vertaistoiminta – kokemuksellista vuorovaikutusta. In: Laatikainen, T. (toim.) Vertaistoiminta kannattaa. Asumispalvelusäätiö ASPA (2010)

Approved Kela standards of outpatient and institutional rehabilitation enacted in 2016. www. kela.fi. Accessed 05 May 2016

Sivunen, A.: Vuorovaikutus, viestintäteknologia ja identifioituminen hajautetuissa tiimeissä. Väitöstutkimus. Jyväskylän yliopisto (2007)

Currell, R., Urquhart, C., Wainwright, P., Lewis, R.: Telemedicine Versus Face to Face Patient Care: Effects on Professional Practice and Health Care Outcomes (Review). The Cochrane Collaboration John Wiley & Sons Ltd, Hoboken (2010)

Suvivuo, P., Asteljoki, S., Kuikkaniemi, A., Kinos, S.: Students' experiences of working on the Virtu Channel. In: Karppi, M., Tuominen, H., Eskelinen, A., Santamäki-Fischer, R., Rasu, A. (eds.) Active Ageing Online. Turku University of Applied Sciences, Reports 155 (2013)

Nummenmaa, L.: Presentation at the Mieli symposium (2015). http://www.mielenterveysseura.fi/ fi/tapahtumavideot/professori-lauri-nummenmaa-mieli-2015-p%C3%A4ivill%C3%A4. Accessed 05 May 2018

Nummenmaa, L.: Tunteiden psykologia. Tammi, Helsinki (2010)

Suvilehto, J., Glerean, E., Dunbar, R., Hari, R., Nummenmaa, L.: Topography of social touching depends on emotional bonds between humans. Proc. Natl. Acad. Sci. U.S.A. 115, 13811–13816 (2015)

Marila, E., Ylinen, A.: Luottamus vuorovaikutuksessa. Teknologiavälitteinen vuorovaikutus ja luottamuksen rakentuminen. Pro gradu –tutkielma. Jyväskylän yliopisto (2002)

Mäkiniemi, J-P., Ahola, S., Peltonen, P.: Verkkokeskustelussa oppimista edistäviä ja ehkäiseviä tekijöitä. In: Myyry, L., Joutsenvirta, Y. (toim.) Sulautuvaa opetusta verkkokeskustelusta ohjaukseen. Helsingin yliopiston valtiotieteellisen tiedekunnan pedagogiset kehittämispalve- lut, Helsinki (2011)

Osman, H.: The virtual project manager: seven best practices for effective communication. Project Management Institute. Virtual Library (2011). http://www.thecouchmanager.com/wp- content/uploads/2011/08/whitepaper_hassan-osman_the-virtual-project-manager_cisco.pdf. Accessed 05 May 2017

Isoherranen, K.: Uhka vai mahdollisuus – moniammatillista yhteistyötä kehittämässä. Väitöstutkimus. Helsingin yliopisto (2012)

Peavy, R.V.: Sosiodynaaminen näkökulma ja ohjauksen käytäntö. In: Onnismaa, J., Pasanen, H., Spangar, T. (toim.) Ohjaus ammattina ja tieteenalana 3. Ohjauksen välineet. PS-kustannus Jyväskylä (2004)

Kim, H.S.: The Nature of Theoretical Thinking in Nursing. Springer, New York (2000) https://www.parkinson.fi/hankkeet. Accessed 05 May 2016

Tenhunen, I., Thynell, V., Österman, M.: Osallistujien kokemuksia verkkosopeutumisvalmennuskursseista – Verkkosova-hanke Opinnäytetyö. Turun ammattikorkeakoulu (2016)

Saari, S.: Kuin salama kirkkaalta taivaalta. Otava Helsinki (2012)

Hiivola, A., Sirkki, A., Viman, L.: Ohjaajan toiminta verkkosopeutumisvalmennuskurssilla. Opinnäytetyö. Turun ammattikorkeakoulu (2016)

Heikelä-Välimäki, A.: Verkko-ohjaaminen sopeutumisvalmennuksen kurssilla. Asiantuntijoiden kokemuksia verkko-ohjaamisesta Verkkosova – projektissa. Opinnäytetyö. Turun ammattikorkeakoulu (2016)

Kaisko, S., Kanerva, M.: Parkinsonin tautia sairastavien tavoitteiden toteutuminen internetissä tapahtuvassa sopeutumisvalmennuskurssissa – Verkkosova –hanke Opinnäytetyö. Turun ammattikorkeakoulu (2016)

Eriksson, A., Lantela, T.: Verkossa vai "livenä" – Suomen Parkinson-liiton sopeutumisvalmennuskurssien Verkkosova-projekti Opinnäytetyö. Turun ammattikorkeakoulu (2016)

Di Mariano, U., Valmunen, J.: Internet sopeutumisvalmennuksen toimintaympäristönä - Kokemuksia Parkinson-Liiton Verkkosova-kursseista. Opinnäytetyö. Turun ammattikorkeakoulu (2016)

Arvola, M.: ICT specialist. Interviewed by Hulkkonen. A. 17 Mar 2016

Kinos, S.: Verkkosova– verkossa tapahtuvan sopeutumisvalmennuksen kehittäminen Hankearviointiraportti. Turun ammattikorkeakoulu (2017)

Marttila, R.: Parkinsonin taudin kulku. In: Rinne, K., Marttila, R., Pasila, A. (toim.) Parkinsonin tauti. Turku: Suomen Parkinson-liitto Ry (2000)

What Happens in Lessons? Risks and Incidents at Schools

Eila Lindfors[✉]

Department of Teacher Education, Rauma Unit, University of Turku,
Seminaarinkatu 1, 2600 Rauma, Finland
eila.lindfors@utu.fi

Abstract. According to a safety paradigm that calls for human factors behind the incidents and emphasizes resilience it can be understood that near-miss cases and accidents are in relation to several physical, social, psychological and pedagogical factors. To be able to develop safety culture at schools there is need to record, monitor and analyze incidents, near-misses, accidents and injuries in learning environments. However there are no systematic procedures in regular use that would allow schools as organizations to learn from incidents and implement alterations in practice to develop their safety culture. It is more a question what schools know about their safety and how they understand their safety culture to develop it proactively. In the paper analysis for 168 incidents from three comprehensive schools in Finland, was executed. On the basis of theory driven analysis the incidents were categorized to physical, social, psychological and pedagogical dimensions. Incidents in pedagogical learning environments are introduced more detailed in this paper. This paper gives prior knowledge of incidents in pedagogical learning environments: what happens, where and to whom.

Based on results there is an obvious need to develop methods of reporting incidents in schools as well as the motivation to report, to be able to develop the safety culture. In the future students' role in recognizing incidents should be emphazised.

Keywords: Incident analysis · Learning environment · School safety

1 Developing Safety in Learning Environments

1.1 Background for School Safety in Finland

Changes in society challenge the safety of schools. The safety challenges are for example accidents and incidents, like school fires, bullying, various kinds of near-miss cases, unintentional injuries, and even intentional injuries like school shootings. Safety is a norm that schools should guarantee for pupils and students based on the Finnish Basic Education Act [1]. Safety at work is a norm also for teachers according to Occupational Safety and Health Act [2]. Safety in its various forms is a main issue when considering criteria for a good learning environment [3]. The latest National Core Curriculum for Basic Education 2014 (grades 1–9, students from 7 to 16 years old) in Finland [4] points out safety procedures for learning environments. However, there are

© Springer Nature Switzerland AG 2018
H. Li et al. (Eds.): WIS 2018, CCIS 907, pp. 79–87, 2018.
https://doi.org/10.1007/978-3-319-97931-1_7

no systematic procedures to collect incident data in regular use in schools. The only obligatory procedure is to document injuries that needed medical treatment to get the insurance cover for the costs. These injuries are registered on national level, but minor incidents and near-misses are not documented and analysed systemically at all.

It is well known that most of the injuries happen in sports lessons and in brakes [5]. Beside sports, home economics, craft, design and technology education, physics and chemistry are considered as safety critical subjects. There are hazards and risks at schools that should have been solved with proactive procedures [6]. However, we can't say that schools as learning environments wouldn't be safe and secure for workers and pupils. It is more a question what schools know about their safety and how they understand their safety culture to develop it proactively. Somerkoski [7] points out that the risks at schools are unpredictable, connected to human factors and caused by students acting against norms and regulations or using structures or products in a way they are not supposed to be used. The definition of safety culture of schools recognizes diversity of actors at schools. The safety culture is seen in educational context as collaborative actions of staff and students as well as implementation of procedures that develop and promote safe and secure learning and working environment. This definition means that all members of school, as an organisation, must understand the importance of their active roles in promoting safety based on their responsibilities. [8] If principals tell that their school is safe without any incidents or injuries we know well based on earlier research [e.g. 9, 10] that it is more a question of not knowing what kind of incidents there has happened than recognizing dimensions of safety culture and preventing incidents proactively and based on evidence. If there are no incidents reported it usually indicates that incidents are not recognized at all. On this basis there is no relevant risk assessment, monitoring or analysis, that would serve as a basis to learn prevention of incidents and preparedness and proactive actions to develop safety culture.

In the EduSafe- and TUKO -projects 2016–2018 [7] the Green Cross digital application was used in schools to allow school staff to report incidents, injuries, accidents and near-miss cases (Fig. 1). This paper will introduce an analysis based on 168 incidents in three comprehensive schools. The paper is a part of the efforts to understand what kind of incidents happen at schools and to get experiences how to gather the incident data to make it possible for schools to develop their safety culture based on evidence. The overall research question is: What kind of incidents happen in schools in comprehensive education during a school year? The analysis of incidents related to physical learning environments indicates that there are falling risks and incidents inside school building, risks and incidents at the schoolyard, risks and incidents with non-functioning or broken facilities, and incidents outside school learning environments as well as incidents with traffic and parking [11]. In this paper the focus is on presenting the incidents that were categorized as incidents in pedagogical learning environments especially related to lessons. Analysis from this point of view is new.

1.2   Safety in Pedagogical Learning Environments

A learning environment is seen as a place, space, community and/or culture for learning that includes tools, materials, equipment and services, e.g. school buildings, classes, schoolyards, sport fields, trips, visits. Safety and security in a learning environment can be considered in physical, social, psychological and pedagogical dimensions. The physical dimension is spaces and facilities with tools, materials, machines and equipment as well as the condition of them. The social dimension is about socially acknowledged values, attitudes and behavior and actions based on them. Psychological dimension includes personal values, attitudes, personality, motivation, knowledge and skills as well as experiences that are the basis for individual actions. The pedagogical dimension is about the organization of teaching and the content and organisation of learning opportunities, participation, affection, rules, justice, responsibilities and peer support. [12] The space and equipment can be safe from a physical point of view but without comprehension of proactive actions in lessons it can be an unsafe and hazardous learning environment. [8] Based on the safety paradigm that calls for human factors behind the incidents and emphasizes resilience [13, 14] it can be understood that near-miss cases and accidents are in relation to several physical, social, psychological and pedagogical factors [10]. This safety paradigm requires recording, monitoring and reporting the incidents and near-miss cases systematically and learning from them and making changes based on evidence. To be able to find out and understand the risks, factors and reasons behind incidents and accidents, there is a need to analyse these on a level that is meaningful for schools, staff and students [15]. The first step is to get prior knowledge of what happens, where and to whom to be able to develop and use methods that can open more detailed reasons behind incidents in the future in school context.

2 Materials and Methods

2.1 Data and Study Context

This paper presents a study on incidents, near-miss cases, accidents and injuries, in three basic education schools with elementary (grades 1–6, pupils age 7–12) and lower secondary (grades 7–9, pupils age 13–16) education. All schools are comprehensive education public schools since there are only few private schools in Finland. The number of staff in these schools is altogether 290 persons and 2360 students. Two of the schools are multicultural city schools and one is a town school with mainly students of Finnish origin. The staff in each school was familiar with research and development projects.

The data consists of 168 reports. Almost all the reports were written in Finnish. These were downloaded into Green Cross application system [16] by school staff during years 2016–2017. The Green Cross is a digital application to be used in a quick documentation of incidents at schools. The idea is to make it easy for school staff, teachers and principals, to report incidents as a part of everyday practice at schools. To be able to report incidents the staff had to sign into the system with a password. The Green Cross is not an application that teachers and principals would use normally as a daily practice. The application was offered to schools for use as a part of the Safe school and EduSafe –research and development projects [17]. The projects and researches encouraged school staff a lot, firstly to understand and notify what is an incident and secondly to recognize that even a near-miss case is worth of a report since the earlier research [18] notifies that all teachers are not committed to promote safety systemically. On a school level it was possible to see all the reported incidents in a monthly view (Fig. 1).

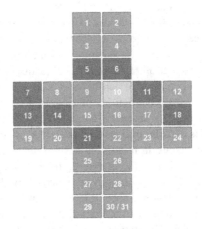

Fig. 1. A monthly view of reported incidents on a school level – Green Cross: School II, October 2016. A green day is a day without reported incidents, yellow colour is a near-miss case day and a red one informs of injuries or accidents. (Color figure online)

While reporting, a short 2–3 min description of the accident, injury or a near-miss case was written into the system. A school safety team or staff responsible for safety had the possibility to analyze reports and implement actions and alterations needed in order to reduce future incidents at their school. However, they treated the incidents like separate cases and did not make any other systemic analysis on their school level. The motivation for the schools to participate in reporting arose from a need to improve safety culture in their school.

2.2   The Analysis

The reports were analysed by qualitative thematic content analysis. The incidents from the reports were collected to a table and coded: a near-miss case or an accident or injury and the school. For example, the incident tagged to the code II/32-NM tells that the incident is report 32 from school II, a near-miss case (Table 1). From all the reported incidents (N = 168) 20% were near-miss cases (n = 33) and 80% were accidents and injuries (n = 135). The seriousness of the injuries varied from light scratches, and/or bruises (minor injury = MI) to accidents in which students or teachers needed ambulance and doctor and hospital visits (serious injury = SI).

The aim was not to compare the schools and incidents. The main aim was to organize the incidents under the themes of theory-driven understanding of learning environment that considers safety and security at school from physical, psychological, social and pedagogical perspective [12]. Content analysis was used to be able to make replicable and valid inferences by coding and interpreting the incidents. After several readings the incidents were organized under the themes. The lower and upper categories were formed under the themes through careful consideration of all the incidents. During this process several incidents were reconsidered and moved to a better fitting category. After all lower and upper categories were finalized, the main categories were formed and named (Table 1).

Based on the analysis four main categories were formulated. These were (1) Risks and incidents in physical learning environments (28% of all incidents), (2) Risks and incidents in social learning environments (36%), (3) Risks and incidents in psychological learning environments (16%) and (4) Risks and incidents in pedagogical learning environments, especially related to lessons (20%). In the main category, which is the focus of this paper, Risks and incidents in pedagogical learning environments, were included the incidents that had direct relation to lessons: teachers were either preparing lessons or teaching, and students were joining in these.

3 Results

In the main category of Risks and incidents in pedagogical learning environments, especially related to lessons included those incidents that were not considered in the physical, social or psychological learning environments point of view. The main category was formed by three upper categories. These are (1) Injuries to teachers while teaching and preparing, (2) Incidents to students during lessons, and (3) Risk management in teaching (Table 1).

Injuries to Teachers While Teaching and Preparing. In the analysis there was noticed incidents that were reported from teachers' part in relation to their own work, either preparing lessons or teaching (Table 1). The reported injuries that happened to teachers in preparing lessons consisted of various types of incidents. Most typical incidents in this category happened as teachers were preparing their lessons and were due to take materials needed using ladders or somehow climbing to reach out to the material boxes. In the incidents teachers either fell down or were hit by falling boxes or other kinds of falling materials. Also, when teachers were carrying teaching materials or equipment in their arms in a way that they could not see their legs was reported to cause falls. *'I had a pile of iPads in my arms on my way to next lesson and could not see my legs properly. That's why I fell down and my ankle was hurt.'* (III8-MI, Table 1), was a typical example. These incidents caused minor injuries. The other lower category was about Injuries to sport teachers during lessons. *'A teacher fell down while skating during a sports lesson. The arm was hurt.'* (I/49-MI). The incident of a teacher falling and hurting oneself represents a typical description of an incident in the category.

Injuries, Accidents and Near-Misses to Pupils During Lessons. The upper category Injuries, accidents and near-misses to pupils during lessons was formed with four lower categories: Injuries in craft, design and technology education lessons, Incidents in home economics lessons and Incidents to pupils during sport lessons. The fourth lower category was Incidents and injuries with things falling from shelfs that was not subject teaching specific than the three first lower categories.

Table 1. Examples of risks and incidents in pedagogical learning environments in lessons in primary and lower secondary education in comprehensive schools: I-III = school, number of the incident, MI = minor injury, MOI = moderate injury, NM = near-miss incident.

Incident	Authentic example of an incident in categorization	Lower category	Upper category	Main category
I/8-MI	A teacher got a cut from a knife while emptying a dish machine before a home economics lesson	Injuries to teachers in preparing lessons	Injuries to teachers while teaching and preparing	Risks and incidents in pedagogical learning environments in lessons
I/24-MI	A teacher reached out to some material from a material box on the upper part of a cupboard. He fell and hit his mouth and teeth to the material box			
III8-MI	A teacher had a pile of iPads in his arms on his way to the next lesson and could not see his legs properly. That's why he fell, and his ankle was hurt			
I/49-MI	A teacher fell while skating during a sports lesson. The arm was hurt	Injuries to sport teachers during lessons		
I/67-MOI	A pupil sawed with a metal saw in CDT lesson. He wounded his hand. There was a need for first aid at the school and doctoral aid at health center	Injuries in craft, design and technology education lessons	Injuries, accidents and near-misses to pupils during lessons	
II18-MOI	A pupil cut a piece of his finger while cutting with scissors and talking with mates at the same time in CDT lesson. First aid was needed and a health center visit after the pupil passed out			
II/14-NM	A pupil put a baking tray into an oven. The baking paper was too close to a heating resistor and the paper went on fire	Incidents in home economics lessons		
II/12-MI	Two pupils collided and fell in sports lesson	Incidents to pupils during sport lessons		
I/25-MOI	In Finnish baseball pupil A caught a ball in his hands while pupil B was trying to hit it. He hit the wrist of the pupil A. The wrist was fractured			
I/13-MI	A basket fell from a shelf while pupils were reaching for something from a shelf	Incidents and injuries with things falling from shelfs		
II/60-NM	Not enough first aid bags for the pupils visiting a forest	Preparedness for incidents	Risk management in teaching	
III/16-NM	Too many pupils in one area at the same time	Prevention of incidents		

The reported incidents in Craft, design and technology were moderate injuries that needed a visit to health center. These incidents were caused by hand tools and were kind of slips and slaps in using hand tools. *'A pupil sawed with a metal saw in CDT lesson. He wounded his hand. There was a need for first aid at the school and doctoral aid at health center.'* (I/67-MOI).

In home economics a small fire in the oven was reported as the baking paper caught fire. This was a near-miss case and did not cause any injury or bigger fire accident. However, the near-miss case is one example of the fire risks that are met in schools.

The lower category of Incidents to pupils during sport lessons was the largest lower category. The incidents were unintentional and happened while doing various exercises in sports lessons. The incidents were near-misses or minor and moderate injuries. An example of a moderate injury is the following: *'In the Finnish baseball a pupil A caught a ball in his hands while pupil B was trying to hit it. B hit the wrist of A. The wrist was fractured.'* (I/25-MOI).

Risk Management in Teaching. The third main category in the analysis of incidents in pedagogical learning environment was named Risk management in teaching (Table 1). These reports to the Green Cross system were near-misses. The teachers reported incidents that they recognised as risks to pupils and teaching. The incidents were related to preparedness e.g. for first aid in outside school building learning environments. Also the big amount of students in certain learning environments was seen as a risk and can be seen as a prevention of accidents and injuries.

4 Discussion

In this paper the category of Risks and incidents in pedagogical learning environments, especially related to lessons presents a systematic incident analysis as an example to be able to discuss how the further research could focus on and how the result could be used in improving safety culture of schools. In this main category three upper categories describe the data: Injuries to teachers while teaching and preparing, Injuries, accidents and near-misses to pupils during lessons and Risk management in teaching. The result of the analysis based on qualitative data from three schools is not generalizable. However, we know about incidents in schools now more than before. In the future study there is a need to monitor more individually, if there could be found groups that are subjects of incidents more or less often than others and why some teachers report the incidents and some don't do. Also focusing on each safety critical subject would reveal the risks of the subject more detailed.

Based on the analysis it is possible to consider the results from teachers and students point of view. The result reveals the analysis that the researcher made but not an analysis that the schools had made. The next step in finding a more detailed knowledge about incidents could be a quantitative data based on qualitative results [11, 19]. The other possibility could be an ethnographic research design that could focus on teachers and students behavior according to incidents.

The incidents with teachers and students are partly different, partly the same. The incidents in safety critical subjects were not a big surprise. Falling things at classes from shelfs were a little surprise as well as the moderate injuries in craft, design and technology even the amount of incidents was the largest in sports. This might have something to do with the unpredictable risks at schools and students behavior to act against norms and regulations or use of structures or products in a way they are not supposed to be used [7].

Nobody says that safety is not important on school level. However, considering the number of the reports (N = 168) and the number of students and staff, it indicates a low rate of reporting despite of the researches' several visits at schools and encouragement of teachers to identify incidents. The individual teachers might consider differently what is worth to report and what is not. This observation together with the fact based on earlier research that all teachers are not committed to promote safety systemically [18], makes the development of safety culture challenging at school level. How would it be possible to learn from near-miss cases and incidents if they are not even reported. On the other hand solutions based on evidence might be simple. For example teachers could use baskets or trolleys in carrying their materials and equipment to learning environments to avoid falling incidents.

One question is the usability of Green Cross application or some equivalent system that could be updated to a more usable mobile application without separate signing to the system [E.g. 19]. The other question is students' role. On the basis of the definition of safety culture in schools [8] students should also have an active role in recording, reporting, monitoring and analyzing incidents and being part of implementation based on lessons learnt.

As a conclusion there is an obvious need to develop methods of reporting incidents in schools as well as the motivation to report to be able to develop the safety culture of schools and lessons learnt from incidents [9]. In research there is also a need to understand more deeply the mechanisms of incidents and human factors around them [13, 14]. Since schools are very unique organisations, diversity with students and staff and altering learning environments make some of the risks unpredictable. The positive from the safety culture point of view this analysis was that some teachers recognized risks in pedagogical learning environments (Risk management in teaching, Table 1) even if they didn't use these terms while reporting the incidents.

References

1. Basic Education Act 628/1998. https://www.finlex.fi/fi/laki/kaannokset/1998/en19980628.pdf, Accessed 14 June 2018
2. Occupational Safety and Health Act 738/2002. https://www.finlex.fi/fi/laki/kaannokset/2002/en20020738_20060053.pdf. Accessed 14 June 2018
3. Piispanen, M.: Good Learning Environment. Perceptions of Good Quality in Comprehensive School by Pupils, Parents and Teachers. Doctoral thesis in Pedagogics. English abstract. University of Jyväskylä, Kokkola University Consortium Chydenius (2008)
4. National Core Curriculum for Basic Education 2014. The Finnish National Board of Education. http://www.oph.fi/download/163777_perusopetuksen_opetussuunnitelman_perusteet_2014.pdf. Accessed 04 June 2018

5. Luopa, P., et al.: Nuorten hyvinvointi Suomessa 2000–2013. Kouluterveyskyselyn tulokset [The wellbeing of adolescents in Finland 2000–2013. The Results of the School Health Promotion study]. Report 25/2014. National Institute for Health and Welfare (THL), Helsinki (2014)
6. Näsi, M., Virtanen, M., Tanskanen, M.: Oppilaitosten turvallisuustutkimus 2016. Helsingin yliopisto. Kriminologian ja oikeuspolitiikan instituutti. Katsauksia 20/2017
7. Somerkoski, B.: Green cross: collecting injury data at schools. In: Tuomi, P., Perttula, A. (eds.) GamiFIN 2017 - Proceedings of the 1st International GamiFIN Conference. http://ceur-ws.org/Vol-1857/. Accessed 14 June 2018
8. Lindfors, E., Somerkoski, B.: Turvallisuusosaaminen luokanopettajakoulutuksen opetussuunnitelmassa [Safety competence in the curriculum of primary teacher education]. In: Pakula, H.-M., Kouki, E., Silfverberg, H., Yli-Panula, E. (eds.) Uudistuva ja uusiutuva ainedidaktiikka [The reforming subject didactics], pp. 328–343. Suomen ainedidaktinen tutkimusseura, Turku (2016)
9. Geller, E.S.: Psychological science and safety: large-scale success at preventing occupational injuries and fatalities. Curr. Dir. Psychol. Sci. **20**(2), 109–114 (2011). https://doi.org/10.1177/0963721411402667. Accessed 04 June 2018
10. Reason, J.: Safety paradoxes and safety culture. Inj. Control Saf. Promot. **7**(1), 3–14 (2000). https://www.tandfonline.com/doi/pdf/10.1076/1566-0974(200003)7%20%3A1%20%3B1-V%3BFT003. Accessed 14 June 2018
11. Lindfors, E., Teperi, A.-M.: Incidents in schools - incident analysis in developing safety management. In: Nazir, S., Teperi, A.-M., Polak-Sopińska, A. (eds.) AHFE 2018. AISC, vol. 785, pp. 462–471. Springer, Cham (2019). https://doi.org/10.1007/978-3-319-93882-0_44
12. Lindfors, E.: Turvallinen oppimisympäristö, oppilaitoksen turvallisuuskulttuuri ja turvallisuuskasvatus – käsitteellistä pohdintaa ja kehittämishaasteita. [The safe learning environment, safety culture and safety education in schools – Concept considerations and development challenges] In: Lindfors, E. (ed.) Kohti turvallisempaa oppilaitosta! Oppilaitosten turvallisuuden ja turvallisuuskasvatuksen tutkimus– ja kehittämishaasteita. [Towards the safer learning institution! Safety and safety education as research and development challenges. The first OPTUKE research and development –symposium, University of Tampere. School of Education], pp. 12–28 (2012)
13. Hollnagel, E.: Is safety a subject for science? Saf. Sci. **67**, 21–24 (2012)
14. Norros, L.: Acting Under Uncertainty - The Core-Task Analysis in Ecological Study of Work. VTT Publications 546, Espoo (2004). http://www.vtt.fi/inf/pdf/publications/2004/P546.pdf. Accessed 04 June 2018
15. Kjellen, U., Albrechtsen, E.: Prevention of Accidents and Unwanted Occurrences: Theory, Methods, and Tools in Safety Management, Second Edition. Chapman and Hall/CRC, Boca Raton. https://ebookcentral.proquest.com/lib/kutu/detail.action?docID=4819335. Accessed 04 June 2018
16. Cloubi, The toolset for publishers to design, produce and operate digital learning material. http://cloubi.com/. Accessed 14 June 2018
17. University of Turku: Oppilaitosten turvallisuuskulttuurin kehittämisverkosto (OPTUKE) [The Developing Network of Safety Culture in Schools (OPTUKE)]. http://utu.fi/optuke_en. Accessed 14 June 2018
18. Waitinen, M.: Safe school? Safety culture in primary and secondary schools in Helsinki and the factors affecting it. Doctoral dissertation. Researches 334. English abstract. University of Helsinki, Helsinki (2011)
19. Somerkoski, B.: Green cross: application for analyzing school injuries. Finnish J. EHealth EWelfare, **9**(4), 322–329. https://doi.org/10.23996/fjhw.65178. Accessed 14 June 2018

Voices of Authorities and Shareholders Affect Voices of Processes

Petteri Mussalo[1(✉)], Virpi Hotti[1], and Hanna Mussalo[2]

[1] School of Computing, University of Eastern Finland,
Microkatu 1, 70200 Kuopio, Finland
mup@iki.fi
[2] Imaging Center, Kuopio University Hospital,
P.O. Box 100, 70029 KYS Kuopio, Finland

Abstract. There are several voices (e.g., needs or requirements) concern the business. In this paper, the voices of authorities, shareholders and processes are defined to be controlled voices the effects of which can be considered within functional domains and enterprise entities. The Voice of the Authority (VoA) is in common controls, the Voice of the Shareholder (VoS) is in corporate controls and the Voice of the Process (VoP) is in process controls. Three constructions are proposed to strength the meaning of the controlled voices. First, common, corporate, and process controls are mapped within two functional domains (i.e., control and operations) of the Industrial Internet Reference Architecture (IIRA) to illustrate the importance of the voices. Second, 11 related entities (i.e., control, course of action, data entity, driver, event, function, goal, measure, process, and service) of the Togaf 9.2 content metamodel are mapped within control and operations domains. Third, the definitions of the entities are mapped within the voices of authorities, shareholders and processes. The Voice of the Authority and the Voice of the Shareholder affect processes via contract, control, and course of action entities. We discuss the meaning of the constructions in the context the healthcare.

Keywords: Voice of the Process (VoP) · Voice of the Authority (VoA)
Voice of the Shareholder (VoS) · Control · Functional domain
Healthcare

1 Introduction

The reform of Finland regional government, health and social services [1] is an example where relationships between enterprise entities have to redefine. Some of the relationships (e.g., customers of services vs. service providers) can be called experience capabilities based on historical knowledge [2]. In general, enterprises control their capabilities over data and information even based on regulatory environments [3]. However, if we do not have any experience capabilities or we will affect the experiences (e.g., customer experience, employee experience, and user experience) then we have to listen to voices of different kinds.

© Springer Nature Switzerland AG 2018
H. Li et al. (Eds.): WIS 2018, CCIS 907, pp. 88–100, 2018.
https://doi.org/10.1007/978-3-319-97931-1_8

The meaning of voice listening can be defined as figuring out either stated or unstated expectations (a.k.a., needs or requirements) of entities [4]. The stated expectations might be process limits, or controlled justifications by authorities and shareholders. For example, the Finnish government sets controlled justifications in healthcare and social welfare reform – it finances the healthcare and social welfare activities of the regional government, and it regulates how the regional governments allocate the funding to the service providers [1]. Moreover, the voices of different kind have to be listening and process limits will be stated because of the aim of the reform is to achieve better coordinated, cost-efficient, customer-oriented, and effective services [1].

Some voices (e.g., the voices of customers and employees) are listening by surveys of different kinds. Some voices (e.g., voices of authorities, processes and shareholders) have to be listening by controls of different kinds. The voices of authorities, shareholders and processes are seen in controls interacting with an environment. Therefore, we research controls of different kinds at the level of functional domains.

The functional domain is "categorized functions that are generally used together" [5]. There are several different functional domains in the subject areas such as Biochemistry, Genetics and Molecular Biology, Immunology and Microbiology, or Medicine [6]. However, we selected the functional domains of the Industrial Internet Reference Architecture [7] because of it offers a generic framework to be taken into the consideration the controlled interactions within an environment.

However, "[s]pecific system requirements will strongly influence how the functional domains are decomposed, what additional functions may be added or left out and what functions may be combined and further decomposed" [7]. Therefore, governance of different kinds (e.g., architecture, corporate and IT) are used to ensure that business is conducted properly [3]. Governances are practices or institutionalized best practices by which entities and their relationships are managed and controlled at an enterprise-wide level. Moreover, some of the entities have to be related properly at architecture level to ensure compliance with authority documents (e.g., regulations, internal and external standards). Therefore, we selected the TOGAF 9.2 content metamodel [3] to specify the management function, as well to demonstrate how related entities will be affected by the voices of authorities, shareholders and processes. The TOGAF content metamodel provides a feature set (i.e., entities and their relationships) that can be either explicitly (e.g., the Government Wide Enterprise Architecture, GWEA) or implicitly (e.g., JHS 179 Enterprise architecture planning and development) mapped on artifacts [8]. Therefore, we will demonstrate how entities and their relationships will be affected by the voices of authorities, shareholders and processes.

Section 2 illustrates the meanings of the voices of authorities, processes and shareholders. Then, we clarify the voices and corresponding controls within the functional domains and enterprise entities (Sect. 3). Furthermore, we discuss the meaning of the voices, controls and functional domains in healthcare (Sect. 4).

2 Controlled Voices - Conceptual Background and Importance

The voices of authorities (Sect. 2.1), shareholders (Sect. 2.2) and processes (Sect. 2.3) are seen in controls that affect functional domains of the business. The Voice of the Authority (VoA) is in common controls, the Voice of the Shareholder (VoS) is in corporate controls and the Voice of the Process (VoP) is in process controls.

2.1 Voice of the Authority

The common controls are used to illustrate requirements or obligations that are derived from the authority documents (e.g., laws and standards) and are controlled by the same party of parties (i.e., by the authorities). The Voice of the Authority is stated requirements that are adapted to the common controls.

There are hundreds authority documents (e.g., best practices, guidelines, regulations and standards) that the organizations have to follow-up. There are the common controls frameworks such as the Common Controls Framework (CCF) by Adobe [9, 10], the Unified Compliance Framework (UCF) by Network Frontiers LLC [11] and the Common Security Framework (CSF) by HITRUST Alliance [12]. The common controls frameworks differ in the selected authority documents and formations of the common controls [13].

We exemplify the Voice of the Authority within the General Data Protection Regulation (GDPR). For example, UCF offers the Common Controls Hub where the GDPR is mapped into 1497 common controls. The GDPR contains 10 chapters and 99 articles as well as 173 recitals [14]. Infringements of the GDPR articles might cause fines. Therefore, safeguards (e.g., encryption or pseudonymisation) are needed to ensure that technical and organizational measures are in place. Furthermore, "appropriate safeguards may consist of making use of binding corporate rules, standard data protection clauses adopted by the Commission, standard data protection clauses adopted by a supervisory authority or contractual clauses authorized by a supervisory authority" [14]. For example, data processing addendum [15] contains data transfer frameworks ensuring that the customers can lawfully transfer personal data to outside of the European Union by relying on either our binding corporate rules, Privacy Shield certification, or standard contractual clauses.

The organizations have to gather and share the authority documents as well decide how to adapt the authority documents. The Voice of the Authority (e.g., the European Union where the European parliament and the council are regulated the GDPR) can be taken into account in many ways. For example, the common controls (e.g., UCF ones) are possible to leverage within the service management system (e.g., [16]) and the guidelines of the authority documents (e.g., [17]) can be used to implement required measures or other requirements. However, even national instructions are needed to interpret the common controls and to implement them.

2.2 Voice of the Shareholder

The Voice of the Shareholder is stated requirements that are adapted to the corporate controls. The corporate controls concern governance of different kinds (e.g., architecture, corporate and IT) that are used to ensure that business is conducted properly at the enterprise-wide level. For example, corporate controls are in accountabilities and responsibilities, as well in the statements of corporate strategy [3].

The term corporate control might refer "to the authority to make the decisions of a corporation regarding operations and strategic planning, including capital allocations, acquisitions and divestments, top personnel decisions, and major marketing, production, and financial decisions" [18]. Therefore, the Voice of the Shareholder might be seen as the Voice of the Authority.

The Voice of the Business (VoB) is influenced by external factors such as regulatory bodies, the economic environment, and legal constraints such as Healthcare Reform [19]. There are three kinds of organization ownerships at the welfare and healthcare sector [20]: the for-profit ownership tries to achieve maximal profits, the government basis organizations pursue the most economical use of given resources, and the nonprofit ownership provides services funded by constitution donors. Based on external factors or ownerships the voice might belong to the shareholder or to the authority. For example, the Finnish government sets controlled justifications in healthcare and social welfare reform which means that the Finnish government is the shareholder and the authority the voice of which is, for example, in regulations how the regional governments allocate the funding to the service providers [1].

2.3 Voice of the Process

Customers feel the variance where "a change in a process or business practice that may alter its expected outcome" [21]. The variation of the process is based on either common causes (a.k.a., noise, chance causes, non-assignable causes, natural patterns, random effects, and random errors) or special causes (a.k.a., signals, sporadic causes, assignable causes, unnatural patterns, systematic effects, and systematic errors).

The Voice of the Process (VoP) is a term used to describe whether the process is under control and what kind of causes are attached to individual measurements. A common cause is a part of natural variation. A special cause needs to be addressed with. We use the term process control is used to illustrate variation ranges (e.g., lower and upper control limits) and individual results that are plotted above and below the average of the process.

The Statistical Process Control (SPC) highlights that there is always variation inside a process and the process are either in or out of control limits [22]. The SPC methods are seen the best possible tool to see if the process is stable or not [23]. Further, Lean and Six Sigma are methods for realizing the continuous process improvement [23]. Six Sigma aims to reduce process variation with data driven methods. Lean eliminates waste and unnecessary project steps. Both of the theorems base theoretically on statistical process control and help the leadership or management to identify and solve the production problems.

Control chart rules (a.k.a., Shewhart control chart rules, out-of-control conditions) for determining assignable cause variation and control charts are a proven technique for improving productivity. There are common types of control chart patterns [24] that are tested, for example, by an Xbar-R-chart, Xbar-s-chart, exponentially weighted moving average (EWMA) control chart, cumulative sum (CUSUM) control chart, state space models or autoregressive integrated moving average (ARIMA) models [25].

3 Controlled Voices Within Functional Domains and Enterprise Entities: Conceptual Constructions

Common, corporate, and process controls are mapped within the functional domains of the Industrial Internet Reference Architecture (IIRA) to illustrate the importance of the voices (Sect. 3.1). The accountabilities and responsibilities of the functional domains are exemplified by the entities of the Togaf 9.2 content metamodel (Sect. 3.2). Finally, the definitions of the entities are mapped within the voices of authorities, shareholders and processes (Sect. 3.3).

3.1 Common, Corporate and Process Controls vs. Functional Domains

The Industrial Internet Reference Architecture (IIRA) provides assistance for the development and utilization of the Industrial Internet of Things (IIoT) and it consists of five functional domains (business, application, control, information, and operations). There are two common sets of the functions of the information domain: analytics and data. The functions of the information domain are complementary to those functions that are implemented in the control domain. There are two common sets of the functions of the application domain: API (application programming interface) and UI (user interface), logic and rules. The functions of the application domain are advisory to those functions that are implemented in the control domain. There are anonymous functions of the business domain that enable end-to-end-operations. Two functional domains (i.e., control and operations) are specified the most accurate [7].

There are seven common functions of the control domain: sensing, actuation, communication, entity abstraction, modeling, asset management, and executor. The sensing function reads data from sensors. The actuation function writes data and control signals to the actuators by which a control system acts upon an environment. The communication function connects edges (e.g., actuators, external entities, and sensors) that are either statistically or dynamically configured. The entity abstraction function serves as the context in which the interactions between the edges and other entities are carried out. The modeling function addresses with the systems under control by the gathered data from the edges and peer systems. The asset management function ensures that policies (e.g., safety and security) are under the authority and responsibility of the edge entities. The executor function ensures that data movement and use of the edges are within the bounds of the policies [7].

There are five common sets of the functions of the operations domain: provisioning and deployment, management, monitoring and diagnostics, prognostics and optimization. Provisioning and deployment consists of a set of functions to provide and bring assets. Management consists of a set of functions to enable the assets to be controlled by the management commands. Monitoring and diagnostics consists of a set of functions to should assist operations by collecting and processing health state of the assets "to reduce the response time between detecting and addressing a problem". Prognostics consists of a set of functions to "identify potential issues before they occur and provide recommendations on their mitigation". Optimization consists of a set of functions to prescribe the assets "by identifying production losses and inefficiencies" [7].

The control and operations domains are building blocks the interactions of which will be seen based on the common, corporate and process controls (Fig. 1).

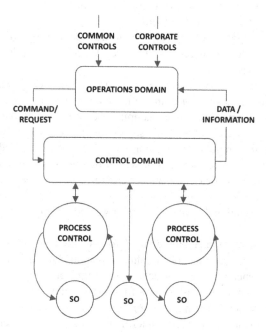

Fig. 1. Common corporation and process controls in the context of control and operations domains, SO = smart object

Both control domain and operations domain contain a set of functions, for example, to manage and respond to the commands/requests. Therefore, the flows (e.g., command/request and data/information) take place in and between the operations domain and control domain. Smart objects (SO) can be humans or physical things such as robots, sensors and software agents. Furthermore, there are several sources (e.g., treatment journals, logs, reports and surveys) to collect quality data either to controlling processes (or quality) or to specifications of the services and other outcomes. The construction is based on common and corporate controls directing by the operations domain and operationalized by the control domain. The continuous loop and sub loops realize the feedback-control system, where processes are controlled and adjusted according to the process output findings [26].

3.2   Enterprise Entities vs. Control and Operations Domains

All controls can be mapped with the management the definition of which is the sets of functions of the operations domain that consists of a set of the functions that enable the assets to be controlled by the management commands [7]. The management commands have to be concrete implementations the controls of different kinds. Therefore, we map enterprise entities [3] within the control and operations domains based on the following entities the definition of which are fulfilled mainly based on the definitions of the ISO Online Platform [27] and the Oxford University Press [28]:

- *Driver.* A factor (external or internal) that contributes to a result or outcome. For example, a change in regulation or compliance rules.
- *Goal.* A statement of intended outcome.
- *Course of Action.* Statements of purposes to the way an organization operates.
- *Function.* A purpose (or an activity) intended for a person and/or thing to deliver business capabilities.
- *Control.* A decision-making step (e.g., business logic or governance gate) for process execution. Business (or domain) logic describes the sequence of operations to carry out the business rule that manipulate data entities. Governance gates are decisions between stages [29] or phases of the process to verify process phases where some form of regulatory or compliance sign-off is required.
- *Process.* A flow of control between or within functions, processes, and/or services performed by roles and/or organization units to achieve a specified outcome (e.g., products).
- *Event.* An organizational state change triggered from inside or outside the organization.
- *Service.* An element of behavior defined for business, information systems, and platforms to provide specific functionality in response to commands or requests.
- *Data Entity.* An encapsulations of data as a recognized thing.
- *Contract.* An agreement that establishes functional and non-functional (e.g., privacy and security) parameters for interaction.
- *Measure.* An indicator or factor to determine success or alignment with goals.

When we clarify roles and charges in functional domains (Table 1) we apply a responsibility assignment matrix, known as RACI matrix. RACI is an acronym derived from Responsible (R), Accountable (A), Consulted (C), and Informed (I). Only one accountable must sign-off (approve) work that at least one responsible provides. Consulted ones are those whose advises or opinions are sought. Informed ones are those who are kept up-to-date of things as agreed.

The accountability of the entities (e.g., assets) and their controls belongs to the operations domain. The responsibility of the relationships belongs mainly to the control domain. The responsibility of the relationships within drivers, goals and courses of action belong to the operation domain because those relationships are mainly statements realized by the relationships within contacts, controls, data entities, events, measures, processes, and services. There are additional entities (e.g., logical and physical components) that fulfill the conceptual ones. However, 11 related entities can be used to concretize the common sets of the functions of the control and operations domains.

Table 1. Related entities vs. control and operations domains

Source Entity	Relationship	Target entity	Control domain	Operations domain
Driver	Creates	Goal	C/I	A/R
Goal	Is realized by	Course of action	C/I	A/R
Course of action	Influences	Function	C/I	A/R
Function	Is realized by/supports	Process	R	A
Process	Is guided by	Control	R	A
Process	Generates/solves	Event	R	A
Process	Decomposes/orchestrates	Service	R	A
Service	Provides governed interface to access	Function	R	A
Data entity	Is accessed and updated through	Service	R	A
Service	Is governed and measured by	Contract	R	A
Measure	Sets performance criteria for	Service	R	A

3.3   Enterprise Entities vs. VoA, VoS and VoP

The enterprise entities will be affected by the voices of authorities, shareholders and processes. We bold and underline the words of the entity definitions to find out the Voice of the Authority (bolded) and the Voice of the Shareholder (bolded and underlined) as follows:

- *Driver.* A factor (**external** or **_internal_**) that contributes to a result or outcome. For example, a change in regulation or compliance rules.
- *Goal.* **_A statement of intended outcome_**.
- *Course of Action.* **_Statements of purposes to the way an organization operates_**.
- *Control.* **A decision-making step** (e.g., business logic or governance gate) for process execution. Business (or domain) logic describes the sequence of operations to carry out the business rule that manipulate data entities. Governance gates are decisions between stages [29] or phases of the process to verify process phases where some form of **regulatory or compliance sign-off** is required.
- *Contract.* An agreement that establishes functional and non-functional (e.g., **privacy** and **security**) **_parameters for interaction_**.

We exemplify the voices with authorities, governing body or process owners. The governing body (e.g., a board of directors) is accountable for the performance and conformity of the organization. The process owners conduct the course of action. The entities the definition of which contain the effects of authorities and governing body are source entities (Table 2). The service entity is governed and measured by the contract entity where both the Voice of the Authority and the Voice of the Shareholders are in the attributes of the contract entity.

The Voice of the Authority and the Voice of the Shareholder affect processes via contract, control, and the course of action entities, for example, by process limits. At the operational level, the event entity is meaningful because it is resolved, for example, by actors (i.e., a person, organization, or system) that initiate or interact with activities of the processes [3].

Table 2. Enterprise entities vs. VoA, VoS and VoP

Source entity	Relationship	Target entity	Authorities	Governing bodies	Process owners
Driver	Creates	Goal	VoA	VoS	
Goal	Is realized by	Course of action		VoS	
Course of action	Influences	Function		VoS	
Control	Ensures correct operation of	Process	VoA	VoS	
Function	Is realized by/supports	Process			VoP
Contract	Governs and measures	Service	VoA	VoS	
Service	Is realized by/supports	Process			VoP
Event	Is resolved by	Actor, Process, Service	VoA	VoS	VoP

4 Discussion

The voices of authorities, shareholders and processes are stated expectations and we proposed constructions to clarify the importance of the voices. The effects of the voices have been illustrated within functional domains or enterprise entities.

The Voice of the Authority. Healthcare is strictly regulated in the meaning of restrictions, data privacy as well roles and responsibilities. In addition to laws and administrative regulations there are huge amounts of common practices, guidelines and instructions called common controls. In addition to the legislation and the administrative instructions there are lots of national, local and discipline specific unofficial instructions and recommendations. Monitoring the regulations and the guideline fulfillment is a complex but important task. For instance, following the medical radiation dose recommendation requires precise recommendation, given dose monitoring and practices to recognize and manage the deviations. The doses between individuals may vary because of patient and target organ properties as well the features of the used device features and local circumstances. Health care operations improvement in large extent requires also changes in way the treatment and service delivery are realized [30]. Common controls-based data extraction and transformation and calculation enable technically easy maintenance. Furthermore, evidence-based tradition in healthcare requires evidences also about the process renewal benefits [31].

The Voice of the Shareholder. The ownership model affects the organization's operational target. Together with VoS the Voice of the Business [19] represents the organization strategic leadership and highest direction to the organization operation target. Both VoS and VoB are steering the planning, interactions and should be notified when realizing the scalability and porting the definitions. As an example the outsourcing agreements with suppliers are controlled with VoA but VoB directs the agreements to support the strategies. VoS provides co trolls for the agreements and instructions to continuously monitoring.

The Voice of the Process. Healthcare quality and process improvement projects follow the Statistical Process Control (SPC) principles [32]. Health sciences and health technology are developing constantly and producing new treatment methods to be used to treat the more complex situations. Care demands are increasing and same time the resourcing is decreasing. New ways to solve the problems are required [33]. Accountability and efficiency of the healthcare organizations with increasing amount of clinical and administrative data increases the focus of statistical data on healthcare regulations. Rating, screening and surveillance will be based on regulations derived from statistical analysis [34]. In addition to the statistical process control, also the process interactions should be monitored. In a complex adaptive multi process environment, like hospital, the monitoring is essential [35]. Monitoring the selected process throughput times may reveal the real crowding sources [36]. For example, crowding in emergency room may be due either local disruptions, increased patient traffic or disruptions at the cooperative units like clinical chemistry or imaging.

Functional Domains and Voices. We selected two functional domains (i.e., control domain and the operations domain) of the Industrial Internet Reference Architecture [7] to illustrate the controlled interactions within an environment. For example, healthcare has parallel and hierarchical functions that have to interact over organizational borders under several controls. Functional domains were the important building blocks to illustrate the context of the common, corporate and process controls and we got a "starting point for conceptualizing a concrete functional architecture" [7]. The control domain realizes the construction measurement and controlling features with smart objects and visualization user interface with the smart objects [7]. However, according to ITIL Information Technology Infrastructure Library (ITIL) the smart objects and control domain realize active, passive and proactive control, surveillance and monitoring [37]. Active monitoring consists of automated regular checks to recognize the failures. Passive monitoring depends on alerts or notifications to find and recognize the different failures. Proactive monitoring predicts future failures with data patterns. In addition to discover the failures the monitoring covers the process status assessment and reporting. Adjusting the terminology may improve the model clarity.

Enterprise Entities and Voices. Our constructions for functional architectures adapt the enterprise entities of the TOGAF 9.2 content metamodel to specify the control domain and operations domain, as well the voices of the authorities, shareholders and processes. It is observable that some entities (e.g., the control and data entity) are related with one another entity. Furthermore, there might be several entities and relationships between two entities. For example, there are five entities (i.e., the goal, course of action, function, process and service) between the driver entity and the data entity. When we researched the entities and relationships against the voices, we realized that the voices of authorities, shareholders and processes concern many entities, even the attributes of the entities such as the attributes of the contract entity. The TOGAF 9.2 content metamodel offers the reasonable entities and relationships to healthcare functional architecture. However, the TOGAF 9.2 content metamodel does not support consistency in information architecture for decision-making [38]. There are even data taxonomies (e.g., ISO/IEC 19944:2017 Information technology—Cloud computing—Cloud services and devices: Data flow, data categories and data use) that adapt, for example, some common controls. However, the data-centric framework is needed. Data, analytics and data driven approaches are seen as revolutionary development for healthcare - future healthcare will be data driven [39]. For example, Curcin et al. [32] proposed Improved Data Model (IDM) for continuous quality improvement, data collection and reporting.

References

1. Finnish Government: Regional government, health and social services reform (2017). https://alueuudistus.fi/en/general-information-reform
2. The International Foundation for Digital Competences: VeriSM^{TM} - a service management approach for the digital age. Van Haren (2017)
3. The Open Group: The TOGAF® Standard, Version 9.2 (2018). http://pubs.open-group.org/architecture/togaf9-doc/arch/index.html
4. The International Organization for Standardization: ISO 13053-2:2011(en) quantitative methods in process improvement—Six Sigma—part 2: tools and techniques (2011). https://www.iso.org/obp/ui/#iso:std:iso:13053:-2:ed-1:v1:en
5. The International Organization for Standardization, the International Electrotechnical Commission: ISO/IEC 26551:2016(en) software and systems engineering—tools and methods for product line requirements engineering (2016). https://www.iso.org/obp/ui#iso:std:iso-iec:26551:ed-2:v1:en
6. Elsevier: Scopus (2018). https://www.elsevier.com/solutions/scopus
7. The Industrial Internet Consortium: The Industrial Internet of Things Volume G1: Reference Architecture (2017). http://www.iiconsortium.org/IIC_PUB_G1_V1.80_2017-01-31.pdf
8. Makola, D., Hotti, V.: Critical success factors for adopting enterprise architecture metamodels in the health sector: literature review. J. Health Inform. Afr. 1(1), 127–132 (2013). https://www.jhia-online.org/index.php/jhia/article/viewFile/43/622013
9. Adobe: Adobe Releases Common Control Framework (CCF) as Open Source (2017). http://blogs.adobe.com/security/2017/05/open-source-ccf.html
10. Adobe: Compliance overview (2017). https://www.adobe.com/con-tent/dam/acom/en/security/pdfs/AdobeCloudServices_ComplianceOverview.pdf
11. Network Frontiers LLC: Unified Compliance Framework (2018). https://www.unifiedcompliance.com
12. HITRUST Alliance: HITRUST (2018). https://hitrustalliance.net
13. Mussalo, P., et al.: Common controls driven conceptual leadership framework. Finnish J. eHealth eWelfare 10(1), 89–101 (2018). https://doi.org/10.23996/fjhw.68821

14. European Parliament: Regulation (EU) 2016/679 of the European Parliament and of the Council of 27 April 2016 on the protection of natural persons with regard to the processing of personal data and on the free movement of such data, and repealing Directive 95/46/EC (General Data Protection Regulation) (Text with EEA relevance) (2016). https://eur-lex. europa.eu/legal-content/EN/TXT/?uri=uriserv:OJ.L_.2016.119.01.0001.01.ENG

15. Salesforce: Data processing addendum (2018). https://www.salesforce.com/content/dam/ web/en_us/www/documents/legal/Agreements/data-processing-addendum.pdf

16. ServiceNow: Use the Unified Compliance Framework (UCF) with Policy and Compliance Management (2018). https://docs.servicenow.com/bundle/helsinki-governance-risk-compliance/page/product/grc-ucf-import/concept/c_UCF-cch.html

17. European Commission: Guidelines (2018). http://ec.europa.eu/newsroom/article29/news. cfm?item_type=1360

18. Advameg Inc.: Corporate Control (2018). http://www.referenceforbusiness.com/ encyclopedia/Con-Cos/Corporate-Control.html

19. De Ana, F.J., Umstead, K.A., Phillips, G.J., Conner, C.P.: Value driven innovation in medical device design: a process for balancing stakeholder voices. Ann. Biomed. Eng. **41**(9), 1811–1821 (2013). https://doi.org/10.1007/s10439-013-0779-5

20. Cho, N.-E., Hong, K.: A kitchen with too many cooks: factors associated with hospital profitability. Sustainability **10**(2), 323 (2018). https://doi.org/10.3390/su10020323

21. General Electric: What is Six Sigma? The Roadmap to Customer Impact (Unknown year). https://www.ge.com/sixsigma/SixSigma.pdf

22. Shewhart, W.A.: Economic quality control of manufactured product. Bell Syst. Tech. J. **9**(2), 364–389 (1930). https://doi.org/10.1002/j.1538-7305.1930.tb00373.x

23. Antony, J., Snee, R., Hoerl, R.: Lean Six Sigma: yesterday, today and tomorrow. Int. J. Qual. Reliab. Manag. **34**(7), 1073–1093 (2017). https://doi.org/10.1108/IJQRM-03-2016-0035

24. Hachicha, W., Ghorbel, A.: A survey of control-chart pattern-recognition literature (1991–2010) based on a new conceptual classification scheme. Comput. Ind. Eng. **63**(1), 204–222 (2012). https://doi.org/10.1016/j.cie.2012.03.002

25. Montgomery, D.: Introduction to Statistical Quality Control. Wiley, Hoboken (2009)

26. Orr, K.: Data quality and systems theory. Commun. ACM **41**(2), 66–71 (1998)

27. The International Organization for Standardization: ISO Online Browsing Platform (OBP). https://www.iso.org/obp/ui#home

28. Oxford University Press: English Oxford Living Dictionary (2018). https://en. oxforddictionaries.com/

29. Cooper, R.G.: Stage-gate systems: a new tool for managing new products. Bus. Horiz. **33**(3), 44–54 (1990). https://doi.org/10.1016/0007-6813(90)90040-I

30. Benneyan, J.C., Lloyd, R.C., Plsek, P.E.: Statistical process control as a tool for research and healthcare improvement. Qual. Saf. Health Care **12**(6), 458–464 (2003)

31. Khoury, M.J., Ioannidis, J.P.: Big data meets public health. Science **346**(6213), 1054–1055 (2014). https://doi.org/10.1126/science.aaa2709

32. Curcin, V., Woodcock, T., Poots, A.J., Majeed, A., Bell, D.: Model-driven approach to data collection and reporting for quality improvement. J. Biomed. Inform. **52**, 151–162 (2014). https://doi.org/10.1016/j.jbi.2014.04.014

33. Bergman, B., Hellström, A., Lifvergren, S., Gustavsson, S.M.: An emerging science of improvement in health care. Qual. Eng. **27**(1), 17–34 (2015). https://doi.org/10.1080/ 08982112.2015.968042

34. Spiegelhalter, D., Sherlaw-Johnson, C., Bardsley, M., Blunt, I., Wood, C., Grigg, O.: Statistical methods for healthcare regulation: rating, screening and surveillance. J. R. Stat. Soc. **175**(1), 1–47 (2012). https://doi.org/10.1111/j.1467-985X.2011.01010.x

35. Mahajan, A., Islam, S., Schwartz, M., Cannesson, M.: A hospital is not just a factory, but a complex adaptive system - implications for perioperative care. Anesth. Analg. **125**(1), 333–341 (2017). https://doi.org/10.1213/ANE.0000000000002144

36. Taner, M.T., Sezen, B., Atwat, K.M.: Application of Six Sigma methodology to a diagnostic imaging process. Int. J. Health Care Qual. Assur. **25**(4), 274–290 (2012). https://doi.org/10.1108/09526861211221482

37. Axelos: ITIL® glossary and abbreviations (2011). https://www.axelos.com/corporate/media/files/glossaries/itil_2011_glossary_gb-v1-0.pdf

38. Hotti, V.: Framework-based data requirements for IT top management. Int. J. Digit. Inf. Wirel. Commun. **4**(3), 299–304 (2014). https://doi.org/10.17781/P001281

39. Rosenberg, L.: Are healthcare leaders ready for the real revolution? J. Behav. Health Serv. Res. **39**(3), 215–219 (2012). https://doi.org/10.1007/s11414-012-9285-z

Mapping Business Transformation in Digital Landscape: A Prescriptive Maturity Model for Small Enterprises

Juhani Naskali[1]([✉]) [iD], Jesse Kaukola[2], Johannes Matintupa[1],
Hanna Ahtosalo[1], Mikko Jaakola[1], and Antti Tuomisto[1]

[1] Information Systems Science,
Department of Management and Entrepreneurship,
Turku School of Economics, University of Turku, Turku, Finland
juhani.naskali@utu.fi
[2] Nordkalk Oy Ab, Pargas, Finland

Abstract. Developing versatile modern ICT is an insurmountable challenge to many small and medium enterprises (SMEs). Resources, such as skills, money, time [1] and knowledge [2], are scarce [3]. This makes the selection and decision of any development project a key business issue. The most important questions for SMEs are (i) where to start and (ii) what to change. While there are hundreds of descriptive maturity models for organizational development [4, 5], these offer little support for organizational decision-making. We developed a prescriptive maturity model that maps a subjective snapshot of the maturity of a business, and identifies the most promising objects for next development steps. This *Business Transformation Map* has three interrelated maturity dimensions: business, technology, and social, that span across past, present and future. We used the model in several test cases, and our results show that the model makes business dimensions visible in a way that makes sense to SMEs. The interviewed SME companies state that depicting company maturity levels in this manner brings clarity to overall business growth options, and it helps transforming this understanding into concrete development steps.

Keywords: Small enterprises · Information systems development
Digitalization · Work informatics

1 Introduction

Modern business development is complicated, and creating a fruitful development plan requires deep understanding of the possibilities of modern ICT. Development actions regarding digitalization are mandatory, but resources, such as skills, money, time [1] and knowledge [2], are scarce [3], limiting the number and content of development actions. This makes the selection and decision of any development project a critical issue affecting all aspects of the small and medium enterprise (SME).

Regardless of scarce resources, companies must strive for a planned digital shift, the use of digital tools and solutions. A successful digital shift allows businesses to run, organize and operate business processes by digital tools. The benefits of this include for

© Springer Nature Switzerland AG 2018
H. Li et al. (Eds.): WIS 2018, CCIS 907, pp. 101–116, 2018.
https://doi.org/10.1007/978-3-319-97931-1_9

instance enabling lower production and labour costs, and creating added value to products and services [6].

> *"Effective process mechanisms involve (a) a comprehensive analysis of the decision problem and the alternative solutions, (b) the use of tailored IT decision making frameworks, (c) strategic experimentation through piloting and "green fields", (d) the involvement of multiple stakeholder constituencies, and (e) mutual understanding, conflict resolution and collaboration among stakeholders."* [7].

Business Process Maturity and the models that depict different maturity levels are for the most part narrow in the sense that they focus on a single aspect of business and typically depict a linear sequence of maturity levels. Hundreds of maturity models have been suggested, and new models are constantly being developed [4, 5, 8]. We claim that organizations, even SMEs, are too complex to be thoroughly understood through a single maturity model or even a set of models. Instead maturity models can and should be used to view a small section of a single organization in the chosen timeframe. Moreover, most of the current models are descriptive in nature. Thus they offer little help, when it comes to deciding what business development activities to do next. More prescriptive models are needed.

The social (people) factors of companies are key to recognizing essential elements of work systems. Technical and economical considerations are traditionally the basis of business development, but the social aspect is crucial [9]. Individuals working in companies make use of their prior experience, interact with customers and partners, and seek support from peers. Social aspect of work does not only come out by participating in collaborative work but is seen also by sharing information and knowledge between individuals at work. The social aspect is increasingly taken into account in modern maturity models [10, 11]. The novel study by [12] suggest that individual work role discussion starts with individual's ideas of one's future work role and actions: desired, imagined, wanted. Hence we suggest that in order to understand the current state of business, it is important to look into the state of processes, systems and individuals simultaneously. In a developing environment where goals for future are set, it's important to understand not only the current state, but also the past of the company, as it is the past that creates the prerequisites for both current existence as well as future possibilities.

In order to maximize the effectiveness in business transformation organizational structure should be aligned with service orientation and IT-governance [13]. To understand better the orientation we look further into the concept of business process re-engineering and business process orientation (BPO) discussed well in [14]. We believe that increased BPO gives a relevant insight on our understanding of business maturity. We utilize the critical success factors (CSF) from a study [15] which discovered 5 CSFs and 27 critical practices. These seem to have an important effect on improving the business process orientation maturity.

The concept of business process has been widely discussed in academics. There are several different kinds of processes that provide value for organization and [16] have generalized the concept well by stating that process is a network of actions to create value for customers. For our purpose this concept is a bit too broad and hence we claim that business action networks should be separated into three action categories. The categories are business actions (e.g. manufacturing of goods or providing services), technology (i.e. the tools, systems and IT used) and social interaction (e.g. customer collaboration, creation and utilization of knowledge capital and both internal and external communication).

2   Different Aspects of Current Maturity Models

2.1   Business Maturity Models

Mapping the developmental stage of businesses is a complicated matter. This is why business maturity models usually focus on a single aspect of business maturity. In growing markets, organizations are constantly looking for competitive advantages against their rivals. This has lead to giving more and more focus on the business processes in the organizations [17]. It is critical for the organizations to determine their business process maturity. Determining process maturity helps businesses in stability, improving and sustainability. Maturity models help organizations see their current maturity level, as well as strengths and weaknesses of their business processes [18]. Maturity models usually include a chain of levels or stages that demonstrate a desired path from current state to maturity. [5].

Business maturity models have also been a target of criticism. Since the Software Engineering Institute launched Capability Maturity Model (CMM) in 1993, hundreds of maturity models have been introduced by researchers and practitioners. Maturity models have been considered as "step-by-step recipes" which lack the empirical foundation and simplify reality [19]. CMM is not focusing on the factors that influence the evolution. Also in regard the suggested improvements, many users rely in the CMM levels to lead in somewhat predefined goals [18].

2.2   Technological Maturity Models

Technology Acceptance Model (TAM) was originally a psychological theory, but has since become a leading information system theory that models how users come to accept and use a technology. Acceptance is a key factor in a technological maturity model. TAM studies how easy to use and how useful the technology is for the user and what kind of relationship there is between the system variables and the potential system usage. Technology users who are more confident in their own abilities are more likely to succeed and more willing to accept new technologies than users with doubts. Additionally, when considering the technological maturity of a business, it is important to pay attention to the different information systems and environments, as well as usability and acceptance factors [20]. Thus the maturity of technological systems is mirrored in their users.

New information systems are usually costly and a long term investment for companies. Still, IS implementation projects have a relatively low success rate [21]. There are several factors that are affecting the success rate and that can be measured. TAM and a newer modification of it are scrutinizing these key factors. For the better maturity state and at the same time technological success and acceptance rate, it has been suggested that TAM could be integrated into a broader maturity model that includes social and organisational factors [21].

2.3 Business Culture Maturity Models

Many maturity models have human and social factors in their evaluation criteria. These models recognize people as key value creators and argue that human and social capital affect business performance. Human capital refers to knowledge, abilities and skills of individuals working in organizations, and social capital is defined as each individual's assets located in networks of relationships from which these assets can be accessed and utilized in purposive actions [22, 23].

However, most models focus on recognizing structural and technical factors rather than behavioural and cultural factors including communication, informed decision-making facilitating, organizational culture establishing and change management [24].

Knowledge management maturity models (KMMMs) consider knowledge within organizations. The human factors include tacit and implicit knowledge, which are types of knowledge that rise from experience and are shared between people and groups within organizations [25]. KMMMs include people, social or human factors, which are the foundation to these maturity models [26]. A rather new maturity model is the Community Maturity Model (CoMM) that can be seen as a sub-model of KMMMs. It was developed on the acknowledgement that very few maturity models are related to community assessment and do not take into account many characteristics of communities; common values, sense of identity, history, among others [27].

2.4 Critique Towards Current Maturity Models

Current maturity models tend to be formal, descriptive and normative. They have been criticized for not enabling future decision-making as they do not prescribe or present actions to perform for overcoming or addressing the identified weaknesses [27]. In real-life business development cases one often has to decide between different development options, as it is seldom possible to change everything at once. Also, there is a call for maturity models of a more prescriptive nature in academia [19, 28].

Additionally, there is a lack of SME oriented maturity models. Existing maturity models oftentimes focus on larger organisations. In SMEs, functions are often not that segregated and organisational structures are more concentrated, and so many maturity models apply poorly [11]. For tools and models to be useful in SMEs, they need to make sense and create understanding among the stakeholders, i.e. company decision-makers. Sensemaking reduces confusion and creates coherence. It affects human behaviour and supports development related decision-making [29]. Hence there is a clear need for a simple prescriptive maturity model.

3 A Prescriptive Maturity Model: Business Transformation Map

Descriptive maturity models give a good overview on the historical development of a company, but they offer little guidance here and now. Organizational maturity can vary a lot between maturity models focusing on different organizational aspects. There is not always a clear step to take for reaching the next maturity level. Hence, the need for a unifying prescriptive model that helps to decide where to start and what to do next is crucial, even though such a model might not give a clear roadmap far into the future. Such a model should help the SME towards upper maturity levels as a continuous development process.

3.1 Requirements of a Prescriptive Maturity Model

A prescriptive business maturity model needs to, by definition, provide actionable plans for developing the business in question. In order to be an effective and valuable tool, it should offer new insights about the company, and take into account all relevant categories of information in the selected field of study.

The main dimensions that need to be mapped are business (or trade), technology and social, as described in Sect. 2. For a complete picture, it has also proven fruitful to touch on past, present and future, in order to understand why the present is as it is (not to change things that work in a certain way due to valid reasons) and where the company representatives wish to go [12].

It is important for the model to resemble reality enough to provide guidance, but it is not necessary to aim for a truly objective view or even a description that is accurate for all purposes. The main point is that the picture is true enough for the actionable conclusions to be valid.

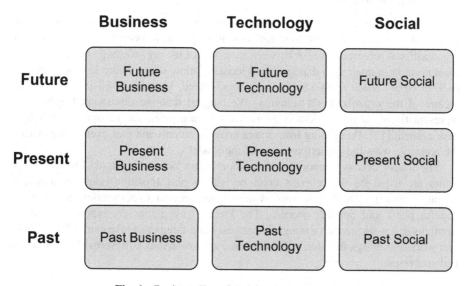

Fig. 1. Business Transformation Map Nine-Field

3.2   Nine-Field Columns - Three Dimensions of Analysis

The columns in our model map (Fig. 1) consist of the different dimensions of organizational analysis: business, technology and social. Business here means things related
to managerial systems, processes and decisions, trade and finance. Technology means
things related to ICT landscape, systems and more generalized tools. Topics that fall
under Social dimension include social interactions and socio-political hierarchy,
organizational knowledge, tacit knowledge, roles and responsibilities, etc.

3.3   Nine-Field Rows - Three Temporal Viewpoints

The three dimensions are analysed from three temporal viewpoints. Many traditional
maturity models map the expected evolutionary stages of a business in a temporal axis,
but the Business Transformation Map is a snapshot in time, and tries to offer a tool to
gather information about past, present and future, as understood in the current moment.

The current situation is perhaps the most interesting part to consider when it comes
to actionable information. However, knowing the future plans and worries of an
organization also give guidance on organizational change. More often than not,
planned changes are reactions to current problems. The plans, and especially how the
company representatives feel about the plans, can give important insight into why
things are happening, and provide opportunities to fine-tune plans.

Knowing the past is also important when making organizational changes. The
current state of affairs is a result of previous actions, and if one doesn't understand why
things are done the way they are, it is highly risk to change things. Also, going over the
past gives more detailed and personal insight into the causal links in the organizational
model's development.

3.4   Using the Model

The model is meant to be used in conjunction with, and not as a replacement for, an
analytical discussion. This is done between an information systems specialist and an
organizational representative, or between members of the organization in question. The
main point is to open up a dialogue, and loosely follow the structure laid out, circling
back to empty fields or things that seem unbalanced, in order to fill in a purposeful
picture of the organization's situation. We suggest that the discussion begins with
representatives' future work and goals, as they are often the reason for initiating
development [12]. Proceeding from future goals to current and past events emphasizes
the narrative way and prescriptiveness of the model.

The model acts as support for discussion and a note-taking tool. The discussed
issues are listed on the relevant columns with a plus (positive issue) or a minus
(negative issue) sign. Future row issues correspond to opportunities and threats,
hopeful plans and possible worries. The Present row issues correspond to current
strengths and weaknesses, or things that are easy and things that take extra effort, things
that work and things that don't. Finally, the Past row issues correspond to past crises
and successes.

The model does not suggest structured interviews. If it is difficult to figure out where to start, one can go over the nine empty boxes starting from past or present. Discussion can progress organically, and come back to topics that have been skimmed over quickly. All fields should be filled to some extent, after the analysis is over.

Figure 2 presents an example of our Business Transformation Map. This fictional organization is planning for rapid growth with a future IT upgrade, but customer support is lagging behind. The nine-field content would seem to support the planned upgrade, but it could be that the social side of customer support needs some development as well. Perhaps the work roles need to be defined more clearly, or they need more sophisticated tools for tracking responsibilities to make customer relations feel less difficult, and to handle the growing number of customers. This situation would merit a deeper probe into the social aspects of customer support, using more specialized tools.

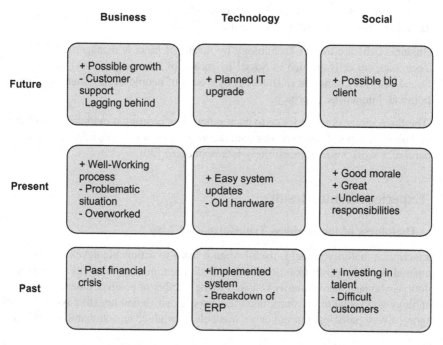

Fig. 2. Examples of Business Transformation Map issues

The three dimensions of Business Transformation Map are interrelated and help to guide discussion along fruitful lines. The function of separating the three dimensions into separate columns is to force discussion to take into account different viewpoints that might otherwise get bypassed. For example, the first thought in this case might be that an organization's current CRM system is not working well, but when prompted to consider the same situation from a social point of view, it is possible that the responsibilities of customer support personnel are not clearly defined, either. Similar correlations occur between Business and Technology, as well as Business and Social, and causal relations are naturally present on the temporal axis.

It is normal for some issues to belong to more than just one column. In these cases one can select the column most suited for the situation or, if two columns feel equally "right", mark the issue on both.

After filling in the model, participants (developers and SME representatives) decide on the next steps together, attempting to find an actionable issue or issues that would produce most benefit to the organization. Often issues cluster around one dimension or a single topic mirrored across all dimensions, signaling fruitful soil for IS development.

3.5   Relationship Between Action Columns

The cells in the model are a collection of relevant items in the business environment and hence create a sort of landscape on how the particular business functions. This landscape view on business does not cover the subtle nuances of actions. Thus it's important to discuss shortly how the different cells connect.

Based on our understanding we claim the following:

1. Business cells are tied to Technology by means of process management
2. Technological cells are tied to Social by means of knowledge management
3. Social cells are connected to Business by means of people management, e.g. socio-political, humanistic approach.

The three dimensions all relate to each other, thus creating a cylindrical landscape instead of a flat plane. This correlates with the general view of work informatics, where all parts of a work system are strongly interconnected [30].

4   Experiences and Results

4.1   Usefulness of the Business Transformation Map

A prescriptive maturity model is useful when it leads to actionable development plans. Compared to descriptive maturity models that often give a clear-cut definition of evolutionary stages, here maturity is linked to the number of positive issues in business, technology and social dimensions, and the ratio of positive and negative issues in each category. Every participant in our cases was able to produce an actionable set of issues into the map.

The number of positive and negative issues is indicative of business maturity. It does not give (or even aim to give) a complete picture. More important is to consider each issue carefully; a few far-reaching and particularly important positive issues can oftentimes trump multiple small problems. The produced picture does, however, point out the relative maturity of different aspects of the company, yet it reveals the main areas that would benefit from development actions. Linking the maturity to the existence of many positive issues (success in the past, well-working present and a future with positive expectations) and a relatively low amount of negative issues (i.e. problems) helps to select viable development actions.

Different issues might not be comparable with each other, and some issues are closer to business core functions than other. The count of positive and negative issues can give indication on which area to focus on - the next viable development target - though this is not always a definite rule.

4.2   Case Examples

Next we present three case examples to illustrate how the Business Transformation Map works, and what potential benefits using it incurs. The case examples are real cases with real organizations. The cases illustrate the possible use of the model in prescribing actionable steps of business digitalization, and give examples on how the model is meant to be used. These examples are not meant to give a complete picture on the strengths and weaknesses of the model, nor prove the validity of the model. Further research is required to empirically validate the model.

Case A: Social Marketing Firm. This case is a social marketing firm, who contacted us to find out about, and possibly implement a prototype of, social media big data tools. They were considering hiring programmers and wanted some consultation. The project was started with a 2-h interview with the main stakeholders using the Business Transformation Map. See Table 1 below.

First, the future plans of utilizing big data were discussed. After going over the different dimensions of A's organization, it was clear that this wish was not due to lack of tools, but a response to not being able to properly articulate their marketing decisions and the benefits of their value-based work processes to their clients.

Results. Organization A ended up ordering an adaptive quality model resembling the PDCA management method [31] that explained and codified their work processes, helping them communicate the benefits and their dedication to quality to their customers. No programmers were hired, but a review of available social media marketing tools was conducted.

Thoughts. Many issues are mirrored between columns: uncoordinated work, business uncertainty and difficulties in articulating benefits to clients seemed to all communicate the same problem on different columns, impacting the organization as a whole.

Although the number of positive social issues was low, they were highly valued and focused on by the company. In general, it is important to note that the issues are not equal, and their context needs to taken into account. This might be expressed better by using multiple plus signs in front of "bigger" positive issues, but the number would also be wholly arbitrary and need interpretation.

The Business Transformation Map successfully mapped the organization's situation, prompting the organization's representatives to say they understood their work better. It also resulted in changing course from big data plans to solidifying the quality processes and overcoming the hurdles in communication.

Table 1. Case A Business Transformation Map

	Business	Technology	Social
Future	+ Experience of content matter + Culture of learning + Adaptability + Growth of sales? − Small number of customers − Limited time resources	+ Big data plans + Automation plans + Process development plans − Fast developing tech − eMarketing experience	+ Plans to participate more deeply in customer operations + Caring of clients − *Difficult to explain the benefits of company values* − Changes in communications culture can be fast
Present	+ Stable customer base + Genuineness + *Quality content (pictures and text)* + *Reputation of quality* − *Uncertainty; focus on right things?* − *Lack of productization* − Lack of sales − *Undocumented processes*	+ Controlled platform (no maintenance or responsibility of hacks) + Good tools − *Uncoordinated work* − Technological know-how	+ *"Deep" customer relations, trust* + Close-knit internal team + *Wish for transparency* − Lack of marketing − Under-utilized contacts − *Articulating gained benefits to clients*
Past	+ Online marketing + Experience in PR and communications + Teaching experience + Long experience in food industry − Slow growth and size of business − Lack of direction	+ Blogging business − Big crisis with hacked Joomla sites (led to change of platform)	+ a large pool of contacts from many fields − terminated clients

Case B: Construction and Renovation Consulting Firm. This case describes a construction and renovation consultant firm which specializes in old and traditional buildings. The firm is ran by an entrepreneur and for this reason the entrepreneur seeks value from external relationships and networks. Based on prior projects with higher education and business development workshops, the firm wanted to better utilize customers' knowledge and to include customers in the decision-making process together with other construction and renovation stakeholders. This is done in order to add transparency to end-to-end construction processes, which has been requested by customer.

The project started with Business Transformation Map based interview with the entrepreneur. The Map narrowed the project scope to mapping out digital platform solutions for enabling transparent decision-making between all stakeholders. This platform thinking was seen as something totally new to the business field and the entrepreneur was willing to investigate possibilities further. See Table 2 below.

Results. All stakeholders and requirements for transparent decision-making were identified. Different digital solutions for enabling efficient decision-making were compared against set business criteria and one solution with automated decision-support functionalities was selected for the firm. The solution provider was contacted and co-operation negotiations were started during the project.

Thoughts. We identified key factors and issues with the Business Transformation Map analysis tool. The firm's willingness to create new methods and ways of working for the entire business field indicated that bold solution proposals could be made. The lack of the entrepreneur's skills in IT resulted in seeking outsourced digital solutions and strategic alliances which is also linked with acknowledging the entrepreneur's role as an solo entrepreneur.

The Business Transformation Map analysis brought insight not only to the entrepreneur, but for the whole project team. The unified model simultaneously visualised the business needs and showed affecting factors. It also led to a change in project scope and topic.

Table 2. Case B Business Transformation Map

	Business	Technology	Social
Future	+ Business growth through increased visibility on market + Growth through reputation; quality, customer value, long-term commitment	+ Through the use of digital tools the end users are enabled to make decisions, opinions and choices + Modern market leader who brings digital tools to the field + Automated decision-making via digital tools will bring new service to business field	+ End user and customer engagement in decision-making in a new way through the use of digital use + Stakeholders are transparently in cooperation (including end customers)
Present	+ Aims to high-quality and high customer appreciation + The new service brand has started to build customer traction	+ Website for the company exists + The technological development plans have been established through previous projects with higher education institute cooperation	+ Actively networked both within the business and with different business development entities (higher education institute cooperation, business accelerators etc.)

(continued)

Table 2. (continued)

	Business	Technology	Social
	+ Long time in business with the now to be built new brand + Active in cooperation with business development entities; is experienced with higher education cooperation − No prior experience of brand building − No prior knowledge of process description building	− New brand with digital technologies to enable decision-making or for communication is not currently online or solutions selected − The need to select digital tools and software is current − No technical experience	+ Active seeker of information, wants to build networks − As a sole entrepreneur finds solo entrepreneurship as a must and thinks many times to be alone
Past	+ Long time in business − Solo entrepreneur (only one person in the company)	− No prior experience of using digital tools in business + Tools in use MS Outlook, MS Office	+ The service relevant and business field knowledge accrued over many years -> high level of content knowledge + Networks have been developed over many years and some are deep in nature

Case C: Cleaning Products Manufacturing Company. Case C company is mature over 40 year-old company which is currently owned by an international conglomerate. The company contacted us for a preliminary analysis and improvement proposal of their current processes concerning employee production reporting which is currently handled through mainly in pen and paper style where employees use personal notebooks to keep track of their production. Although using manual reporting with pen and paper, the company is also mature in IT use on other business sections. Currently they use two separate enterprise resource planning (ERP) systems with which they handle warehouse, orders, manufacture and most of the reporting. The information system landscape of two ERPs contains the old ERP being legacy system from prior to acquisition by the international conglomerate and the new ERP is used and supported by the new owner. The new owner is leaving the decision on which ERP system to use on manufacturing for the local company but wants reporting on the company used system. See Table 3 below.

The discussion with case company C started with Business Transformation Map analysis tool interview. Although the target of the company was clear (to reduce the amount of paper-based reporting and duplicate reporting work performed by manufacturing employees and factory floor manager), the Business Transformation Map presented the need in a more vast scale. The aim of the project was set to finding ways of improving work methodologies and creating efficient working environment, which would also decrease the number of printed work cards and personal notebooks.

Results. The project resulted in suggesting a large-scale module implementation to their existing ERP system that is used by the new owner. With this module the company would be able to handle employee reporting through systems interfaces which could be added to each workstation. The module would also support future development towards for example IoT (internet of things) which would connect each manufacturing equipment to the ERP system. The Business Transformation Map provided the company with information with which it could present their business and information technology need to the new owner.

Thoughts. This case shows that the Business Transformation Map Nine-Field is scalable also to larger SME companies employing more than 50 persons and it presents business factors and landscape of a larger company equally comparing to smaller company sizes. The nine-field can also present more complex business environments which are international and represent multiple corporate entities. The nine-field view of this case company includes, takes into account and connects entities from individual manufacturing employees to larger international company requirements.

The Business Transformation Map also presents a snapshot-like view that captures factors regarding internal and external relations and the maturity of the company, which are factors needed to take into account in development projects by the consultant.

Table 3. Case C Business Transformation Map

	Business	Technology	Social
Future	+ Increase in manufacture through relieved work force from manual reporting + Effective and comprehensive reporting + Good level transparency and corporate requirement response	+ Unified and conglomerate compatible IT infrastructure + Efficient work methodologies + Manufacturing traceability fully operated with digital tools + Automated reporting in vast use	+ Engaged employees from all levels in digital development/work + Efficient and sustainable work environment through digitalization
Present	+ Established business with a long history + Defined products + International market share with customers from 20+ countries + Own Ltd company although main ownership shifted to an international conglomerate − Employee hourly reporting done by pen and paper	+ Uses currently two separate ERP systems + One ERP in efficient use (willing to use more) + Vast IT and ICT knowledge in company management − Other ERP system is business crucial but in non-full use − No traceability via digital tools	+ Roles and responsibilities clear with the company management + Employees are a valued asset whom are wanted to give insight to business process development + Employees are wanted to make part of digitalization project + Seeks and wants to continue cooperation with local companies, such as

(continued)

Table 3. (*continued*)

	Business	Technology	Social
		− Employee reporting adds additional work to process as done to system after recorded via pen and paper − Building access control system outdated	the factory access control system service provider
Past	+ History as a family company before acquired by the international conglomerate − The base for salary is by piece rated which doesn't correspond to current way of working and base for salary	+ Old ERP has been in greater use in past + New ERP introduced by conglomerate company + IT experience on high level from previous work	+ Good long term relationships between employees and management

4.3 Findings

These three cases were the most fruitful among our 13 test cases, in that the use of Business Transformation Map clearly resulted in new actionable understanding that guided the following development projects' content. There were no cases where the model didn't result in actionable information, though in some cases it only validated the already prescribed development plans.

It might be that the simple use of plus and minus signs is not descriptive enough. Many issues are not equal in scope or value, and it might be necessary to denote this with, for example, multiple plus or minus signs. However, the decision of such an 'impact factor' would be totally arbitrary, and might not lead to better prescriptions. As it is impossible to completely normalize the issues, it is in any case recommended to use the number of issues as a guideline and not as a rule, when deciding on a course of action.

5 Conclusion

SMEs need simple prescriptive tools for identifying fruitful targets for business development. We presented the Business Transformation Map as a possible solution for the initial analysis preceding the decision of actual business development projects, and described three small company cases.

Our findings suggest that our model is a viable tool that helps in the arduous process of selecting actionable development steps in the work system for a business to take. It is simple enough for SMEs to utilize, though they still might require someone with experience of business development projects to discuss the situation with them. It is descriptive enough to provide a current snapshot of the business for identifying areas ripe for development, and seems non-restrictive enough to fit the needs of an organization in any field.

Further study is required on several fronts: Is the model clear enough for people who are less experienced with business development? Is it descriptive enough to prescribe an actionable development course in all, or at least most, situations? How exactly does the model compare to alternative tools for initial analysis? The tool can hopefully be developed further after such questions are answered.

The next step for developing the model is to test the long-term results of business development projects where the Business Transformation Map was used. A prescriptive maturity model is only as good as the results of its use. The end-result should be a better work system, meaning better productivity and wellbeing. The proposed model shows promise, but a more extensive study is required to prove the validity of the Business Transformation Map.

References

1. Jones, O., Macpherson, A., Thorpe, R., Ghecham, A.: The evolution of business knowledge in SMEs: conceptualizing strategic space. Strateg. Change **16**, 281–294 (2007)
2. Holsapple, C.P., Joshi, K.D.: An investigation of factors that influence the management of knowledge in organizations. J. Strateg. Inf. Syst. **9**, 235–261 (2000)
3. Atherton, A.: The uncertainty of knowing: an analysis of the nature of knowledge in a small business context. Hum. Relat. **56**(11), 1379–1398 (2003)
4. Becker, J., Knackstedt, R., Pöppelbuß, D.W.I.J.: Developing maturity models for IT management. Bus. Inf. Syst. Eng. **1**(3), 213–222 (2009)
5. Röglinger, M., Pöppelbuß, J., Becker, J.: Maturity models in business process management. Bus. Process Manag. J. **18**(2), 328–346 (2012)
6. Nguyen, T.H., Newby, M., Macaulay, M.J.: Information technology adoption in small business: confirmation of a proposed framework. J. Small Bus. Manag. **53**, 207–227 (2015)
7. Ribbers, P., Parker, M.M.: Designing information technology governance process: diagnosing contemporary practices and competing theories. In: Proceedings of the 35th Hawaii International Conference on System Sciences (2002)
8. De Bruin, T., Freeze, R., Kaulkarni, U., Rosemann, M.: Understanding the main phases of developing a maturity assessment model. In: Australasian Conference on Information Systems (ACIS), 30 November–2 December (2005)
9. Kumar, K., Van Dissel, H.G., Bielli, P.: The merchant of Prato-revisited: toward a third rationality of information systems. MIS Q. **22**(2), 199–226 (1998)
10. Schumacher, A., Erol, S., Sihn, W.: A maturity model for assessing industry 4.0 readiness and maturity of manufacturing enterprises. Procedia CIRP **52**, 161–166 (2016)
11. Igartua, J.I., Retegi, J., Ganzarain, J.: IM2, a maturity model for innovation in SMEs. IM2, un Modelo de Madurez para la innovación en PYMEs. Dirección y Organización **64**, 42–49 (2018)
12. Tuomisto, A., Kaukola, J., Koskenvoima, A.: Sensitive development of work systems – the story of dandelions. In: Conference paper: Information Systems Research Seminar Scandinavia (IRIS) 38 (2015)
13. Chatzoglou, P.D., Diamantidis, A.D., Vraimaki, E., Vranakis, S.K., Kourtidis, D.A.: Aligning IT, strategic orientation and organizational structure. Bus. Process Manag. J. **17**(4), 663–687 (2011)
14. Zhang, Q., Cao, M.: Business process reengineering for flexibility and innovation in manufacturing. Ind. Manag. Data Syst. **102**(3), 146–152 (2002)

15. Škrinjar, R., Trkman, P.: Increasing process orientation with business process management: critical practices. Int. J. Inf. Manag. **33**(1), 48–60 (2013)
16. Bergman, B., Klefsjö, B.: Quality from Customer Needs to Customer Satisfaction, 3rd edn. Studentliteratur AB (2010)
17. Looy, A.: Does IT matter for business process maturity? A comparative study on business process maturity models. In: Meersman, R., Dillon, T., Herrero, P. (eds.) OTM 2010. LNCS, vol. 6428, pp. 687–697. Springer, Heidelberg (2010). https://doi.org/10.1007/978-3-642-16961-8_95
18. Albliwi, S.A., Antony, J., Arshed, N.: Critical literature review on maturity models for business process excellence. In: IEEE International Conference on Industrial Engineering and Engineering Management (2014)
19. Pöppelbuß, J., Röglinger, M.: What makes a useful maturity model? A framework of general design principles for maturity models and its demonstration in business process management. In: ECIS 2011 Proceedings, p. 28 (2011)
20. Marangunić, N., Granić, A.: Univ. Access Inf. Soc. **14**(1), 81–95 (2015)
21. Legris, P., Ingham, J., Collerette, P.: Why do people use information technology? A critical review of the technology acceptance model. Inf. Manag. **40**(3), 191–204 (2003)
22. Jansen, R.J.G., Curşeu, P.L., Vermeulen, P.A.M., Geurts, J.L.A., Gibcus, P.: Information processing and strategic decision-making in small and medium-sized enterprises: the role of human and social capital in attaining decision effectiveness. Int. Small Bus. J. **31**(2), 192–216 (2011)
23. Hernández-Carrión, C., Camarero-Izquierdo, C., Gutiérez-Cillán, J.: Entrepreneurs' social capital and the economic performance of small businesses: the moderating role of competitive intensity and entrepreneurs' experience. Strateg. Entrep. J. **11**, 61–89 (2017)
24. Bititci, U.S., Garengo, P., Ates, A., Nudurupati, S.S.: Value of maturity models in performance measurement. Int. J. Prod. Res. **53**(10), 3062–3085 (2015)
25. Fabio, L.O.: Knowledge management barriers, practices and maturity model. J. Knowl. Manag. **18**(6), 1053–1074 (2014)
26. Khatibian, N., Hasan gholoi pour, T., Jafari, H.A.: Measurement of knowledge management maturity level within organizations. Bus. Strategy Ser. **11**(1), 54–70 (2010)
27. Boughzala, I.: A Community Maturity Model: a field application for supporting new strategy building. J. Decis. Syst. **23**(1), 82–98 (2013)
28. Tarhan, A., Turetken, O., Reijers, H.A.: Business process maturity models: a systematic literature review. Inf. Softw. Technol. **75**, 122–134 (2016)
29. van der Hoorn, B., Whitty, S.J.: The project-space model: enhancing sensemaking. Int. J. Manag. Proj. in Bus. **10**(1), 185–202 (2017)
30. Heimo, O.I., Kimppa, K.K., Nurminen, M.I.: Ethics and the inseparability postulate. In: Proceedings of Ethicomp (2014)
31. Deming, W.E: Elementary Principles of the Statistical Control of Quality: A Series of Lectures (1950)

The Impact of Multidimensionality of Literacy on the Use of Digital Technology: Digital Immigrants and Digital Natives

Shahrokh Nikou[✉], Malin Brännback, and Gunilla Widén

Åbo Akademi University, 20500 Turku, Finland
{snikou, malin.brannback, gwiden}@abo.fi

Abstract. Considering the speed at which new digital technologies are evolving, it is the aim of this paper to assess the impact of multidimensionality of literacy on intention to use digital technologies. An empirical research, using antecedent factors of adoption, is executed to investigate the relationships between factors influencing digital immigrants and digital natives' intentions to use digital technology. By using a survey data of 118 and 127 digital immigrants and digital natives, Structural Equation Modelling (SEM) and Fuzzy-set Qualitative Comparative Analysis (fsQCA) are applied. The results of the analyses while show some similarities, reveal that these two groups are different in many aspects and their intentions to use technology are influenced by different factors. Moreover, fsQCA results, while supporting the SEM findings, show that there are multiple configurations of conditions leading to the outcome of interest.

Keywords: Digital natives · Digital immigrants · Digital literacy
Information literacy · Digital transformation · Digital technology

1 Introduction

Digital transformation is a groundbreaking and ongoing revolution in our contemporary society. Due to digitized characteristics of 21st century, many industries, organizations and educational environments, including schools and universities, are tremendously investing to transform their current operational and activities to comply with the shifts forced by the digitalization. Today, most of our daily tasks and activities are done with the digital devices and services (smartphones, laptop, PC and applications). Literacy means the condition of being literate and a literate person should have the basic ability to read and write. In other words, a literate person has the basic ability to read, write and is able to understand her native language. As new dimensions of literacy have emerged (e.g., information literacy, digital literacy, technical literacy, cognitive literacy, social-emotional literacy, media literacy, visual literacy and financial literacy to name just a few), the dominance of digital medium introduces a revolution in the use and effects of literacy. It has been argued that different dimensions of literacy have critical roles in achieving objectives and success in whatever task individuals perform in their workplaces, such as in lecture hall, retail store, government agency [3]. Therefore, individuals' abilities to locate and evaluate information from multiple

© Springer Nature Switzerland AG 2018
H. Li et al. (Eds.): WIS 2018, CCIS 907, pp. 117–133, 2018.
https://doi.org/10.1007/978-3-319-97931-1_10

sources, using digital technologies and tools, solving complex problems and thinking critically play important roles in achieving success in digitized society of the 21st century.

We argue that individual's intention to use digital devices and tools is affected by their literacies capabilities. In this paper, individuals are divided into groups, digital immigrants and digital natives. Digital immigrants refer to individuals who were born before 1990 and are considered to be the users of digital technologies, content and tools [1]. Their counterpart generation refers to digital natives, individuals who were born roughly after 1980 [2] or according to Prensky, digital natives are individuals who were born after 1990 [1]. This generation is given other labels such as "Millennials" described as a new generation with distinct characteristics, optimistic, team-oriented achievers, talented with technology and Internet has always been part of their lives [4]. In contrast to their parents, digital natives have always been surrounded with digital technologies, computers, digital music, mobile (smartphones) and are considered to be the creator of digital content [1, p. 1].

Literature informs us that the current research on literacy often focuses on either digital natives or on digital immigrants. In this study, while we acknowledge the relevance of these attempts, we focus on both groups. The aim of this study is therefore, to understand how multiple dimensions of literacy impact digital immigrants and natives' attitudes and consequently their intentions to use digital technologies. The context of this study is chosen to be a university and the subjects are selected from university staff (digital immigrants) and university students (digital natives) from one of the main universities in Finland. In particular, the research question guiding us throughout this research is *"what antecedent factors influence digital immigrants and digital natives' intention to use digital technology"?*

This paper is organized as follow. Section 2 presents literature review. Section 3 describes the theoretical background and development of the hypotheses. Section 4 introduces the research methodology, followed by discussion of the results in Section 5. Section 6 presents the discussions and concluding remarks.

2 Related Work

A literate person is expected to have the basic ability to locate, retrieve, assess, evaluate information in addition to possession of some basic competences and skills to use and reproduce the information in an appropriate manner [5]. Considering the speed at which digital information is currently produced, the ability of individual to evaluate and use information in an appropriate manner has become a critical issue [6]. Eshet-Alkalai argued that evaluating information appropriately has always been central to successful learning [7]. In digital society, people are exposed to unlimited digital content and information, as such a multiliterate person can successfully produce, publish and modify information in an appropriate and efficient way. Multiliteracies ability for evaluating and assessing information and using digital tools and devices appropriately has become a *"survival skill"* [7]. As already mentioned, there are many new dimensions for contemporary literacy [8], but this research particularly focuses on information literacy and digital literacy. Broadly speaking, information literacy is defined as the ability to recognize information needs and identify, evaluate and use information effectively [5]. Gilster defines digital literacy as the ability to understand and use information in multiple formats from a wide range of sources when it is available and presented through computers [9, p. 1]. Martin states that digital literacy is the awareness, attitude and ability of individuals to operate and use digital tools and devices in an appropriate way [10, p. 135]. It has been argued that multidimensionality of literacy impacts differently individual's intention to use digital technologies for achieving objectives in whatever task they perform in their workplaces [11]. Moreover, it has been stated that compared to their counterpart, digital technology impacts digital natives' education differently as they are active experimental learner, proficient in multitasking, hugely dependent on digital technologies for interacting and communicating with others [12, p. 776]. The difference between digital immigrants and digital natives has been the focus of [13] and the authors argued that these two groups fundamentally differ from each other when it comes to the use of technology as digital natives have grown up in a digital environment that has shaped how they think, operate, behave, and act (p. 329).

In this paper, we argue that depending on how these two groups use technology and how important they perceived it to be, their intentions to use digital technology are influenced by different factors. We assume that digital natives have higher self-perceptions on their ICT skills compared to digital immigrants. Digital immigrants perceive digital technology as a tool to perform tasks and for them self-efficacy and different dimensions of digital skills are the most important factors for forming their attitudes and intentions to use technology. Other researchers, such as [14, 15] have conducted empirical research focusing on digital immigrants and found that confidence, competence, and attitudes are the most important antecedent factors for technology adoption in classrooms. Moreover, [13] asserted that digital natives' intention to use technology is significantly affected by social influence, personal factors and belief on technology use. In another study, Teo investigated the role of subjective norm, perceived ease of use, perceived usefulness, facilitating condition and attitude toward use on teachers' intention to use technology in Singapore and found that except social norms, all other factors impact decision to adopt and use technology [16]. Moreover, [17] investigated teachers' intention to use technology by using factors such as computer self-efficacy and perceived usability and found both of these constructs to be important.

3 Theoretical Model and Hypotheses

In this section, according to the following observation, theoretical model is explained (see Fig. 1). We start with the definition of digital literacy from a broader scope and provide a detailed overview on the information literacy. Finally, three technology acceptance factors, i.e., social norms, self-efficacy and attitude toward using technology are discussed.

3.1   Digital Literacy

A digital literate person is expected to have technical and operational competences to use digital technology for different purposes in everyday activities [8]. In addition to technical and operational competences, a digital literate person is expected to be a critical thinker, able to use Internet responsibly for communicating, able to select appropriate a software program and use his or her ICT skills in searching and evaluating digital information for learning or performing a task [8, p. 1068]. In a broader perspective, digital literacy can be considered as an intersection of three dimensions of technical, cognitive and social-emotional [8].

The *technical dimension* involves technical and operational skills for using ICT for learning and in everyday activities. In other words, it includes the ability; for example, to connect an Ethernet cable for using wired networks or the ability to troubleshoot by reading digital manuals. Moreover, a digitally literate person is expected to possess the ability to operate technologies adequately, for example, through understanding file structures; finding, downloading and installing applications; setting up and using communication and social networking tools; sending and retrieving attachments via email [8]. In context of this study, we expect the university employees (digital immigrants) and university students (digital natives) to have the basic technical literacy ability and based on that they form a positive attitude to use digital devices and tools to perform their daily tasks, hence:

H1: *Technical literacy has a positive effect on attitude toward using digital technology for both digital immigrants and digital natives.*

According to [8] *cognitive dimension* of digital literacy model involves the abilities such as being a critical thinker while searching and evaluating digital information. IT cognitive dimension of digital literacy requires a digitally literate person to be knowledgeable with the ethical, moral and legal issues associated with online trading and content reproduction (e.g. copyrights and plagiarism). Eshet-Alkalai [7] argued that cognitive dimension of digital literacy involves hyperlinking capabilities to navigate intelligently through hypermedia environments to construct new knowledge using appropriate online or offline tools, thus:

H2: *Cognitive literacy has a positive effect on attitude toward using digital technology for both digital immigrants and digital natives.*

Social-emotional dimension of digital literacy involves the ability to use Internet responsibly for socializing, learning and communicating with others using an appropriate language and words to avoid misinterpretation and misunderstanding. It also involves protecting individual safety and privacy by keeping personal information as private as possible and not disclosing personal information more than what is necessary. A digital literate person is expected to be able to recognize when (s)he is being threatened and be capable of knowing how to deal with it, for example whether to ignore, report or respond to the threat [8]. Obviously, critical thinking ability is central in all three dimensions of digital literacy. In the context of this study, we expect individual's ability to use Internet responsibly for socializing, learning, teaching and communicating influences the attitude of both groups to use digital technology at their work and study places, hence:

H3: *Social-emotional literacy has a positive effect on attitude toward using digital technology for both digital immigrants and digital natives.*

3.2 Information Literacy

Information literacy refers to ability for searching, locating, assessing, e.g., Web-based information and content and an information literate person is expected to be a critical thinker [8]. The widespread Internet use has made the access to information easy and inexpensive, therefore, this dimension of literacy involves not only profound abilities to locate reliable information, but also to use information effectively and efficiently. It has been argued that in digital society, information literacy is a key ICT skill due to sheer amount of unlimited digital information and content, as people can easily publish and manipulate information without difficulty [7]. Some authors, such as [6] argued that the ability to effectively evaluate and assess information properly largely determines the attitude toward using the technology and also the quality of the decisions. An information literate person is expected to be able to assess the credibility, originality and source of information, we argue that information literacy is closely associated with attitude toward using digital technology, hence:

H4: *Information literacy has a positive effect on attitude toward using digital technology for both digital immigrants and digital natives.*

3.3 Attitude Toward Using Technology

Attitude toward using technology is defined as an individual's overall affective reaction to use a system and has shown to be one of the strongest predictors of behavioral intention [18]. Some authors stated that teachers' (digital immigrants in this paper) attitude to use computer is positively associated with their ICT skills [19]. Teachers with higher ICT skills show more positive attitudes toward using ICTs in the classrooms [20]. Students' attitudes towards using technology for learning purposes has been investigated by [21] and strong positive relation between the degree to which students use a technology and the degree to which they endorse its use in their studies at university was found (p. 116). In this paper, we argue that the more confident digital natives and digital immigrants are with their ICT skills, the more positive their attitude toward using digital technology will be, hence:

H5: *Attitude toward using technology has a positive effect on intention to use digital technology for both digital immigrants and digital natives.*

3.4   Social Norms

It has been found that social norms positively impact intention, e.g., intention to use technology. Social norms refer to extend to which the pressure of others impacts one's decision, for instance using or not using a technology [22]. Venkatesh et al. argued that the effect of social norms will be stronger in mandatory setting compared to voluntary settings (may impact only perception about the technology) [18]. In the context of this study, we argue that the use of technology for learning or performing daily tasks heavily relies on the pressure of other peers and colleagues, therefore, the effect of social norms could be attributed to compliance in mandatory settings. Therefore, we argue that in response to social pressure, social norms influence individuals' intention to use technology, thus:

H6: *Social norms has a (positive) effect on intention to use digital technology for both digital immigrants and digital natives.*

3.5   Self-efficacy

Self-efficacy refers to "one's ability to organize and execute the courses of action required to manage prospective situations" [23, p. 2]. This construct has extensively been used in various studies to assess its impact on individual's intention to use technology. For example, the use of Web 2.0 technology at university [24] or university students' behavioral intention to use an e-learning system [25]. In the context of digital technology use [26] define self-efficacy as "an individual judgment of one's capability to use a computer". We use self-efficacy to assess how digital immigrants and digital natives' self-assessments about their digital skills influence their intention to use digital technology, thus: we hypotheses:

H7: *Self-efficacy has a positive effect on intention to use digital technology for both digital immigrants and digital natives.*

3.6   Intention to Use

In this paper, intention to use is used as a proxy of digital immigrants and digital natives' intention to use digital technology, therefore it is our dependent variable. This construct has widely been used to predict the future technology use. In fact, in many prior studies this construct has shown to be the strongest predictor or determinant factor for future use of technology and making decision to take specific action or not [13, 27]. Some authors have used this construct to investigate the intention to adopt Web 2.0 technologies among higher education [24]. The results showed that it is an appropriate factor for investigating one's intention of using technology. As such, this construct is used in this study to assess digital natives and digital immigrants' intention to use digital technology. Based on the above discussion, we propose the following research model, see Fig. 1.

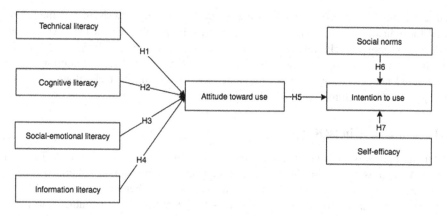

Fig. 1. Conceptual model

4   Research Methodology

Fuzzy-set Qualitative Comparative Analysis (fsQCA v.3.0) and Structural Equation Modelling (SEM) using SmartPLS v.3.0 have been applied as two distinct methods to analyze data. These two methods have recently been used in parallel in recent studies, such as [30]. In the following, we first discuss the fsQCA method and then SEM.

4.1   Fuzzy-Set Qualitative Comparative Analysis

FsQCA was introduced by Ragin [33] and since its conception has been widely used in various domains and disciplines, and more recently in business and Information Systems studies [e.g. 30, 34]. This method is an analytic technique that uses Boolean algebra for creating logical comparison and can be used in variable-oriented as well as case-oriented research. FsQCA presents each case as a combination of causal conditions by logically simplifying each combination through construction a truth table [35]. Logical minimization technique is then used for showing different combinations of variables (conditions in terms of fsQCA analysis) leading to the outcome of interest. Crisp-set QCA and fuzzy-set QCA are two variants of Qualitative Comparative Analysis [36]. Crisp-set presents the memberships in binary format, meaning that a case can only be either "in" or "out" of the set and fsQCA presents the membership in terms of interval between 0 and 1.

4.2   Necessity and Sufficiency Analysis

One of the main distinctions of this method compared to other statistical methods is that fsQCA analysis returns only necessary and sufficient conditions leading to the outcome of interest. Before, running the main part of fsQCA, which is the sufficiency analysis, we need to assess the necessity analysis. The necessity analysis enables to examine whether there are any conditions (variables) which could be considered as necessary for the outcome [37]. A condition is necessary when it must be present for the outcome and sufficient condition when it can produce an outcome by itself. Consistency value can be used for indicating the relevance of the necessity relationships. Consistency value over .90 means considerable relationships [36]. In our necessity analysis, none of the conditions had values greater than .90, so it can be concluded that no condition can be considered necessary for the outcome (intention to use digital technology) for both groups, i.e. digital immigrants and digital natives.

4.3 Procedures in fsQCA Analysis

After the necessity analysis, the main part of fsQCA analysis is performed. The first step is known as calibration, which means we need to transform all continuous scales into fuzzy sets ranging from 0 to 1. Fully out or no set membership gets value of 0 and fully in or full set membership gets value of 1 [38]. Calibration of variables into fuzzy sets uses three anchors: fuzzy score = .95 for full membership, fuzzy score = .05 for full non-membership and fuzzy score = .51 for cross-over point to show the degree of membership for each condition [34]. Then, a truth table of 2^k rows where k is the number of predictor conditions is constructed to indicate possible combinations of conditions in each row [40]. Ragin [38] recommended to set the consistency levels to (>.75). The fsQCA analysis generates three sets of solutions: parsimonious, intermediate, and complex. We use intermediate solutions for interpreting the findings [38]. The following notations will be used to illustrate the results. Black circles (●) show the presence of a condition and blank circles (○) show its absence. Blank spaces show "do not care" [39]. A binary condition, i.e., gender is presented as follow: black circles (●) indicate "males" and blank circles (○) show "female", see Table 3.

4.4 Measures

In this study, all items have been selected from previously validated scales. Social norms were measured by three items, intention to use was measured by six items and self-efficacy was measured by eight items, all were adopted from [18]. Moreover, information literacy was measured by seven items, technical literacy was measured by six items, cognitive literacy was measured by two items, social-emotional literacy was measured by two items and attitude toward using technology was measured by five items, all were adopted from [8, 28, 29]. Moreover, gender is considered as a control variable to measure potential variations in individuals' intention to use digital technology.

4.5 Data Collection

Two separate questionnaires, one for the digital immigrants and one for the digital natives have been designed, pre-tested with 15 potential respondents and experts and distributed. We invited students, professors, administrative and non-administrative employees to get their feedback on the clarity of the items listed in the questionnaire to avoid any ambiguous expressions and statements. The final version of the questionnaires was administered in one of the well-known universities in Finland. For the digital immigrants group, respondents were selected from e.g., university employees, professors and administration and for the digital natives group, the potential respondents were selected from university students at the different levels. After distributing the questionnaires on March 2018, a reminder was sent after two weeks. Over the course four weeks, 125 questionnaires were returned from digital immigrants group and 134 from digital natives group. After cleaning the datasets from missing data, the final datasets consisted of 118 and 127 complete responses for digital immigrants and digital natives, respectively.

The digital immigrants' sample consisted of employees at different levels, such as Professors, Senior Lectures, Senior Researchers, Administrative personnel. Digital natives' sample consisted of students at Bachelor, Master and Ph.D. levels. We paid a careful attention to recruit participants that fit only into one category (immigrants or natives). In order to obtain valid and reliable responses, we required respondents to indicate that they have basic knowledge on using different digital tools and services relevant to their work and study. This university is well-known for its employee training programs for using the latest digital (specially information systems) applications and programs for performing daily tasks. English language was used in both questionnaires. The questions were measured using a seven-point Likert-type scale that ranged from "strongly disagree 1" to "strongly agree 7". For both groups a non-response bias test following [31] approach was performed, we compared the first 25% of the respondents and the last 25% of the respondents on all variables using chi-squared test. The test results showed no major differences between groups; thus, we concluded that non-response bias was not an issue in this study.

5 Results and Analysis

5.1 Descriptive Statistics

As data was collected from a single source, we ran the common method bias test to make sure that the validity of the findings is not affected by this issue. To do so, first, we ran Harman's one-factor test on the items using a principal component factor analysis [32]. The test results showed that none of the obtained factors accounted for more than 50% of the total variance, thus common method bias was not an issue. The seven factors had eigenvalues greater than 1.0 accounting for 78.76% [digital natives = 69.45%] of the variance.

Digital Immigrants
With respect to digital immigrants, 57% were females, 37% were males, and 6% preferred not to say. Of the respondents, 14% were professors, 29% university employee (administration), 23% (researcher and lecturer), 6% (teaching and supervision), 6% (research and supervision), 13% Ph.D. candidates and 9% were ICT and technical employees. The majority of the respondents (97.64%) indicated that they use smartphones several times each day. Digital devices and tools such as desktop PC

(59.84%), Tablet (25.2%), Laptop (69.29%), and digital technologies such as Broadband Internet (78.74%) and WiFi (92.13%) are being extensively used on daily basis for performing different daily tasks. The use frequency of software and applications was relatively high, for instance, 88.19% indicated that they use MS-word processor, spreadsheet 55.91%, sharing applications (e.g., Dropbox & Google drive) 28.61%, once or several times each day. However, the low proficiency was visible in the use of digital technologies which are apparently not instrumental to the job performance, such as website management. The proficiency of using exclusive educational-related software and applications such as Peppi and Moodle (course management platforms) and travel system was surprisingly very low, only 3.94%, 12.7% and 9.52% respectively.

Digital Natives

In the digital natives group, 59% of the respondents were females and the rest were males, 50% of the respondents were Bachelor, followed by 49% Master students and only 1% Ph.D. candidates. The majority of the respondents (96.15%) indicated that they use smartphones several times each day. Digital devices and tools such as: desktop PC (31.5%), Laptop (62.31%) and Tablet (13%), and digital technologies such as Broadband Internet (47.69%) and WiFi (85.38%) are being extensively used on daily basis for performing daily educational and learning tasks. The use frequency of software and applications was relatively high, for instance, 68.45% indicated that they use MS-word processor, presentation (PPT) 4.62%, spreadsheet 24.6%, sharing applications (e.g. Dropbox & Google drive) 39.23% once or several times each day. With regard to proficiency of using these technologies, nearly 32% have indicated that they are very proficient in using MS-word, 17% Excel spreadsheet, and 24.62% sharing applications. However, there were some low proficiency in the use of digital technologies which are apparently not instrumental to the study performance (e.g., video editing applications). The proficiency in using exclusive educational software and learning-related applications such as MinPlan (study plan management tools) and Moodle (course management platform) was rather low, 23% and 9% respectively.

5.2   Measurement Results

In the following, we present all the SEM findings for digital immigrants and in the square brackets the SEM results for the digital natives. Confirmatory factor analysis was used to assess the measurement model, first convergent and discriminant validity were assessed for the validation. Convergent validity was assessed through composite reliability and the average variance extracted. The results showed that the CR values for both groups ranged from .82 to .93 [digital natives = .83 to .96], all above the threshold level of .70, and the AVE values ranged from .62 to .87 [digital natives = .60 to .83], all above the threshold level of .50. In addition, all the Cronbach alphas (α) and items loadings were above the minimum accepted levels (>.70), see Table 1.

Table 1. Reliability and validity: digital immigrants [digital natives]

Construct	Loading	t-stat	α (Alpha)	CR	AVE
Attitude toward use (4 items)	.838–.871 [.759–.873]	28.96–31.74 [14.82–32.08]	.896 [.886]	.927 [.916]	.762 [.688]
Cognitive literacy (2 items)	.928–.939 [909.–.912]	34.09–57.68 [22.84–7.84]	.853 [.794]	.931 [.907]	.871 [.829]
Self-efficacy (8 items)	.743–.873 [713.–.867]	12.12–41.12 [10.95–38.01]	.914 [.919]	.930 [.932]	.623 [.632]
Information Literacy (4 items)	.702–.869 [715.–.820]	9.91–30.83 [8.73–20.03]	.841 [.838]	.892 [.883]	.675 [.601]
Intention to use (5 items)	.856–.952 [766.–.940]	20.01–40.07 [11.04–30.14]	.957 [.949]	.867 [.960]	.855 [.800]
Social-emotional literacy (2 items)	.793–.869 [842.–.851]	14.34–20.99 [17.91–29.62]	.659 [.604]	.818 [.835]	.692 [.717]
Social norms (3 items)	.799–.914 [819.–.880]	9.79–24.96 [4.92–8.17]	.801 [.792]	.882 [.878]	.714 [.706]
Technical literacy (6 items)	.797–.909 [714.–.888]	16.94–56.53 [11.12–39.43]	.921 [.913]	.838 [.933]	.718 [.699]

Discriminant validity was assessed through the square root of the AVE. Table 2 shows the square root of the AVE values for all constructs. The values are greater than the correlations among constructs, thereby confirming the discriminant validity.

Table 2. Discriminant validity: digital immigrants [digital natives]

	ATT	COG-L	SELF	INOL	INT	SOEL	SN	TLIT
Attitude toward use	**.873** **[.829]**							
Cognitive literacy	.427 [.451]	**.933** **[.911]**						
Self-efficacy	.557 [.598]	.471 [.502]	**.789** **[.795]**					
Information literacy	.493 [.520]	.647 [.672]	.431 [.462]	**.822** **[.775]**				
Intention to use	.372 [.516]	.416 [.532]	.389 [.379]	.351 [.432]	**.925** **[.894]**			
Social-emotional literacy	.566 [.602]	.417 [.343]	.427 [.463]	.409 [.340]	.231 [.351]	**.832** **[.846]**		
Social norms	.218 [.210]	.226 [.349]	.319 [.352]	.259 [.361]	.321 [.320]	.171 [.142]	**.845** **[.840]**	
Technical literacy	.529 [.452]	.632 [.642]	.527 [.615]	.602 [.569]	.387 [.427]	.371 [.329]	.409 [.320]	**.847** **[.836]**

5.3   Structural Results

The measurement model was assessed through Structural Equation Modelling (SEM) using SmartPLS v3.0. As indicated in Fig. 2, intention to use digital technology was explained by a variance of 23% [31%]. Attitude toward using technology was explained by variance values of 46% [49%]. The SEM analysis revealed that technical literacy has a significant relation with attitude toward using digital technology, $\beta = .30$, $p < .001$ [$\beta = .13$, $p < .05$], thus H1 is supported for both groups. The SEM analysis revealed that cognitive literacy has no influence on attitude toward using digital technology, thus H2 is rejected for both groups. It was found that social-emotional literacy has a significant effect on attitude toward using digital technology $\beta = .41$, $p < .001$ [$\beta = .46$, $p < .001$] for both groups, thus accepting H3 for both groups. The SEM analysis revealed that information literacy has a significant relation to attitude toward using digital technology, $\beta = .18$, $p < .05$ [$\beta = .27$, $p < .001$], thus H4 is supported for both groups. Moreover, The SEM analysis showed that attitude toward using technology has a significant relation to intention to use digital technology, $\beta = .21, p < .001$ [$\beta = .45, p < .001$], thus H5 is also supported for both groups. Social norms positively effect intention to use technology for both groups, $\beta = .21, p < .05$ [$\beta = .21, p < .01$], thus H6 is supported for both groups. Finally, self-efficacy has a significant relationship with intention to use technology ($\beta = .20, p < .001$) for digital immigrants, thus, H7 is supported for this groups. However, the results showed that this path is not significant for digital natives, thus H7 is rejected for this group.

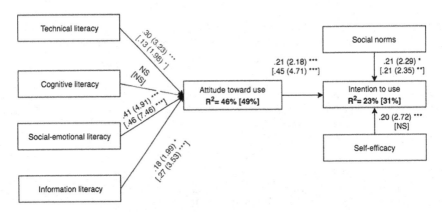

Note: *, **, and *** show significance at the 0.05, 0.01, and 0.001 levels, respectively.

Fig. 2. Structural model results

5.4   Moderating Effect

The gender of the respondents was used as a control variable and the following results were obtained. For digital immigrants, we found that the path between self-efficacy and intention to use technology is significant for males ($\beta = .38, p < .001$), but not significant for females. We also found that for females the path between social norms and intention to use is significant ($\beta = .18, p < .001$), but not for males. Information literacy to attitude toward using technology is significant for males ($\beta = .38, p < .001$), but not for females. For digital natives, the following differences were found. The path between attitude toward using technology to intention to use, surprisingly was found to be significant for females ($\beta = .56, p < .001$), but not for males. The path between social norms and intention to use is significant for females ($\beta = .21, p < .05$), but not for the males.

5.5 Fuzzy-Set Qualitative Comparative Analysis Results

The fsQCA analysis for intention to use digital technology revealed five solutions (configurations) for digital immigrants. In most of the configurations, the presence of cognitive literacy is noticeable (see Table 3) suggesting that this condition might be necessary—but not sufficient—for the outcome of interest. Solution 1 shows that the presence of cognitive literacy and the negation of technical literacy and attitude toward use lead to the outcome of interest. Solution 2 shows that the presence of cognitive literacy, information literacy, social norms and attitude toward using technology lead to the outcome of interest. Solution 3 shows that the presence of cognitive literacy, social norms, self-efficacy and attitude toward using technology lead to the outcome of interest. This solution is applicable to females only. Solution four is the most important solution from consistency value perspective and shows that the negation of social-emotional literacy, technical literacy and attitude toward using technology lead to the outcome of interest and applicable only to males. However, from coverage perspective, this solution covers only 9% of the cases. Solution five shows a configuration that the presence cognitive literacy, information literacy, social norms and self-efficacy in addition to negation of social-emotional literacy lead to the outcome of interest. Overall solution consistency is .955 and overall coverage is .469, meaning that these five configurations covers 47% of the cases.

Table 3. Configurations for intention to use digital technology

#	Configurations: digital immigrants					Configurations: digital natives				
	S1	S2	S3	S4	S5	S1	S2	S3	S4	S5
Cognitive literacy	●	●	●		●	●	●	●		●
Social-emotional literacy				○	○	○				
Technical literacy	○			○					○	○
Information literacy		●			●			○		
Social norms		●	●		●		●			●
Self-efficacy		●			●	○	○		●	
Attitude toward use	○	●	●	○			●	●	●	●
Gender			○		●	○	○	○	●	○
Consistency	0.97	0.97	0.96	0.98	0.97	0.99	0.98	0.98	0.99	0.99
Solution coverage	0.31	0.38	0.15	0.09	0.33	0.21	0.26	0.28	0.13	0.26
Unique coverage	0.01	0.03	0.01	0.01	0.06	0.03	0.01	0.03	0.13	0.01
Overall solution consistency	0.955					0.983				
Overall solution coverage	0.469					0.477				

As per digital natives, the fsQCA analysis revealed also five solutions. Solution 1 shows that the presence of cognitive literacy and negation of social-emotional literacy and attitude toward using technology lead to the outcome, this solution is only applicable of females. Solution 2 shows the configuration that the presence of cognitive literacy, social norms and attitude toward use in addition to negation of self-efficacy lead to the outcome of interest, again this solution is only applicable for females. Solution 3 shows that the presence of cognitive literacy and attitude toward use in addition to negation of information literacy lead to outcome interest and applicable for females. Solution 4 is the only solution in digital natives group that is applicable for males and indicates that the presence of self-efficacy and attitude toward use in addition to absence of technical literacy lead to the outcome. Finally, solution 5 shows a configuration for females that the presence of cognitive literacy, social-norms and attitude toward use and the absence of technical literacy lead to the outcome of interest. Overall solution consistency is .983 and overall coverage is .477, meaning that these five configurations covers 48% of the cases. IT is interesting to note that, cognitive literacy is considered to be an important condition. Moreover, for digital natives, four out five obtained configurations are geared toward females, whereas for digital immigrants the gender of respondents plays a role only in two solutions.

6   Discussions and Conclusion

This paper investigates how different dimensions of literacy such as information literacy and digital literacy impacts digital immigrants (individuals born before 1990) and digital natives' (individuals born after 1990) intention to use digital technology. A conceptual model of antecedent factors of intention to use technology is proposed and tested. The data was analyzed using two different methodological approaches, namely Structural Equation Modelling (a regression-based method) and fuzzy-set Qualitative Comparative Analysis (a configurational thinking method). The SEM results reveal that for digital immigrants, in addition to digital literacy and information literacy, social norms and self-efficacy play important role. Whereas, for digital natives, self-efficacy is not important. It is plausible to state that for this group of individuals who have always been exposed to digital technologies and Internet has been part of their lives, their perception towards own ability of using digital technology are significantly influenced by other indicators to build beliefs on own competence, e.g., their feelings and expectations rather than self-efficacy. An interesting finding is that, SEM analysis shows that cognitive literacy, a dimension of digital literacy, has no impact on attitude toward using digital technology for both digital immigrants and natives.

The fuzzy-set Qualitative Comparative Analysis results; while, reinforced the SEM findings, show that there are multiple paths for reaching the outcome of interest. Moreover, the fsQCA results show that different combinations of conditions (variables) impact digital immigrants and digital natives' intention to use technology. One of the major findings of fsQCA analysis is that, cognitive literacy, a variable that based on the SEM results found to have no impact on attitude toward using technology, appear to have a major role in many configurations, such that its presence in 8 out of 10 solutions is noticeable. If we would have relied only on the SEM findings and would not have investigated further, we would not be able to gain this valuable insight. This is an important observation and contribution, because fsQCA produces solutions based on the combined effect of conditions (i.e., variables) in contrast to SEM analysis where linear relationships (one-to-one) is considered.

This paper contributes to the literature of literacy research by including both digital immigrants and natives into one study, comparing their intentions to use technology. The findings of this paper have some practical implications. For instance, policymakers and high-level executives at the universities can use the findings of this study to make better and informed decisions on digital transformation and to enhance the processes of digitalization in more efficient ways. Moreover, the findings of this paper are helpful to understand the possibilities and what policies and investments are needed during digital transformation at the different educational environments. The findings also help policymakers to understand the implications of multidimensionality of the literacy for the economic and social development. Moreover, the findings have the potential for impact on practice by showing that we may have to develop and implement different training programs for digital immigrants and digital natives who are not quite familiar with digital tools and services at the educational environments.

As per limitation, it should be noted that this study has been conducted only in one university, and future studies are recommended to use the proposed conceptual model in other, perhaps expanding the context and see if similar findings can be found. Another limitation is that in this study digital literacy (cognitive, social-emotional and technical) and information literacy have been used. We recommend to use other dimensions of literacy in future studies to assess the difference between digital immigrants and digital natives.

Acknowledgement. The first author of this paper would like to thank the generous financial support by Säästöpankkien Tutkimussäätiö [Research Foundation of Savings Banks] in Finland. This research was also partially supported by Academy of Finland for DiWIL funded project (No: 295743). We thank our colleagues from Åbo Akademi University who provided comments, feedback and expertise that greatly assisted our research, although they may not agree with all of the interpretations/conclusions of this paper.

References

1. Prensky, M.: Digital natives, digital immigrants part 1. Horizon 9(5), 1–6 (2001)
2. Prensky, M.: Digital natives, digital immigrants part 2: do they really think differently? Horizon 9(6), 1–6 (2001)
3. Gui, M., Argentin, G.: Digital skills of internet natives: different forms of digital literacy in a random sample of northern Italian high school students. New Med. Soc. 13(6), 963–980 (2011)
4. Howe, N., Strauss, W.: Millennials Rising: The Next Great Generation. Vintage, New York (2000)
5. Bruce, C.S.: Workplace experiences of information literacy. Int. J. Inf. Manag. 19(1), 33–47 (1999)
6. Kerka, S.: Consumer education for the information age. Practice Application Brief 4, 12–15 (1999)

7. Eshet-Alkalai, Y.: Digital literacy: a conceptual framework for survival skills in the digital era. J. Educ. Multimed. Hypermed. **13**(1), 93–106 (2004)
8. Ng, W.: Can we teach digital natives digital literacy? Comput. Educ. **59**(3), 1065–1078 (2012)
9. Gilster, P.: Digital Literacy. Wiley, New York (1997)
10. Martin, A.: DigEuLit–a European framework for digital literacy: a progress report. J. eLit. **2** (2), 130–136 (2005)
11. Eisenberg, M.B.: Information literacy: essential skills for the information age. DESIDOC J. Libr. Inf. Technol. **28**(2), 39–47 (2008)
12. Bennett, S., Maton, K., Kervin, L.: The 'digital natives' debate: a critical review of the evidence. Br. J. Educ. Technol. **39**(5), 775–786 (2008)
13. Gu, X., Zhu, Y., Guo, X.: Meeting the "digital natives": understanding the acceptance of technology in classrooms. J. Educ. Technol. Soc. **16**(1), 392–402 (2013)
14. Bingimlas, K.A.: Barriers to the successful integration of ICT in teaching and learning environments: a review of the literature. EURASIA J. Math. Sci. Technol. Educ. **5**(3), 235–245 (2009)
15. Hew, K., Brush, T.: Integrating technology into K-12 teaching and learning: current knowledge gaps and recommendations for future research. Educ. Technol. Res. Dev. **55**(3), 223–252 (2007)
16. Teo, T.: Factors influencing teachers' intention to use technology: model development and test. Comput. Educ. **57**(4), 2432–2440 (2011)
17. Holden, H., Rada, R.: Understanding the influence of perceived usability and technology self-efficacy on teachers' technology acceptance. J. Res. Technol. Educ. **43**(4), 343–367 (2011)
18. Venkatesh, V., Morris, M.G., Davis, G.B., Davis, F.D.: User acceptance of information technology: toward a unified view. MIS Q. **27**(3), 425–478 (2003)
19. Buabeng-Andoh, C.: Factors influencing teachers' adoption and integration of information and communication technology into teaching: a review of the literature. Int. J. Educ. Dev. Inf. Commun. Technol. **8**(1), 136–155 (2012)
20. Rozell, E.J., Gardner, W.L.: Computer-related success and failure: a longitudinal field study of the factors influencing computer-related performance. Comput. Hum. Behav. **15**(1), 1–10 (1999)
21. Kennedy, G.E., Judd, T.S., Churchward, A., Gray, K., Krause, K.L.: First year students' experiences with technology: are they really digital natives? Australas. J. Educ. Technol. **24** (1), 108–122 (2008)
22. Thompson, R.L., Higgins, C.A., Howell, J.M.: Personal computing: toward a conceptual model of utilization. MIS Q. **15**(1), 124–143 (1991)
23. Bandura, A.: Self-efficacy in Changing Societies. Cambridge University Press, New York (1995)
24. Ajjan, H., Hartshorne, R.: Investigating faculty decisions to adopt Web 2.0 technologies: theory and empirical tests. Internet High. Educ. **11**(2), 71–80 (2008)
25. Park, S.Y.: An analysis of the technology acceptance model in understanding university students' behavioral intention to use e-learning. J. Educ. Technol. Soc. **12**(3), 150–162 (2009)
26. Compeau, D.R., Higgins, C.A.: Computer self-efficacy: development of a measure and initial test. MIS Q. **19**(2), 189–211 (1995)
27. Wang, Q.E., Myers, M.D., Sundaram, D.: Digital natives and digital immigrants. Bus. Inf. Syst. Eng. **5**(6), 409–419 (2013)
28. Hargittai, E.: Survey measures of web-oriented digital literacy. Soc. Sci. Comput. Rev. **23** (3), 371–379 (2005)

29. Hargittai, E.: An update on survey measures of web-oriented digital literacy. Soc. Sci. Comput. Rev. **27**(1), 130–137 (2009)
30. Nikou, S., Mezei, J., Brännback, M.: Digital natives' intention to interact with social media: value systems and gender. Telemat. Inform. **35**(2), 421–435 (2018)
31. Armstrong, J.S., Overton, T.S.: Estimating nonresponse bias in mail surveys. J. Mark. Res. **14**(3), 396–402 (1977)
32. Podsakoff, P.M., Organ, D.W.: Self-reports in organizational research: problems and prospects. J. Manag. **12**(4), 531–544 (1986)
33. Ragin, C.C.: The Comparative Method: Moving Beyond Qualitative and Quantitative Strategies. University of California Press, Berkeley (1987)
34. Woodside, A.G.: Moving beyond multiple regression analysis to algorithms: calling for adoption of a paradigm shift from symmetric to asymmetric thinking in data analysis and crafting theory. J. Bus. Res. **66**(4), 463–472 (2013)
35. Ragin, C.C.: The Comparative Method: Moving Beyond Qualitative and Quantitative Strategies. University of California Press, Berkeley (2014)
36. Schneider, C.Q., Wagemann, C.: Qualitative Comparative Analysis (QCA) und fuzzy Sets. Barbara, Budrich (2007)
37. Ragin, C.C.: Set relations in social research: evaluating their consistency and coverage. Political Anal. **14**(3), 291–310 (2006)
38. Ragin, C.C.: Redesigning Social Inquiry: Fuzzy Sets and Beyond. Chicago University Press, Chicago (2008)
39. Ragin, C.C., Fiss, P.C.: Net effects analysis versus configurational analysis: an empirical demonstration. In: Ragin, C.C. (ed.) Redesigning Social Inquiry: Fuzzy Sets and Beyond, pp. 190–212. University of Chicago Press, Chicago (2008)
40. Mikalef, P., Pateli, A.: Information technology-enabled dynamic capabilities and their indirect effect on competitive performance: findings from PLS-SEM and fsQCA. J. Bus. Res. **70**(2017), 1–16 (2017)

Data Federation in the Era of Digital, Consumer-Centric Cares and Empowered Citizens

Tiina Nokkala[✉] and Tomi Dahlberg

Turku School of Economics, University of Turku, Turku, Finland
{tiina.nokkala, tomi.dahlberg}@utu.fi

Abstract. Breast cancers, similar to any other types of cancers or diseases, need treatments and other actions that generate medical and patient data. As the owner of the data about him-/herself, a patient has the right to get and inspect all basic, treatment and other data recorded about her/him. However, this data is typically in the form of inconsistent data entries, such as medical reports, x-ray and other images, blood test admission notes and results, medication history and diagnoses, and is provided to the patient "as is". The structure, format and meanings of these data entries differ enormously. Thus, when a patient is given access to all data stored about her/him, (s)he usually lacks capabilities and tools to handle the data, and to use the data for her/his benefit. Still, patients are expected to be able to act on the basis of the data available to them, for example, to make appointments or to bring laboratory test results with them. In a previous study, we made the data of similarly different medical and patient ISs interoperable to the cancer specialists of breast cancer cases by using shared attributes as the linkage between data storages. In this conceptual article, we apply our federative approach to contemplate from the patient's point of view, how data available to a patient could be made interoperable. We explain the theoretical background of the federative approach and related tools within the mentioned breast cancer case and in general. We then describe how the federative approach could be used in the context of digitalized citizen/patient services, empowered citizens and patient/citizen-centric care. With this article we contribute to research by developing the federative approach further and by explaining how (medical and patient) data can be made interoperable to patients/citizens. Our results suggest means to support citizens and digitalized healthcare service intermediaries as well as patient empowerment.

Keywords: Governance of data · Data federation · Patient health register
Data ontology

1 Introduction

Two different sources of motivators led to the research idea of this study. We helped the information and cancer specialist of a university hospital to find a practical data federation approach to make data from multiple data storages interoperable. The characteristics of the data storages differed significantly, such as data types, data

© Springer Nature Switzerland AG 2018
H. Li et al. (Eds.): WIS 2018, CCIS 907, pp. 134–147, 2018.
https://doi.org/10.1007/978-3-319-97931-1_11

sources and data dimensions. This led us to ask the question, could we help citizens to make the (medical and social welfare) data available to them interoperable in a similar way? Secondly, the national healthcare and social welfare system in the country of this study (Finland) undergoes currently the biggest reform of the system during the 100-years of the country as an independent republic. One of the most critical issues of the reform is, how to integrate or federate data between the data storages in the thousands of medical and social welfare information systems (IS) so that the data is made interoperable to both professionals and citizens? We asked ourselves, is our federative approach able to offer practical means to make data interoperable?

In Finland, the number of positive breast cancer diagnoses has grown rapidly during the recent decades. The current annual number of positive diagnoses (mainly women but also some men) is almost 5000 (almost one per a thousand citizen). However, 90% of patients are alive 5 years after a confirmed positive diagnosis [1]. Due to the grown number of breast cancers it is a common death cause in all the age groups of Finnish women. Breast cancers are diagnosed and treated in various types of healthcare institutions: public healthcare centers, occupational healthcare, private healthcare centers and university (central) hospitals. Sieving studies are performed periodically and women are reminded to regularly check their breasts. The aim is to detect breast cancers in their early stage, to be able to treat the cancer immediately and to prevent the formation of rapidly spreading tumors.

Radiotherapy, cytostatic treatments and surgeries are typical treatments for diag-nosed breast cancers and other types of cancers, as well. The specialized units of university hospitals mainly give these treatments. Laboratory tests, X-rays, pathology examinations and ultrasound scans are typical pre-treatment events. There could also be medicine prescriptions. The execution of examination and treatment events result in enormous amounts of data entries such as cover letters, medical statements, reports, test results and images. Medical devices and personnel like nurses, doctors, cancer spe-cialists and clerical personnel create these entries into diverse ISs. After diagnoses and treatments rehabilitation data and follow-up reports are added to ISs.

A breast cancer patient is in the center of all events, and is either directly or indirectly the subject of all data entries. In the era of digitalization and consumer-centric business, many patients have experiences about data collection. Patients expect that healthcare professionals use data about them and their treatments with patients' consent, be transferred electronically between professionals and ISs so that they do not have to repeat the same data. Patients also expect that data are kept safe and secure and used only to purposes described in data storage register definitions. Laws, such as the general data protection register (GDPR) act, are important part of data security.

Despite of alignment thinking and attempts to place patients/citizens/customers into the center of healthcare treatment processes, the prevailing way is still to look at patient care from a physician's viewpoint, and consequently ISs are organization and/or profession-centric [2]. ISs are designed so that each (organizational) unit has their own ISs that support their operations (silos). The data of separate unit specific ISs are linked – made interoperable - through a patient identification and/or some other key data attributes. They are used to compile data available about a patient.

A more patient centric approach has resulted in attempts to give patients more (digital) tools to access their own health data. So far, the focus has been on "giving access" to data entered by healthcare professionals. In Finland, Kanta (www.kanta.fi) is a register that healthcare service providers use to enter summaries, test results and medicine prescriptions. A citizen is allowed to access her/his own Kanta data after strong identification. Currently only healthcare professionals are allowed to enter and update data in the Kanta register. Patients are unable to add entries, such as the results blood pressure or diabetes measures executed at home (with devices that healthcare professionals gave them), statements of perceived conditions after treatments, or even to correct errors in data. Communication is entirely one-way. Furthermore, at the moment, the Kanta register contains a limited set of stored data. The fact that the ISO approved Health-Level 7 (HL7) data standard is used in all medical ISs in the country potentially facilitates extended future opening up of healthcare data.

On the other hand, patients are expected to be prepared when they meet healthcare professionals, to communicate effectively data about their health condition, and even to actively monitor their health status and recovery. To execute tasks falling to them patients use various sources of more or less reliable information. Typical unreliable sources include relatives having personal opinions and experiences and online discussion forums, articles, platforms and applications. Doctors, nurses and other professional may provide more reliable advice and/or consultation via phone, messaging or Internet. The consequence is that from a citizen's perspective health information is scattered and left to the citizen to compile and use. Citizens need help to manage their personal health data and to make available data interoperable [3]. We see a research gap here, that is, in how to provide healthcare data to citizens. In a previous research, we used the federative approach to make cancer data interoperable to medical experts. The purpose of this article is to investigate could the federative approach be used to provide interoperable (healthcare) data to citizens as well. From a practical point of view, our article aims to describe, what benefits the federative approach is able to deliver to citizens by making healthcare data interoperable, and how those benefits empower citizens to take better care of their own health.

Tang and Lansky [4] reported several positive consequences from the sharing of patient data between physicians and patients with any (electronic) means. According to them patients started to describe themselves as "team members in their own care" as they perceived that they had better visibility to data about them. The concept of personal health record (PHR) was proposed as the tool to make patients empowered in relation to their diseases and treatments [e.g. 2, 5]. The concept of patient empowerment has evolved over time. Bos et al. [6] described "patient 2.0 empowerment" already a decade ago. Information and communication technologies were seen as the tools to offer a citizen means to participate interactively into one's healthcare. On the other hand, Detmer et al. [5] and Archer et al. [7] suggested that the lack of data standards and ISs interoperability, and the high complexities and costs of data integration hamper the development and adoption of PHR. We address these issues.

We developed the federative approach over several years [e.g. 8, 9] and have used it in addition to the cancer case to help companies to manage their product and customer master data. In the breast cancer case, the objective was to detect malignant breast cancer cases as early as possible and to help to analyze the effectiveness of various cancer treatments. Even to our surprise cancer data became interoperable through the identification of four shared attributes only and through the descriptions of their metadata. Thus, in the breast cancer case, we were able to address and solve similar challenges that Detmer et al. [5] and Archer et al. [7] described as the challenges of PHR adoption. The realization of that motivated the present study. Against the discussed backdrop we outlined the following research questions for this research:

RQ1: How should federative data interoperability be described to citizens when they have access to patient and healthcare data?

RQ2: What benefits are federated interoperable data able to offer to breast cancer (and other) patients?

RQ3: Is data federation able to help citizens to cope with healthcare digitalization, especially with digital patient and healthcare data?

The rest of the article is organized as follows. In next section, we explicate different ontological stances on how to achieve data interoperability as well as the reasoning behind the federative approach and its tools. Then, in Sect. 3, we revisit the breast cancer case from methodology perspective. Section 4, results, discusses how the cancer case findings were transformed to the personal health record (PHR) use contexts as well as how our tools help to address some typical PHR adoption problems. We end the article with a discussion and conclusions Section.

2 Theoretical Background

2.1 The Justification of the Federative Approach and Related Tools

We advocate our federative approach to data interoperability and related tools. The theoretical basis of this approach responds to the challenge caused by the transformation from closed IS and data storage environments to open systems environments. Until about 20 years ago, digital data was predominantly structured internal data that was created inside of organizations and stored into their internal information systems. ISs were built in-house, and even if they were outsourced or purchased, data models behind them were owned by the organizations using these ISs. Almost all data were created internally, and due to that their history and data models were known. Consequently, organizations understood the semantic contextual meaning of the data stored into their ISs as well as the data entry, maintenance and usage processes. Different data models in the various ISs an organization used for different purposes were not a problem, as those differences were known and could be managed due to their small number. Data types included master data, reference data and metadata that were linked to transactional data, reports, documents and contents [10, 11]. Data integration and interoperability challenges in their current meaning and severity did not exist. These features characterized the era of closed systems environments.

In open systems environments, organizations buy software packages and services from external IS vendors, and the number of different ISs has grown enormously. For example, a typical hospital has several hundred ISs and applications. In addition to traditional transactional and clerical data, digital data is increasingly unstructured, including, e.g., videos, images and sensor data. The majority of data could even be external to an organization with constantly changing data models. The sources and dimensionality of data have exploded as well. Organizations use social media data and message contents. Many kinds of analysis are done on data, like health care text mining or the automated processing of X-ray images. Timespan and locational span of data and events have become valuable, like the time series of blood tests. A citizen's data usage has gone through similar changes. Data is created with diverse applications and googled or searched with other tools from numerous data storages that have different unknown data models. Several applications available to citizens allow data integrations, for example the attachment of various files to messages or emails.

In closed systems environments, it was easier to integrate and to make data interoperable because the meanings of data and data models in various ISs were known, including their IS technical metadata like field lengths and formats. Organizations were able to plan the data models of their internal ISs so that there was little overlapping. In open systems environments, data integration requires much more and could be limited to data federation with limited data interoperability only, for example having access to various data storages instead of true data integration. Informational and social meta data are needed if the expectation is to do more than just provide access to data storages. IS technical meta data (= location and access meta data) is sufficient for that. Informational and social meta data explain what data mean in each IS, from which the data are federated. Data federation between the data of ISs is done by identifying the shared attributes of these ISs together with the three types of s meta data in each IS. The role of informational and social metadata is to capture and to make understandable differences between the values of shared attributes. This kind of data federation offers access and interoperability to data that are needed to create a full understanding or picture about a situation, for example a patient's health.

Data integration and interoperability has become one of the key data management issues as the consequence of the transformation to open systems environments and data explosion. For example, the first version of DMBOK (data management book of knowledge) published in 2009 treated this issue narrowly and from a different ontological stance than the second version published in 2017. In general, data federation requires a lot of knowledge about the data to be federated. Dahlberg and Nokkala [8] proposed a list of data properties that must be defined for data governance and federation, such as data source types, structural properties of data, internality-externality of data, life-cycle phases of data and most importantly the contextual meaning of data. We used that list to develop the federative tools discussed in this article.

2.2 Data Ontology in Data Integration and Interoperability

From data management perspective, the data of organizations split into dozens or hundreds of overlapping and fragmented ISs in open systems environments. It could be unclear to data users, which of the ISs are trustworthy in specific situations, as the meaning of data is unclear due to hazy origins and insufficient metadata. Knowledge about available data sources, the meanings of original and processed data in each data source and the quality of data is needed to ensure that data is used effectively.

In situations with fragmented and controversial data, it is necessary to understand the data management consequences of two main ontological stances to data interoperability: canonical and contextual. According to the canonical stance it is possible to agree one "version of truth" for shared data attributes with "golden values" for each record between the various ISs integrated and made interoperable. This builds on the assumption that data has the same meaning and interpretation in all data use contexts [10, 12–14]. The data management consequence is that data interoperability is achieved by replacing IS specific anomalous values with golden values. The contextual or federative stance proposes that data is contextual. Canonical stance is needed in each specific use context to implement an unambiguous data model to that context. Data interoperability, however, means the federation of various use contexts with data about the same persons, objects, concepts or locations without replacing the original record values of various contexts, since that leads to the loss of (critical) data. Context-determined data is made interoperable with meta data as described above [15].

There is no agreement among academics or practitioners that one of the two ontological stances is preferable. Rather they suit to different situations and environments. In our opinion, "one version of the truth" was, and is, a possible data interoperability solution in closed systems environments, where the number of ISs was limited and their data models were known and controllable. Thereby it was/is possible to understand the differences between real world and the data world modeled with ISs. In open system environments, the number of data contexts and related data models has exploded. It is impossible to know all data usage contexts and an organization is seldom even able to know and control data models. Our federative approach builds on Wand and Wang [15], who explained that real world is seen through the lens of the context. An organizations typically has a specific IS for each specific context. In open systems environments, such context specific ISs are usually purchased from outside IS suppliers who also own the data models of the purchased ISs. More over, the data model of an IS does not model the reality of any specific organization but a generalized organization. During the implementation of the IS, e.g. SAP r/3 or S/4, an IS integrator modifies the generic data model into the real world of the user organization. This means that only the integrator has knowledge about the modified data model.

The user who directly observes the real world may have another view (perceived mental model) about the specific real world context than the IS supplier or the IS integrator. Data deficiencies are born, when the user's view of the real world context differs from the interpreted world context of the IS represented in its data model. During the era of open systems, the number of possible contexts and thereby also the number of possible data deficiencies grows within ISs and between ISs. The contexts of healthcare ISs include professionals' and patients' real worlds. Since their views on real worlds are probably dissimilar the probabilities of data defects increase. The real world contexts of healthcare ISs, that is, their data models most often represent the real world of healthcare professional and then that is presented to patients. Patient capabilities to interpret data differ and usually their real world context as well.

Real world changes constantly and the events changing the real world are represented in the data of an IS [16]. That is the ontological premise of an IS. Ontologies are means to describe the meaning of the data in an IS representing the real world context of the data. Even though the real world changes, the ontology of data explains the purpose of data creation, use and storing and what is the meaning of data in each phase of its life cycle. Ontologies representing patients' real world could help patient understanding in situations, where they are given healthcare ISs data (to interpret and use) that healthcare professionals have entered into ISs by using their real world representations. If a patient understands the premises, under which data were created, processed and used, that may decrease the number of perceived data deficiencies.

In our data federation tools, the role of ontologies is to explain the meaning of data in each federated data context, that is, in each federated IS or IS module. In the federation of data, the data set of each IS (module) being expected to have its own technical, information processing and social characteristics that are described with meta data ontologies. Technical characteristics, (i.e. meta data), include data attribute formats, lengths and cardinalities (i.e. is the attribute mandatory and/or a search key) and other similar meta data. Information processing meta data defines the processing of the attribute and social meta data the meaning of the attribute. Seemingly similar attributes of two ISs may have different processes and their real world context may change non-similarly over time. To sum up, discussion here describes our ontological stance.

2.3   Consumer-/Citizen-Centric Healthcare and PHR

Both patients and healthcare professionals/service providers benefit from understanding better data about patients' diseases and treatments. Similarly, a comprehensive understanding about a patient's situation helps a healthcare professional to provide better service. Personal health records (PHR) are one means to support such understanding. The purpose of electronic PHRs is to make patient information readily available to patients and to healthcare professionals. Patients may use PHR data to improve self-managed care [7]. PHRs have recently been linked also to so-called shared decision making (SDM) concept as a means to enhance healthcare outcomes positively [17, 18]. SDM is a citizen-centric healthcare means where a patient is engaged into shared decisions made about his/her health.

Literature presents various types of PHRs. A wide variety of PHR products from commercial to self-kept (by hospital, hospital district, patient, some other actor) archives are available in tethered and untethered versions [7]. We do not distinguish diverse PHR product types but discuss, how our data federation tools are able to support any type of PHR. PHR is just one angle to consumer-centric healthcare. Healthcare expenses and consequences monitoring of chronic diseases, lifestyle surveillance tools, personal wellness management, wellness diaries and assisted living for elderly are other concepts discussed in the connection of consumer-centric care. Consumer-centric care builds on such ideas that the ways to provide healthcare services must change as the consequences of digitalization, the development of mobile technologies and connectivity technologies [2].

Ultimately consumer-centric healthcare is about concentrating on a patient instead of the procedures and treatments that various healthcare unit provide. Consumer-centricity and PHR mean that relevant information about a patient is connected and compiled from all possible angles and sources, not only from data that hospitals and healthcare units offer. In Varshney's [19] figure several pervasive healthcare applications are connected so that both the sources and usage situation of data are shown together with facilitating technological tools. Varshney's figure illustrates the wide variety of data types, meanings and use situations of data, and leads to the conclusion that the integration and interoperability of all relevant information is a difficult task.

Varshney's research describes the starting point of our federative approach crafting [8] and the later development of related tools [9]. We used the crafted tools to make integrated customer and product master data interoperable and later used similar tools to make heterogeneous cancer data interoperable.

IoT (Internet of Things) data, the data of other sensor types and wearable data are also connected to PHR. Islam et al. [20] explained how these technologies can be linked to customer-centric care to complement traditional legacy healthcare data. Islam et al. claim that the usage of IoT technologies offers significant potential to improve healthcare services, to increase the efficiency of those services, to develop proactive services that lower the need of expensive cures and to empower citizens.

3   Methodology and the Cancer Data Case Revisited

The aim of the cancer case research [9] was to demonstrate how data on breast cancer patients and their treatments could be made interoperable with our federative approach in a university hospital. The benefit objectives were: by using federated data the specialists of the hospital should able to detect widely spread breast cancer cases earlier, to estimate better the survival rates of patients that had been diagnosed with this form of breast cancer and to predict more precisely the efficiency of treatments. In the case research, data federation was investigated only from the perspective of data specialists, that is, how they could achieve benefit objectives of data federation. In this article, we revisit the case from the perspective of empowered citizens and customer-centric health care. The objective is to reason, could the same data federation tools be used to solve also the data federation and interoperability of PHRs [5].

In the cancer case study, we followed the guidelines of Yin [21] in the planning and execution of the case and Eisenhardt [22] in theory building from the findings of the case. Since our research was a single case study in one single hospital in one country, our study had obvious limitations, most notably in theory building [22].

3.1   Case Study

Yin [21] offers guidelines for data collection in a case study, which we followed. To begin with, we wrote a formal case study protocol. Data collection was executed in the form of workshops, by preparing material to the workshops and in discussions with the data specialists after workshops. As Yin [21] advices, it is possible to obtain a richer set of data by using and combining several sources of evidence, like interviews, observation and archival material. We did not use direct observation data of cancer treatments but used all the five other data described by Yin [21, pp. 105–117].

The case study was conducted in January–March 2016. Planning meetings with data specialists were held to introduce the data federation matrixes (presented in Figs. 1 and 2) and their use. We organized several workshops to collect data. In each workshop, the participants were the experts of one breast cancer treatment area, such as pathologists or surgeons, two data specialists of the hospital and us. Experts first identified ISs with most valuable data to them (matrix 1) and then described the shared attributes of those ISs (matrix 2). They explained how, by whom and when the data was processed as well as what do those attributes mean in their tasks. We also discussed data quality and data defect issues.

3.2   The Case

The university hospital offers special healthcare services, e.g. cancer treatments. It cooperates with the municipal healthcare stations, private healthcare service providers and healthcare districts of its special enactment area and shares data with them. Within the hospital there are several data professionals responsible for data governance and information services that are offered to both medical and research staff.

Patient IS is the main healthcare IS. All departments of the hospital use it. This backbone IS has all basic data about a patient: name, social security identification, address, phone number, occupation as well as data about diagnoses, given treatments, allergies, consents given, medical risks. The patient IS is divided into two subsystems to execute resource governance and treatments reporting. The results of laboratory tests, medication and other treatments are integrated to patient and events in this IS.

In addition to the patient IS the hospital has dozens of unit, disease and treatment specific ISs. For example, laboratory, pathology, surgery and radiotherapy units have their own systems, which need to be integrated to the patient IS. The diversification of data types, formats and sources is a challenge in master data, reference data, meta data, transactions, content and reports. Data formats vary from strictly formatted to unformatted, such as free text based diagnosis and treatment reports, X-ray and other images and dictated audio data. Data are transferred electronically between some ISs, whereas users must re-enter even the basic data of a patient into some other ISs. Some ISs use reference data to control the correctness of data entries like social identification codes, postal codes, diagnosis codes, and medication names. Other ISs use reconciliation reports comparing the data of two ISs at a time to control data quality.

Data governance addresses also other challenges. Some old legacy ISs have been developed in-house, whereas most ISs have been purchased from IS suppliers. The data of some ISs have been accumulated for decades, while some other ISs covered data from the last five years or even shorter period of time. ISs and data have been merged and harmonized. Due to this the values of some attributes are not used. Data entry practices and rules have changed over time. There is variety in units follow data entry practices and rules. Units may use the same attributes in divergent ways.

In the case study, we helped the data specialists of the hospital. They had been mandated to compile data from the various ISs with the objective to identify widely spread breast cancers as early as possible and to analyze the effectiveness of various cancer treatments. In the beginning, we discussed data governance in general to establish shared understanding of concepts used. By doing this we gradually understood the data interoperability challenges of the data specialists. We also had to learn the basic terminology of breast cancer diagnostics to be able to fill the two matrixes in the workshops with various breast cancers medical and treatment specialists.

3.3   Data Federation Matrixes

The data federation matrixes we have developed and used are based on the governance of data framework proposed in Dahlberg and Nokkala [8]. The two matrixes shown as Figs. 1 and 2 are simplified from the actual matrixes to illustrate their ideas. Figure 1 presents the 4 shared attributes we used to federate data from the various breast cancer ISs. ISs are listed in the title row of the matrix and attributes in listed in title column. Social security identification is used to identify the patient. The cancer diagnosis code was used to ensure that the patient had breast cancer. Tumor node metastasis (TNM) code told us the size and extent of cancer tumor (T), how widely that tumor has spread lymph nodes (N) and a distinct metastasis (M). That code had to be reasoned on the basis of meta data since the code value indicating malignant breast cancer did not exist prior to a positive confirmation. Dates of events that reported either cancer diagnosis or TNM code were used to ensure that only data of related events are made interoperable.

	Patient IS	Laboratory IS	Surgical IS	Radiotherapy IS	Pathology IS	Information System N
Social security identification	X	X	X	X	X	X
(Cancer) diagnosis code	X	X	X	X	X	X
Tumor node metastasis (TNM) code	X	X	X	X	X	X
Date of events	X	X	X	X	X	X

Fig. 1. Tool to identify shared attributes from the various IS

By using the content of Fig. 1 we filled the cell values of the table shown in Fig. 2 for each of the four attributes. Here we just show an empty matrix with no shell values. The metadata of Fig. 2 was collected to federate data from the various ISs without "mixing apples and oranges". To simplify Fig. 2 we show only part of metadata properties (= rows with additional meta data characteristics were dropped). Figure 2 gives an idea of what kind of meta data characteristics were collected about the shared attributes. We collected IS technical meta data, information processing meta data and socio-contextual meta data. Meta data was used to specify the IS technical properties, data lifecycle properties and the meaning of shared attributes in the original ISs. Metadata was stored into a metadata repository for further use.

The purpose of our tools is not to suggest that all relevant data should be compiled into one data storage for reporting, which obviously is possible, but to create links to establish interoperability. By using those links and the meta data repository it is possible to federate data sets by letting data to reside in the original ISs. The metadata repository also stores federation rules, mappings between data attributes including the mappings about the meanings of data attributes, descriptions of data processing that are used to improve the control of data quality, and other meta data definitions. The shared attributes used to federate data are called interoperable shared attributes.

Our federative approach differs significantly from the canonical approach to data integration. We do not even try to collect all the data for reporting into a single IS, although that would be possible. Instead of that meta data repository is describing data made interoperable.

Personal ID / Diagnosis / TNM code	Patient IS	Laboratory IS	Surgical IS	Radiotherapy IS	Pathology IS	Information system N
IS Technical metadata						
- Description						
- Field name/length etc.						
Information processing metadata						
- Place of initial data entry creation						
- Creator of data entry						
- Responsible for data storage						
Socio-contextual metadata						
- Meaning when saving patient data						
- Meaning for treatments						
- Meaning in diagnosis						
- Meaning for medication						

Fig. 2. Tool to describe the metadata of shared attributes in various ISs

4   Using the Data Federation Matrixes for PHR

Nykänen and Seppälä [2] claim that due to the growing number of stakeholders and actors (e.g. sensors and advanced technological solutions) in the healthcare field or ecosystem, the development of a comprehensive system to collect data created by all stakeholders and actors is challenging. According to them both the structure and the meaning of data must be defined to facilitate the development of such a system. True interoperability between ISs requires the existence of such definitions. Tang and Lansky [4] suggest that full interoperability of data is achieved through coded data exchange standards instead of data silos, since healthcare is not either given in silos.

Earlier research, e.g., studies cited above advocate strongly the benefits of data interoperability but also recognize that the implementation of interoperability needs be easy and inexpensive. Similarly to us, they doubt that only the compiling of (healthcare) data into one data storage, e.g., a data lake, is possible due to technical and capacity limitations - or enough unless the meaning of various data set are known. Our data federation tools are useful in establishing the needed links between various (healthcare) data storages, similarly as in the breast cancer case discussed above. With our tools the integration of patient data from several systems means that shared attributes are agreed and their metadata is described and stored into a meta data repository. Physical (= software code level) integration and interoperability is implemented with the help of the metadata repository. Meta data repository may also be used to agree the content and format standardized messages used to exchange data automatically between healthcare ISs. Should our tools have been used as in the cancer case that helps to do the same for citizen data as the same shared attributes could be viewed from the citizen perspective, that is, their meaning to patient would be described.

For a PHR, healthcare data are compiled from the electronic health records of various healthcare and other actors and from other applications, such as IoT. A patient may is one possible PHR input data provider and may provide, for example, home measurements of blood pressure or blood sugar levels. Patient data entries need to be defined similar to other data sources. That is, the IS technical, information processing and socio-contextual metadata need to be described to establish trust in the data.

In our opinion, the data federation tools depicted here fit well to PHR data federation, and may even provide the missing link to doing such federations. Also for a PHR, the data matrixes are filled with the descriptions of shared attributes and their meta data. If our tools are used in several cases, the matrixes of various cases could be compared. Those attributes that are similar – and already described in details – between two or more cases could be used to increase the scope of data federation if needed. This approach could even be used to solve the data federation of complex PHR. Divide it into smaller parts and combine them after each part is solved. This Section provides our answers to the three research question outlined in Section one.

5   Discussion and Conclusions

Cancer patients who are effectively able to manage their own data have more positive feelings about their cancer treatments and are better able to adjust to stress [23]. This finding indicates that interoperability, which data federation typically offers to healthcare professionals, is potentially highly beneficial to patients as well. This is our specific response to RQ2. Data federation enables more efficient use of data and better understanding regarding the meaning of the data. Citizens should be made aware about these opportunities. We offer this the specific answer to RQ1.

Federative data interoperability means that data can reside in the original data storages as is, and still be used for usage purposes. IS technical, informational and socio-contextual meta data are needed to do this safely. From the patient perspective nothing changes in data collection, whereas access to data is able to provide data related benefits to citizens. The use of federated data may even help healthcare professionals to save time and to order less laboratory tests, as trusted meta data on how test data was created and what they mean are available. Information processing and contextual meta data help the users of data to evaluate whether data can be trusted. With the advancement of technology, measurement devices can be used to collect data about the environment where the data was collected. This is our detailed response to RQ3.

Customer or citizen centric healthcare appears as the concept that healthcare professionals crave for. The use of federated interoperable PHR data is one potential solution. Data federation does, however, not solve all barriers of PHR adoption described in literature [5, 7], but offers tools to deploy technical standards for interoperability and may also help to reduce data integration costs.

Digitalization is seen both as the enabler of better services and as something that demands the learning of new competencies. Citizens are encouraged to take more responsibility of our own healthcare. To a citizen this means the adoption of several new (digital) healthcare, well-being and other services. As the revisited case study showed, our data federation tools suited well to situations where data from several data storages were made interoperable to provide a holistic picture, e.g., of one's life. Our tools are able to federate the data of these services and to empower citizens to use healthcare data and correspondingly. This is our complementary response to RQ3.

A similar data federation PHR study as we conducted in the breast cancer case is an amenable venue of future research. For this study we did not collect new evidence. This is the main limitation of our speculative study. However, this limitation is possible to remove in future studies. Our advice to researchers and practitioners is to carefully consider the ontological nature of federated data.

References

1. Finnish Cancer Registry. https://cancerregistry.fi/statistics/cancer-statistics/
2. Nykänen, P., Seppälä, A.: Collaborative approach for sustainable citizen-centered health care. In: Wickramasinghe, N., Bali, R.K., Sumoi, R., Kirin, S. (eds.) Critical Issues for the Development of Sustainable E-health Solutions. HDIA, pp. 115–134. Springer, Boston (2012). https://doi.org/10.1007/978-1-4614-1536-7_8
3. Pratt, W.: Personal health information management. Commun. ACM 49(1), 51–55 (2006)
4. Tang, P.C.: The missing link: bridging the patient-provider health information gap. Health Aff. 24(5), 1290–1295 (2005)
5. Detmer, D., Bloomrosen, M., Raymond, B., Tang, P.: Integrated personal health records: transformative tools for consumer-centric care. BMC Med. Inform. Decis. Mak. 8(1), 45 (2008)
6. Bos, L., Marsh, A., Carroll, D., Gupta, S., Rees, M.: Patient 2.0 empowerment. In: SWWS, pp. 164–168(2008)

7. Archer, N., Fevrier-Thomas, U., Lokker, C., McKibbon, K.A., Straus, S.E.: Personal health records: a scoping review. J. Am. Med. Inform. Assoc. **18**(4), 515–522 (2011)
8. Dahlberg, T., Nokkala, T.: A framework for the corporate governance of data - theoretical background and empirical evidence. Bus. Manag. Educ. **13**(1), 25–45 (2015)
9. Dahlberg, T., Nokkala, T., Heikkilä, J., Heikkilä, M.: Data federation with a governance of data framework artifact as the federation tool: case on clinical breast cancer treatment data. Front. Artif. Intell. Appl. **292**, 31–42 (2017)
10. Mosley, M., Brackett, M., Earley, S., Henderson, D.: The DAMA Guide to the Data Management Body of Knowledge: DAMA-DMBOK Guide, 1st edn. Technics Publications, LLC, Bradley Beach (2010)
11. Cleven, A., Wortmann, F.: Uncovering four strategies to approach master data management. In: Proceedings of the Annual Hawaii International Conference on System Sciences 2010, pp. 1–10 (2010)
12. Dreibelbis, A., Hechler, E., Milman, I., Oberhofer, M., van Run, P., Wolfson, D.: Enterprise Master Data Management: An SOA Approach to Managing Core Information. Pearson Education, London (2008)
13. Loshin, D.: Master Data Management. Morgan Kaufmann, Burlington (2010)
14. Berson, A., Dubov, L.: Master Data Management and Customer Data Integration for a Global Enterprise. McGraw-Hill, Inc., New York (2007)
15. Wand, Y., Wang, R.: Anchoring data quality dimensions in ontological foundations. Commun. ACM **39**(11), 86–95 (1996)
16. Wand, Y., Weber, R.: An ontological model of an information system. IEEE Trans. Softw. Eng. **16**(11), 1282–1292 (1990)
17. Shay, L.A., Lafata, J.E.: Where is the evidence? A systematic review of shared decision making and patient outcomes. Med. Decis. Mak. **35**(1), 114–131 (2015)
18. Davis, S., Roudsari, A., Raworth, R., Courtney, K.L., MacKay, L.: Shared decision-making using personal health record technology: a scoping review at the crossroads. J. Am. Med. Inform. Assoc. **24**(4), 857–866 (2017)
19. Varshney, U.: Pervasive healthcare and wireless health monitoring. Mob. Netw. Appl. **12**(2), 113–127 (2007)
20. Islam, S.R., Kwak, D., Kabir, M.H., Hossain, M., Kwak, K.: The Internet of Things for health care: a comprehensive survey. IEEE Access **3**, 678–708 (2015)
21. Yin, R.K.: Applications of Case Study Research. Sage, Thousand Oaks (2011)
22. Eisenhardt, K.M.: Building theories from case study research. Acad. Manag. Rev. **14**(4), 532–550 (1989)
23. Auerbach, S.M.: Should patients have control over their own health care?: Empirical evidence and research issues. Ann. Behav. Med. **22**(3), 246–259 (2000)

Chasing Professional Phronesis in Safety and Well-Being: Teacher Education Curriculum as a Case

Brita Somerkoski[✉]

Department of Teacher Education, Turku School of Economics,
University of Turku, Turku, Finland
brita.somerkoski@utu.fi

Abstract. Enhancing the safety culture in school context sets new challenges to prospective teachers, their need for safety skills and for the teacher education. This paper discusses firstly, how skill and knowledge oriented safety and well-being contents in the teacher education curriculum could be distinguished. Further on, it is explored, how these two repertoires are presented in the curriculum text of one teacher education unit and how they reflect the Aristotelian ideal of achieving phronesis, practical wisdom. The data pointed out that safety was included in the curriculum and could therefore be seen as a value in teacher education, hence the focus was very strongly in the interactive skills and the group dynamics.

Keywords: Safety risks · Well-being · Safety culture · Learning environment
Phronesis · Safety competence · Skills · Teacher education

1 Introduction

Safety and well-being in general, have received growing attention in recent years, but the research is still for the most part focusing on health education, with little attention paid to the safety risks confronting pupils, teachers, teacher students or school staff. The extreme violence in schools as well as the unintentional injuries and incidents have changed the safety culture in schools [1–3]. Enhancing safety culture demands knowledge of both organizational and individual risks, however, practical training should also be considered [4, 5]. These competencies demand sustainable measures, both proactive and reactive, carried out in the organization [4, 6]. Enhancing the safety culture in school context sets new challenges to prospective teachers, their need for safety skills and for the teacher education. Content of teaching, pedagogy and school practices should be reviewed and renewed in relation to the changes in the learning environment and skills [7]. This paper discusses firstly how skill and knowledge orientated safety and well-being contents in the teacher education curriculum could be distinguished. Further on, it is explored how these two repertoires are presented in the curriculum text of one teacher education unit and how they reflect the Aristotelian ideal of achieving phronesis, practical wisdom.

© Springer Nature Switzerland AG 2018
H. Li et al. (Eds.): WIS 2018, CCIS 907, pp. 148–161, 2018.
https://doi.org/10.1007/978-3-319-97931-1_12

2   Curriculum Content, Phronesis and Discourses

According to Phelan [8], teachers are responsible for specific actions and concrete decisions. The concept of phronesis is introduced in Nicomachean Ethics [9–11] and the text includes that between theory and practice, knowledge and experience there is a constant interplay. Phronesis is an academically recognized concept describing the definition of *practice*. It is one of the key definitions of this study as well [12, 13]. Phronesis is here seen from situational perception, the capacity to discern particulars and judgements about how to act in different contexts and situations [8]. Aristotle states, that in teaching, *techne* includes the kind of reasoning and activity that we see in the use of instructional techniques, whereas *phronesis* centres on making judgments about what to do and taking action as part of these ethical deliberations for human being [14, 15]. Firstly, the Aristotelian concepts phronesis and *episteme* cannot be totally or always distinguished –the concepts are related to each other. It is stated that for Aristotle, phronesis is a way of thinking that can only be demonstrated in moral action. Making moral decisions involves identifying what is right in the given situation and then acting on this decision [16]. Yet in the educational context, phronesis cannot be taught directly — the curriculum should provide possibilities that make learning from practical situations possible and phronesis may develop by itself [17]. Teachers need practical wisdom, sense of justice, temperance and courage. These virtues make the teacher profession a social practice [18], especially in the safety context, teachers and teacher educators make decisions in the absence of information and sometimes also in the presence of conflicting information [19]. Phronesis is needed just in these kinds of sudden and surprising situations by consideration, judgment and choice. This reminds of the definitions used by Dewey [20] who mentions phronetically acting as whole-heartedness and open-mindedness. Acting phronetically is both intellectual and moral work [20]. Chistie [21] proposes phronesis as embodied, situated practical judgement that involves tacit knowledge and discursive constructions that influence subject formation. The most of the researchers agree, that phronesis is a complex concept and a form of rationality or knowledge, and that it is distinguishable from technical and theoretical information. In these terms phronesis is revealed in the teachers' ability to act correctly, not only in a technical sense, but also more impor-tantly in a moral sense [22]. However, not all researchers do quite share Aristotle's idea of episteme being universal and unchanging. Neither do they agree that phronesis is closer to episteme than techne. For instance Flyvbjerg [23] sees episteme as being formed through the practical rationality and actions of scientists. Finally Chistie [21] comes to the conclusion that the boundaries between phronesis and episteme are not as clear as their original conceptions imply.

Higgs [25] discusses close concepts around phronesis. She states that practice is doing, knowing, being and becoming, based on values and grounded in assumptions rather than conscious decisions, whereas wisdom is born of multiple ways of knowing through experiences, learning and reflecting. Practice is characterized by complexity, uncertainty and diversity and it occurs within social contexts that are framed by the professional experience, yet Vaara and Whittington [25] state that practice is embodied, materially mediated arrays of human activity centrally organized around shared practical understanding. The other central definition close to practice and skills is competence. Competence is here understood as the ability to perform a specific set of skills related to the tasks that are partly constitutive of that particular professional practice. Competence in the broad sense means that a person has the ability to fulfill a task or solve a problem and that he or she has the values and attitudes, knowledge and skills [26] and ability to use these in an innovative way [27]. In safety context that would mean for instance a teacher's ability to take care of the group dynamics in the classroom in emergency situations, monitoring and actively preventing unintentional injuries and violence, being able to solve school bullying cases or being able to use the machinery in an appropriate way. Sellman takes the definition further by stating that competence acts as a precursory for professional phronesis. It has to be noted that the teacher is not only expected to be technically competent in fulfilling the responsibilities of curriculum delivery but he or she is to exemplify a moral person and to act in an ethical manner consistent with that morality [28]. The basic values of the core curriculum in Finland [29] for comprehensive schools include also citizenship skills, one of them being responsibility and ability to take care of oneself. Teacher education should prepare and support the prospective teachers in teaching the skills according to the curriculum aims and goals. It is also stated that teachers need, more than before, skills for interaction and teaching multicultural groups in various learning environments [27, 30]. Theser can be considered as safety skills.

This study does not directly reflect Aristotle's thoughts on phronesis, practical wisdom. Yet Aristotle's thoughts on phronesis are here seen as the teacher's safety competence, such as an ability to react, notice and respond to the risks, ability to prevent accidents, violence and self-harm, ability to act in emergency situations, and interaction knowledge and skills. This study explores the curriculum texts and safety discourses in the teacher education curriculum. The aim was to understand the practical and knowledge-based safety and well-being discourses in the teacher education curriculum and find out what kind of safety and well-being related repertoires are found to find out and whether the curriculum supports the prospective teachers to become safety competent phronimos [30] wise professionals.

3 Safety Skills in the Context of Education

The educational system of Finland is based on trust in teacher education. In general, all teachers are required a Master's degree (4–6 study years). The master level teacher education offered at universities should provide the teacher students with capabilities, skills and knowledge to guide the learning of students. The high level of training and practical skills are seen necessary as teachers in Finland are very autonomous professionally. Teachers have the possibility to decide for instance which teaching methods and learning materials they want to use [31]. Safety is mentioned as a value in the school legislation. Students' right to safety, security and welfare is also mandated: "A pupil participating in education shall be entitled to a safe learning environment" [32]. This means that the education provider shall draw up a plan, in connection with curriculum design, for safeguarding students against violence, bullying and harassment; execute the plan and supervise adherence to it and to enhance interaction skills and human relations in the learning environment. To fulfill the safety as a value, it is necessary for the teachers to make immediate judgements when trying to protect the students from harm. These, sometimes also ethical, questions are solved for instance when a teacher has a reason to believe that a student carries a weapon in school or is breaking the law or norm in another way [18].

According to the WHO, safety is a condition where factors that are a threat to a society are managed in such a way that citizens have the opportunity to gain welfare and well-being. Safety is also seen as a condition where one is free from danger. In English, the concept 'safety' has two separate meanings. 'Safety' implies a human aspect and freedom from accident or injury, while 'security' implies deliberateness or intent, and being protected from dangers. The word 'safety' is frequently used in connection with accidents and the word 'security' is used to refer to protection against undesirable threats [33, 34]. Niemelä and Lahikainen [35] state that safety and security include for instance economic, social, cultural, infrastructural or criminal dimensions. The definition of safety does not only include knowledge but also competence such as survival from risks, for instance traffic or fire, with decent and appropriate behavior. These competencies demand sustainable measures, both proactive and reactive, carried out in the organization [4, 6].

It is also stated, that the health and safety services are fragmented across a variety of operators such as authorities, organizations and the private sector. To understand safety can be challenging also because it is acting with non-events - events that never happened. Sometimes the subjective dimension of personal safety is better understood through the definition of insecurity that affects the most vulnerable groups and can be related to gender, age, ethnicity or victim experience [34, 36]. In this study, safety is seen as a broad concept, one form of well-being and a basic value of life. Although an individual's values may change during the life, safety is considered as a basic value [37]. Further on safety can be seen as life satisfaction and fulfilment. Student support, school safety and academic achievements are often discussed separately, but researchers state that the concepts are interactive, for example, school safety is one correlate of attendance and academic achievement [38]. Both safety theories and learning environment research distinguish [35] physical, mental and social dimensions of safety. These dimensions create the framework for this curriculum content study.

From former results of the research we know that the pupils need safety related skills and that the learning environment should be developed to prevent school injuries and violence. The safety should be part of the every-day measures and the culture of well-being [39], because the curriculum always reflects the values of the surrounding society [40] and safety can be seen as one of the basic values [37]. To fulfill the law a teacher needs knowledge and skills on various dimensions of safety. Curriculum related safety education includes learning about hazards, risk management, personal health and safety as well as interpersonal skills and emotions related to risk-taking and problem solving. These are included in most of the safety education programs. On the whole, safety education programs aim to bridge the gap between knowledge and behavioral transformation. Safety education programs consist basically of three objectives: awareness raising, social skills and behavior modification approaches that aim to reduce risk-taking [19]. The safety skills are needed to enhance and sustain safety at school. Also in case of unintentional injuries teachers need appropriate safety skills for first aid. In emergencies at the learning environment the teacher is sometimes the only adult to respond. In addition, the teacher also needs safety knowledge as a content of teaching. University teachers as well as prospective teachers make ongoing, conscious or subconscious, decisions about how to adjust the curriculum content to the classroom reality as teachers work as a messenger between the written and the enacted [41, 42] curriculum. Many researchers state that there is a theory-practice gap in the area of professional development [43]. Teacher education should prepare prospective teachers for professional skills. In order to guide teaching, explicit objectives for skills should be set. The group of experts state firstly that both knowledge and skills should be ensured [26] and secondly that citizen skills will be defined as part of the general national objectives by the new basic education decree. In Finland the citizen skills will be included in the objectives of multi-disciplinary subject groups and of separate school subjects. Safety contents may be included in the group of "Self-awareness and personal responsibility" [27].

4   Teacher Education Curriculum as a Context of This Study

The description of teacher education curriculum is presented here, firstly, because it is the most important strategic guiding document in the teacher education studies, and secondly, because here it serves as the basic data being an essential part of the context description. Curriculum is here seen as a document of official (state) and expert (academic) discourses. Curriculum theory sees teacher education as engaging and practicing teachers in interdisciplinary studies located at the intersections of self and society, the school subjects and everyday life [44]. At the university the curriculum represents the aims and contents of what the students should learn. Written curriculum is often seen instructive as it represents the official status of an institution and what it stands for. In addition it binds the students to the contents of teaching [8, 45]. Curriculum has a dual representation in the educational system, of which also the teacher education is an essential part. Firstly, it is a strategic guiding document with a legislative background and secondly the curriculum is considered to be a tool for teaching with pedagogical background, pedagogical thinking and activities. The curriculum in teacher education is understood as a mediating construction between teacher educators and the social context and it includes characters of global discourses and local actors [45]. What it comes to teacher education, the curriculum is often seen as a part of prospective teacher's professional growth. The curriculum is considered to be a major guideline for teacher education and it is based on the legislation that gives a pedagogic frame for teacher education. From previous studies we know that there is considerable variation between teacher education institutions since the universities in Finland hold academic autonomy when establishing the written curricula. Depending on the administration of the university the curriculum is approved within the university. Both the approval and the pedagogical content are based on the expertise of professors, academics or faculty members. Also part of the autonomy is the specialization of expertise depending on the university. The ethos in Finnish schools and also in teacher education is very much one of professional accountability. Values and an understanding of what is best for the learners and teacher students are shared and embedded into the school or university culture, thus making formalised evaluation unnecessary. It has to be noted that also the definitions around the curriculum may vary, for instance some teacher education units call the curriculum a study plan whereas others name it as a study guide, study program or general degree requirement [46, 47]. The study material in this study is the comprehensive studies content of the written curriculum in one teacher education unit in Finland.

As mentioned before, enhancing safety in educational context means not just theoretical background and attitude, but also ability to act [48] On the national level in Finland there are various multi-sectoral target programs promoting safety and security, for instance *Programme for preventing injuries at home and in leisure 2014–2020* that strengthens the regional and local work on the prevention of injuries. In the target program, special attention is paid on acts and measures. For instance the municipalities and the Association of Finnish Local and Regional Authorities and NGO's are expected to carry out a total of 92 actions on injury prevention. These measures include for instance injury prevention education as part of the basic and supplementary training of the teachers [49]. The other crucial strategic program is *The national action plan for injury prevention among children and youth.* It discusses what should be done to reduce health problems in key arenas of the everyday lives of children and young people, such as preventing unintentional injuries in the school environment, providing safety education and enhancing safety in schools [50] It can be quite clearly stated that Finland has a strong leadership to support the existing infrastructure, learning and values on children's and adolescents' safety. In addition, in the field of education, one of the problems is the dominance of the knowledge-focused school subjects [27]. Also at the strategic level, there is an urgent need for implementation that supports the idea of practical measures taken towards phronesis in safety, which in this study is seen as a variety of safety related knowledge that is based on competence, but includes the ability to respond in emergency situations and acts in the prevention. On the whole teacher's safety competence demands theoretical and contextual knowledge, but also skills and abilities as well as beliefs and moral values [51]. The attainment of theoretical and contextual knowledge continues to be essential for teachers, and a broad concept of competence as inclusive of knowledge and understanding, skills and abilities is adopted, as well as of teachers' beliefs and moral values.

This study explores the curriculum safety discourses with three questions: How can the skills and knowledge be distinguished at the teacher education curriculum texts? What kind of safety discourses are found in the teacher education curriculum? and secondly, How well do these discourses serve the idea of phronesis, the practical wisdom in safety?

5   Methods

The discourse presented in the teacher education curriculum of one teacher education unit, is here seen from the viewpoint of neo-Aristotelianism that recognizes traditional knowledge, *episteme*, pragmatic variable, *techne*, and further on *phronesis*, practical wisdom. The focus in this study is how the curriculum supports the prospective teacher's developmental aims towards phronesis, which is an Aristotelian concept emphasizing deliberation and moral action [9]. The teacher education curricula are renewed in each of the teacher education units in Finland about after every three years to be able to adapt to the change of the surrounding society and in a best possible way to respond to the new challenges and changing learning environment. As stated earlier the universities and the faculties hold their academic autonomy also when designing the curriculum. The practical power in the university is wielded by the faculty council. In Finland the faculty council consists mostly of the academics such as professors and other faculty members and of administration staff and it decides about the curriculum and student intake [51]. Here, the curriculum of one teacher education unit is analyzed with methods of discourse analysis.

Discourse analysis is often used in the qualitative studies to analyze texts and as a method, it is seen as a social process. The method is the study of the ways in which language is used in texts or discussions. Discourse analysis focuses on language as the primary instrument through which dominant understandings are transmitted, enacted and reproduced According to Fairclough and Wodak [52] "discourse analysis sees itself not as dispassionate and objective social science, but as engaged and committed". Rogers [53] suggests that there is no formula for conducting discourse analysis. Van Dijk [54] states that there cannot be a complete discourse analysis, because there are so many relevant units, dimensions, strategies, and other structures of discourse. Discourse analysis focuses on language as the primary instrument through which dominant understandings are transmitted, enacted and reproduced [see also 53]. In this study, the discourse analytic model is not strictly followed, yet using the concept of discourse analysis it can be studied where the exact focus exists in the teacher education curriculum texts.

The data for the survey consisted of 80 (N = 80) curriculum courses written for the class teacher education program in one teacher education unit, including bachelor and master level studies. Out of these, 33 study courses were voluntary or minor subject studies. The data consisted of study courses representing a total of 247 study points when minor subject studies were excluded. The data analysis was carried out in several phases being typical in qualitative approach studies, since the research material is here qualitative and there are no previous this type of research of the documents. The data was written in a form of initial matrix with all the course descriptions of the teacher education. The study material consisted of the aims and contents of the teacher education curriculum texts in comprehensive studies. The study material, such as or further readings or any other text presented at the teacher education curriculum was excluded from the data. In the data, the meaning units that were counted as safety related, were courses with the word or word cluster concerning safety, security, protect, bullying, risk, harassment, first aid, injury, group dynamic, interaction and the proper use of materials or machinery were used.

The data was progressed from singular units towards meaning systems and was based on repetitive meanings in the documents. The case study here was to analyze the teacher education curriculum texts and how safety in a practical manner is emphasized in the curriculum. A special attention was paid to verbs of the curriculum texts. In the very first phase the data was collected by reading the curriculum texts carefully and the matrix was drawn to find the characteristics of safety contents. In the second phase the collection of verbs was analyzed and categorized. Further on the data was divided in two sections for the purposes of this study. Attention was paid especially to the verbs of the text, which were divided in two groups whether the verb referred to the cognitive dimension (knowing) or practical skill-related activities (doing). The meaning units were translated into English. The meaning units were organized to two matrixes, one with the knowledge (K) and the other with the skills (S).

In the third phase these two groups were analyzed separately to get a deeper picture of the curriculum content. The analytic unit was either a word (e.g. *understands, argument*) or few words together, word cluster (e.g. *practice working methods, orientate to interaction skills*).

6 Results

The case study here was to analyze the teacher education curriculum texts and how safety in a practical manner is emphasized in the curriculum. A special attention was paid to verbs of the curriculum texts (see Table 1). Out of 80 (N = 80) study courses offered 23 included words or meanings related to safety. There were total 41 (f = 41) meaning units found in the data, 66% (17) referring to knowledge (K) and 34% (14) for the practical skills (S).

Table 1. Examples of the meaning units related to knowledge (K) and skill (S) dimensions in the teacher education curricula.

Knowledge (K)	Skills (S)
to analyze	to enhance
to argument	to practice
to evaluate	to practice working methods
to discuss	to develop
to perceive	to develop the use
to master knowledge	to learn
to consider	to learn to design practices
to describe	to take into account
to realize	to support the participation
is able to interpret	to orientate to conduct
is able to consider critically	to orientate to working methods
to get acquainted	to orientate to interaction skills
to deepen	to get acquainted with
to consider	to try to enhance
to recognize	to construct action
to have readiness to take into account	to apply
to have readiness to design	the readiness to use
to understand	the readiness to support
to understand the meaning of skills	
to project	

Meaning units in knowledge based contents contained verbs such as *analyze, argument, evaluate, discuss, perceive*. All these meaning units indicated the knowledge

(K) dimension that the prospective teacher would gain by learning the curriculum. In the other group the meaning units that indicated connections to practical doing or skill (S) dimension were distinguished, such as to practice, enhance, develop and get acquainted.

These verbs indicated that prospective teacher should learn to do something.

Further on, the safety discourses of the curriculum texts were analyzed to find whether there were repetitive meanings in the data. In the overlaps, the same kind of text was found in many courses, and during the analysis, it became evident that some expressions of language appeared in the most of the data. This was the key to formulate the discourses.

The content of the knowledge-based curriculum texts represent prospective teachers' safety competencies in the light of interaction and group dynamics. In the curriculum texts prospective teacher *"recognizes the social, group dynamic and cultural phenomenon"*; *the student is able to "reflect the interaction and group dynamics and socio-cultural phenomenon and reflect them in the light of the theoretical knowledge"* and the prospective teacher *"is able to recognize the group dynamic phenomena and reflects them"*. He or she is able to reflect the group dynamics and interaction critically. The prospective teacher is also able to research and document the interaction in the classroom.

The texts emphasize the interaction towards the class, the school, colleagues and society, even media and other social surroundings in school context. This hegemonic repertoire of the curriculum discourse was part of the practical training as well as seminar and courses offered as comprehensive to all elementary teachers at the unit.

The other part of the data consisted of meaning units that were based on practical skills. Also these contents were strongly emphasized by the interaction and group dynamics. In the seminar and practical training activities the curriculum text pointed out that *"the student is able to build a positive teacher-student interaction"* or in the pedagogic seminar *"the student is able to use observation of interaction and group dynamics as a research method"*. The data included that the prospective student gets acquainted with web-based interaction. Also the student *"gets acquainted with the mediating society and what it means for the psychological well-being of an individual"*. In the skills based safety discourse the interaction was emphasized as well: the student *"is getting acquainted with the group dynamics"* and *"is able to conduct flexible behavior in the interaction situations in the classroom"*. The skills related curriculum discourse focused on interaction in multiple ways and levels: in between the prospective teachers, teacher-students, teacher-class, teacher-school and teacher-society, such as media and the web. In addition the practical skills were mentioned in the crafts education: the student *"is able to use the machinery safely"*. This was mentioned in both textile and technical craft courses.

Very clear discursive practice, interaction and group dynamics, was revealed in this case study where the data consisted of class teacher education studies. Based on this study it seems evident that Finnish teacher education has its knowledge basis in the educational and behavioral sciences that are strongly tied to social processes, such as interaction and group dynamics. This repertoire was found in both the dimensions, knowledge and skills.

7 Conclusions

Teacher education should prepare and support the prospective teachers according to the curriculum aims and goals. It is also stated that teachers need skills for interaction in various learning environments [27]. The aim of this qualitative study was also to understand the knowledge and skills based safety discourses in the teacher education curriculum to enhance the safety and well-being in the school context. The safety content of the curriculum was analyzing the verbs of the curriculum texts by classifying the meaning units in two dimensions. The two groups that were established were knowledge and skill dimensions. Teacher education in Finland has its roots in academic principles and therefore it is understandable that 2/3 of the meaning units found were knowledge based. These two groups were studied separately to find out what kind of safety discourses could be found at the curriculum text.

Practice is, as Higgs put it [24] doing, knowing, being and becoming, yet *wisdom* is more knowing through experiences, learning and reflecting. In this study the social dimension was strongly focused in all the curriculum texts indicating that interaction skills and group dynamics are an integral part of teacher professionalism what it comes to safety. The analysis showed that at the both groups the curriculum used substantially more text to describe group dynamics and social issues than safety competences in the other areas.

In the light of this study on teacher's safety competence to catch phronesis, it can be drawn a conclusion that the safety discourse in the teacher education curriculum is dominated by interaction and group dynamics discourse. In the curriculum contents, the prospective teacher needed interactive skills in various forms, for instance in the class room, in the society and with the media. If the Neo-Aristotelian point of view in safety is seen, like here, as a practical competence that means ability to react, notice and respond to the risks and ability to prevent accidents and violence, teacher education curriculum does support to catch the phronesis only partially. The data pointed out that safety was included in the curriculum and could therefore be seen as a value in teacher education [40], hence the focus was very strongly in the interactive skills and the group dynamics.

The view presented here is not meant to be privileged or replace other views, but to enrich our understandings of the complexity of science teacher knowledge and practice and the central role of teacher judgment. Phronesis and virtue epistemology can provide a framework for understanding the moral dimension of science teachers' knowledge and their intimate relation to content knowledge and pedagogical knowledge. Phronesis gives us ideas of professional development and practice, yet the knowledge base for teaching whether a teacher or a teacher student, is not final. The view presented here is not meant to replace other views, but anyway it may enrich our understanding the complexity of the teaching practices [55]. It may also be true that phronesis is not the answer to the central professional dilemmas. However, to support prospective teachers to fulfill the value of safety [37], practical issues should be taken into account. Official documents are instructive as they represent the public face of an institution and what it stands for and on the other hand, the study program handbook is one of the rare documents that bind the students to the contents of teaching [8]. This analysis suggests that both knowledge and skills in the written curriculum were connected to social dimensions of safety and well-being, such as group dynamics or interaction.

The safety and well-being discourse in the curriculum was presented well what it comes to competence in interaction and group dynamics and therefore it is evident that the curriculum gives the prospective teacher a possibility to achieve the phronesis in this dimension. However, safety discourse remained somewhat one-sided and incomplete. It seems that teacher education curriculum and the requirements in target programs for promoting and enhancing the safety culture differ in focus. Safety and well-being as a broad concepts consist of various points of views, for example economic, cultural, technical, infrastructural or criminal. The curriculum being a strategic, conducting and guiding document should serve contents of safety broader. There were no meaning units found on fire or traffic safety, safety in buildings, sexual harassment, self-harm, cyber safety or violence in the comprehensive studies in the teacher education curriculum in one of the ten teacher education units in Finland. To serve and support the prospective teachers better, teacher education units should provide safety courses that are focused also on practices and skills, for instance how to respond injuries, such as emergency call or first aid, injury and near-miss case reporting, traffic safety, safety management or structural safety and to conduct fire-drills or lock-downs at school facilities. In addition, the content of the curriculum should be based on the safety issues where monitoring the risks and injuries, injury prevention and decent respond abilities and finally – achieving phronesis in safety, would become possible.

8 Limitations

The current survey, focuses on and is limited to the written curriculum of only one teacher education unit as a case. Since the universities and teacher education units hold their autonomy, this study may not represent the whole picture of the area in the country. However, in the teacher education curricula more attention should be paid to the safety discourse and to the safety skills to bridge the gap between skills and knowledge and to better support prospective teachers to catch the phronesis.

Acknowledgements. The writer of this article wants to thank for the Finnish Fire Protection Fund for the support of this study.

References

1. BJS. Bureau of Justice Statistics. Indicators of School Crime and Safety: 2012. National Center of Educational Statistics. NCES 2013-036. U.S. Department of Education (2012)
2. Helsingin Sanomat, Helsinki times: Gunman sprayed bullets in classroom and corridor, and threw petrol bombs. http://www.helsinkitimes.fi/. Accessed 24 Sept 2008
3. BBC News: Fatal shooting at finnish school. BBC News, 07 November 2007. http://news.bbc.co.uk/2/hi/europe/7082795.stm. Accessed 13 Apr 2016
4. Reiman, T., Oedewald, P.: Turvallisuuskulttuuri [Safety Culture]. VTT Publications, Espoo (2008)

5. Waitinen, M.: Turvallinen koulu? Helsinkiläisten peruskoulujen turvallisuuskulttuurista ja siihen vaikuttavista tekijöistä. Doctoral dissertation: Safe School: Safety culture in basic education. University of Helsinki/Unigrafia, Helsinki (2011)
6. Somerkoski, B.: Learning outcome assessment: cross-curricular theme safety and traffic in basic core curriculum. J. Mod. Educ. Rev. **5**, 588–597 (2015)
7. Halinen, I. (2015). www.oph.fi/download/151294_ops2016_curriculum_reform_in_finland.pdf
8. Phelan, A.: Curriculum Theorizing and Teacher Education: Complicating Conjunctions. Routledge, London (2015)
9. Aristoteles: Nikomakhoksen etiikka [Nikomakheans Etics] (S. Knuuttila, Trans.). Gaudeamus, Tampere (1989)
10. Tiberius, V.: The Reflective Life: Living Wisely with our Limits. Oxford University Press, Oxford (2008)
11. Tiberius, V., Swartwood, J.: Wisdom revisited: a case study in normative theorizing. Philos. Explor. **14**, 277–295 (2011)
12. Gunder, M.: Making planning theory matter: a lacanian encounter with phronesis. Int. Plann. Stud. **15**, 37–51 (2010)
13. Jansson, N.: Discourse phronesis in organizational change: a narrative analysis. J. Organ. Change Manag. **27**, 769–779 (2014)
14. Aristotle: The Nicomachean ethics (T. Irwin, Trans.). Hackett, Indianapolis (1999)
15. Jope, G.: Grasping phronesis: the fabric of discernment in becoming an ethical teacher. Doctoral Dissertation. The University of British Columbia, Vancouver, Canada (2014). http://circle.ubc.ca/bitstream/handle/2429/46659/ubc_2014_september_jope_gilmour.pdf?sequence=1
16. Bradley, B.: Rethinking experience in professional practice: lessons from clinical psychology. In: Green, B. (ed.) Understanding and Researching Professional Practice, pp. 65–82. SensePublishers, Rotterdam (2009)
17. Loftus, S., Higgs, J.: Health professional education in the future. In: Loftus, S., Gerzina, T., Higgs, J., Smith, M., Duffy, E. (eds.) Educating Health Professionals: Becoming a University Teacher, pp. 323–334. SensePublishers, Rotterdam (2013)
18. Ellet, F.: Practical rationality and a recovery of Aristotle's phronesis. In: Kinsella, E., Pitman, A. (eds.) Phronesis as Professional Knowledge. Practical Wisdom in the Professions, pp. 13–33. SensePublishers, Rotterdam (2012)
19. Schearn, P.: Teaching practice in safety education: qualitative evidence. Res. Pap. Educ. **21**, 335–359 (2006). http://www.tandfonline.com/doi/abs/10.1080/02671520600793799
20. Hibbert, K.: Cultivating capacity: phronesis, learning, and diversity in professional education. In: Kinsella, E., Pitman, A. (eds.) Phronesis as Professional Knowledge. Practical Wisdom in the Professions, pp. 61–71. SensePublishers, Rotterdam (2012)
21. Chistie, F.: Phronesis and the practice of science. In: Kinsella, E., Pitman, A. (eds.) Phronesis as Professional Knowledge. Practical wisdom in the Professions, pp. 101–114. SensePublishers, Rotterdam (2012)
22. Jones, C.: Care and phronesis in teaching and coaching: dealing with personality disorder. Sport Educ. Soc. **22**(2), 214–229 (2015)
23. Flyvbjerg, B.: Making Social Science Matter: Why Social Inquiry Falls and How it can Succeed Again. Cambridge University Press, Cambridge (2001)
24. Higgs, J.: Realising practical wisdom from the pursuit of wise practice. In: Kinsella, E., Pitman, A. (eds.) Phronesis as Professional Knowledge. Practical wisdom in the professions, pp. 73–86. SensePublishers, Rotterdam (2012)
25. Vaara, E., Whittington, R.: Strategy-as-practice: taking social practices seriously. Acad. Manag. Ann. **6**, 285–336 (2012)

26. Loughran, J.: Enacting pedagogy of teacher education. In: Russel, T., Loughran, J. (eds.) Values, Relationships and Practices. Enacting Pedagogy of Teacher Education, pp. 1–15. Routledge, Oxon (2007)
27. OKM: Ministry of Culture and Education. Perusopetus 2020 – yleiset valtakunnalliset tavoitteet ja tuntijako. [Core Curriculum and Aims in Basic Education] Opetus- ja kulttuuriministeriön työryhmämuistioista ja selvityksiä 2010:1. Yliopistopaino, Helsinki (2010). www.minedu.fi/export/sites/default/OPM/Julkaisut/2010/liitteet/okmtr01.pdf?lang= En. Accessed 13 Apr 2016
28. Pitman, A.: Professionalism and professionalization: hostile ground for growing phronesis. In: Kinsella, E., Pitman, A. (eds.) Phronesis as Professional Knowledge. Practical wisdom in the Professions, pp. 131–146. SensePublishers, Rotterdam (2012)
29. FNAE a Finnish National Agency for Education. Core Curricula and Qualifications. http://www.oph.fi/english/curricula_and_qualifications. Accessed 13 Apr 2016
30. Spence, S.: phronesis and the student teacher. J. Educ. Thought (JET)/Revue De La Pensée Éducative 41(3), 311–322 (2007). http://www.jstor.org/stable/23765525
31. FNBE: Finnish National Board of Education. www.oph.fi/download/154491_Teacher_ Education_in_Finland.pdf. Accessed 23 Apr 2017
32. Basic Education Act Section 29. http://www.finlex.fi/en/laki/kaannokset/1998/en19980628. pdf. Accessed 11 Nov 2017
33. WHO: World Health Organization. Safety and Safety Promotion. Conceptual and Operational Aspects (1998). www.inspq.qc.ca/pdf/publications/150_SecurityPromotion.pdf . Accessed 15 Nov 2017
34. Somerkoski, B., Lillsunde, P.: Safe community designation as quality assurance in local security planning. In: Saranto, K., Castrén, M., Kuusela, T., Hyrynsalmi, S., Ojala, S. (eds.) Safe and Secure Cities. Communications in Computer and Information Science, vol. 450, pp. 194–202. Springer, Cham (2014). https://doi.org/10.1007/978-3-319-10211-5_20
35. Niemelä, P., Lahikainen, A.: Inhimillinen turvallisuus [Human Safety and Security]. Kirjakas, Tallinna (2002)
36. Welander, G., Svanström, L., Ekman, R.: Safety Promotion - An Introduction, 2nd edn. Karolinska Institutet, Stockholm (2004)
37. Helkama, K.: Suomalaisten arvot: Mikä meille on oikeasti tärkeää? [Finnish values: What is really important for us?] Suomalaisen Kirjallisuuden Seura, Helsinki (2015)
38. Barton, P.: Parsing the Achievement Gap: Baselines For Tracking Progress. Educational Testing Service, Princeton (2003)
39. Jukarainen, P., Syrjäläinen, E., Värri, V.-M.: Kohti turvallista ja hyvinvoivaa koulua – Valvontaa, vastuuta ja elämää erilaisuuden kanssa [Towards safety and wellbeing in the school – monitoring, responsibility and living with difference]. Kasvatus 43, 244–253 (2012)
40. Yrjänäinen, S.: Koulu ja vastuulliseen kansalaisuuteen kasvattaminen [School and bringing up citizenship]. In: Mäkinen, J. (ed.) Asevelvollisuuden tulevaisuus, vol. 9, pp. 118–132 (2013)
41. Törnroos, J.: Curriculum, textbooks, and achievement – grade 7 mathematics achievement under assessment. Doctoral dissertation. University of Jyväskylä, Jyväskylä. Institute for Educational Research. Research Reports 13, pp. 19—25 (2005). https://jyx.jyu.fi/dspace/ bitstream/handle/123456789/37534/978-951-39-3226-8.pdf?sequence=1. Accessed 15 Jan 2018
42. Pinar, W., Reynolds, W., Slattery, P., Taubman, P.: Understanding Curriculum: An Introduction to the Study of Historical and Contemporary Curriculum Discourses. Peter Lang Publishing, Bern (1995)

43. Ross, W., Mathison, S., Vinson, K.: Social studies curriculum and teaching in the era of standardization. In: Ross, W. (ed.) The Social Studies Curriculum. Purposes, Problems, and Possibilities, 4th edn, pp. 25–49. State University of New York Press, Albany (2014)
44. Pinar, W.: What is curriculum? (2004). http://www.khuisf.ac.ir/DorsaPax/userfiles/file/motaleat/0805848274.pdf
45. Hökkä, P., Eteläpelto, A., Rasku-Puttonen, H.: Recent tensions and challenges in teacher education as manifested in curriculum discourse. Teach. Teach. Educ. **26**, 845–853 (2010)
46. Universities Act Finlex (2009). https://www.finlex.fi/en/laki/kaannokset/2009/en20090558.pdf
47. Vitikka, E., Salminen, J., Annevirta, T.: Opetussuunnitelma opettajankoulutuksessa [Curriculum in the teacher education]. Opetushallitus. Muistiot 2012:4 (2012)
48. Somerkoski, B.: Turvallisuus yläkoululaisen kokemana [Safety from the perspective of secondary students]. In: Mäkinen, J. (ed.) Asevelvollisuuden tulevaisuus, vol. 9, pp. 133–143. Maanpuolustuskorkeakoulu, Helsinki (2013)
49. STM Koti- ja vapaa-ajan tapaturmien ehkäisyn kansallinen tavoiteohjelma vuosille 2014—2020 [The national programme for preventing injuries at home and in leisure activities 2014—2020]. Publications of the Ministry of Social Affairs and Health 2013:16 (2013). www.stm.fi/julkaisut
50. THL: Providing a safe environment for our children and young people Finland's national action plan for injury prevention among children and youths. In: Markkula, J., Öörni, E. (eds.) Turvallinen elämä lapsille ja nuorille (2009). https://www.julkari.fi/bitstream/handle/10024/80158/bcda07c2-aa23-4faa-a59d-55a60fdc6764.pdf?sequence=1
51. University of Lapland Opinto-opas. [Curriculum for the University of Lapland]. Kasvatustieteiden tiedekunta 2012—2013. Lapin yliopistopaino, Rovaniemi (2012)
52. Fairclough, N., Wodak, R.: Critical discourse analysis. In: van Dijk, T. (ed.) Discourse as Social Interaction: Discourse Studies, vol. 2, pp. 258 – 284. Sage, London (1997, 2012)
53. Rogers, R.: An introduction to critical discourse analysis in education. In: Rogers, R. (ed.) An Introduction to Critical Discourse Analysis in Education. Lawrence Erlbaum Associates, Mahwah (2004)
54. van Dijk, T.: Critical discourse analysis. In: Tannen, D., Schiffrin, D., Hamilton, H. (eds.) Handbook of Discourse Analysis, pp. 352–371. Blackwell, Oxford (2001)
55. Salloum, S.: The place of practical wisdom in science education: what can belearned from Aristotelian ethics and a virtue-based theory of knowledge. Cult. Stud. Sci. Educ. **12**, 355 (2017). https://doi.org/10.1007/s11422-015-9710-8

Digital Disability Divide in Finland

Anne-Marie Tuikka[1]([⊠]), Hannu Vesala[2], and Antti Teittinen[2]

[1] University of Turku (Turun yliopisto), 20014 Turku, Finland
anne-marie.tuikka@utu.fi, amstou@utu.fi
[2] Finnish Association on Intellectual and Developmental Disabilities FAIDD,
Helsinki, Finland

Abstract. The modern societies have become more and more digitalized during recent years. Owning a digital device and accessing internet at home are part of everyday life, while many essential services, such as banking, are offered through internet. However, advances in digital technologies have not affected everybody similarly and there can still be groups of people who do not use internet on daily bases. Hence, we concentrates on studying the digital divide from specific viewpoint – the one of people with disabilities. Prior studies indicate that their possibilities to access and use internet are lower than for people without disabilities. This gap is referred as digital disability divide.

This study employs a quantitative approach to analyse digital disability divide in technologically advanced society. Our data is retrieved from a nationwide survey, which was conducted in Finland during years 2012–2015 by National Institute for Health and Welfare. The data was analysed regarding two main aspects: access to internet and use of internet. The analyses focused on people with disabilities and their family members. The results indicate that both access rate and usage of internet are lower among them than the rest of the population.

Keywords: People with disabilities · Disabled people · Digital divide
Disability divide · Digital disability divide · Finland

1 Introduction

Usage of internet and digital devices are normal things in today's developed societies. Most of the citizens in these societies except that they can access the world's biggest repository of knowledge on any given time. Governments have also been interested in getting benefits from these new technologies for few decades, which has led to different plans and projects to digitalize governmental services including public administration and social services. Digitalization have also spread to health care and education sectors, which are part of governmental services in Nordic welfare states.

In developed countries, these services are generally organized through digital mediums, although not all efforts to digitalize them have been successful. There are also more and more services, which citizens can access directly through internet. If a citizen joins some activity organized by governmental services provider (such as school) they may need to use digital devices to perform that activity. As such, it seems possible to say, that digital societies already exists today. However, this raises the concern, whether all citizens have equal access to services and possibilities offered by these societies.

H. Li et al. (Eds.): WIS 2018, CCIS 907, pp. 162–173, 2018.
https://doi.org/10.1007/978-3-319-97931-1_13

This is an important topic from the viewpoint of people with disabilities. According to previous studies, people with disabilities have faced challenges in independent use of internet [1]. Because people with disabilities often need to use internet through personalized devices and user interfaces, they may be restricted to use computers at home. For the same reason, the set-up cost is higher and there may be need for special technical support. When people with disabilities are able to access internet, it can affect their experiences of agency [2]. Digitalization of the society also affects the parents whose children have disabilities. Højberg and Jeppesen [3] found out that parents of children with disabilities benefitted from virtual networking.

Without access to internet, person cannot benefit from the services and engagement possibilities offered by it. Availability, accessibility and usage of internet among people with disabilities are of interest for research on digital divides. In Nordic countries, such as Finland, internet access is generally high among population [4], however the research on the internet access among people with disabilities and their families remains scarce. According to European Union level studies, Finland has an apparent gap between people with disabilities and people without disabilities in relation to accessing internet at home [5]. For this reason, this study aims to expand our knowledge on the digital disability divide in Finland. To study this topic, we have used data from a nationwide survey, which was conducted by National Institute for Health and Welfare. Data from this survey gave us opportunity to study the access to internet and the use of digital services among people with disabilities and their families. Hence, our research question is: "does access to internet and use of internet differ between people, who need disability service, and the rest of the population?"

2   Literature Review

2.1   Digital Divides

Digital divides have been studied for a long time and prior research has shown that there are different types of digital divides. From one perspective, a digital divide can be understood as a phenomenon, which exists between countries that differ in their level of technological advancements and access to ICT. Such a gap can also be found between the member states of European Union [6]. Cruz-Jesus et al. [4] have identified five clusters of countries which differ in their digital development in relation to ICT infrastructure, adoption of ICT among population and the cost of e-business and internet access. Finland, Denmark, Sweden, the Netherlands, and Luxembourg represent the digital leaders where ICT infrastructure is in good level, most of the population has adopted ICT and the cost of e-business and internet access is low. Romania and Bulgaria represent the polar opposite of these countries and are defined as the digital laggards of European Union.

However, digital divides can also exist within countries between groups of people who may differ in their ethnicity, age, education or economical resources. Cruz-Jesus et al. [7] have studied the relationship between digital divide and education level within European Union. They found out that digital divide is lowest between medium and low education levels in Finland and in Romania, whereas the lowest digital divide between high and low education levels is found in Denmark and in Sweden.

The research on digital divide is shifting from studying "the haves" and "the have nots" to studying different type of users, who differ in their internet usage and online participation [8].

2.2   Digital Disability Divide

Prior studies have shown that people with disabilities use internet and own ICT less often than people without disabilities. This gap is one of the digital divides and it can be referred as digital disability divide [10] or as disability divide [9]. Digital disability divide has been observed in different countries during last ten years. In European Union, people with disabilities have 65% lower chance of having internet access at home than people without disabilities [5]. Living with other people increased internet access for people with disabilities more than for people without disabilities. The gap was narrowest in Sweden, Denmark, and the Netherlands, and widest in Greece, Portugal, and Romania. Finland has generally high levels of internet access, however only 61% of people with disabilities have internet access at home where as 88% of people without disabilities have it. Similar type of findings have been made outside Europe. In South Korea, people with disabilities have computers (74.1%) and smart devices (41.0%) less often than people without disabilities of whom 85.5 have access to computer and 74.4% to smart devices [11]. According to their results, people with disabilities also have lower skills to use computer than people without disabilities however in both groups people have better skills to use internet and perform tasks with smart phones.

One reason why people with disabilities may experience more barriers to access and use ICT compared with people without disabilities is that they may need assistive technologies to use them. For this reason, a person with disabilities may need to have more economical capital than a person without disabilities in order to access assistive technology in addition to accessing the required digital technology. People with disabilities also need disability-specific cultural digital capital to have the needed awareness of the assistive technology available for their needs [12].

In the case of people with intellectual disabilities, one reason for lack of access to ICT may be related to their housing arrangement such as living in the residential homes. In Sweden, there is a gap in the ownership and use of ICT between people living in residential homes and the rest of the population [13].

Despite the challenges of accessing and using ICT, internet usage has arisen among people with intellectual disabilities. They most commonly use it for leisure and social engagement [14]. Duplaga [15] have studied that people with intellectual disabilities use internet most often to check and send emails, and to use internet communicators. ICT has an important role in supporting empowerment and social participation especially for the young people with intellectual disabilities [16].

3   Research Method

The data (n = 89 777) used came from the Finnish national survey "The Health and Wellbeing of Adults" conducted by the National Institute for Health and Welfare in years 2012–2015 [17]. The survey was posted to random samples of adults of 20 years old or older. In 2015, the response rate was 53%.

Our study focused on the people with disabilities. However, the questionnaires did not include questions about the disability status of the respondent. Instead, the questionnaires included one question that we could use to identify our target group: "Have you during the last 12 months needed … Services for the disabled?" All those who answered this question by selecting one of the following alternatives were identified as part of our target group:

i. Would have needed, but service not received
ii. Have used, service was inadequate
iii. Have used, service was adequate

2357 (estimate; 2.7%) of the respondents were in need of the disability services. However, we do not know whether these respondents were themselves persons with disabilities or persons, who had other persons with disabilities in their household. We define this group as "people who live in households with the need of disability services." The number of respondents belonging to this group is not a representative sample of people with disabilities and their family members, because other data source indicate that approximately 6% of Finnish people receive disability benefits [18]. Data was analysed by using SPSS Complex Samples – method.

4   Results

Our analysis focuses to explore the access and use of internet among people, who live in households with the need of disability services (DS), and those who do not need these services. We named these two groups accordingly as "DS Needed" and "No DS". We are also examining differences within these groups based on gender, age, marital status, education, employment and economic situation.

The survey had two questions which were used to explore the access and use of internet:

1. Do you have an internet connection at your household?
2. Do you use internet connection for the following? (i) e-transactions; (ii) finding information.

As a whole, 83.4% of respondents says they have an internet connection at their household. Further, 81.5% says that they use internet either to e-transactions or to finding information. When we combine these, we find that in addition to those, who have an internet connection, 2.6% of all respondents are using internet. Probably they are using mobile devices or are using internet in public services, where internet is free, such as libraries. This means that 85.9% are internet users (have an internet connection and/or are using internet) and the rest 14.1% are non-users (do not have an internet connection and/or do not use internet).

Comparison of the internet usage between those who have needed services for disabled (DS Needed) and those who have not needed (No DS) reveals that there is a big difference between these groups (see Fig. 1). Among those who have needed services for disabled, only 69.9% are using internet compared to the 86.4% of the rest of respondents. This also means that almost one-third of the people needing disability services are outside the internet or do not have access to internet.

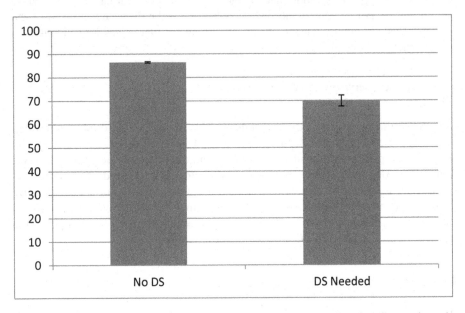

Fig. 1. Comparison of internet usage in groups according to the need for disability services: the percentages of internet users and 99% confidence intervals. (Chi square = 528,38, p < .001)

Next, we examine these group differences in subgroups based on gender, age, marital status, education, employment and economic situation. An overview of the background information of the respondents is available in Table 1.

4.1   Gender

In both groups (DS Needed and No DS) there is a significant gender-difference: men are more often using internet than women (see Fig. 2). Among men there seems not to be statistically significant difference between those who have needed disability services and those who have not, although the percentage of internet users is a little bit lower among those needing disability services. Among women there is a statistically significant difference between groups: women who have needed disability service use less internet than other women.

Table 1. Background information

	No. DS	DS needed
Gender: male	48.2%	43.9%
Age: 20–54 years	57.4%	41.4%
Age: 55–74 years	32.0%	34.4%
Age: 75 years or older	10.6%	24.3%
Lives in a relationship	80.6%	69.5%
Education level: low	44.1%	52.4%
Education level: medium	30.0%	25.5%
Education level: high	25.9%	22.1%
Employed (full-time or part-time)	49.0%	19.1%
Economic situation: covering costs easy	68.1%	53.1%

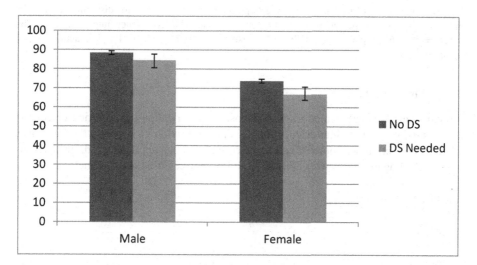

Fig. 2. Comparison of internet usage in groups according to the need for disability services among men and women: the percentages of internet users and 99% confidence intervals. (gender: Chi square = 32,62, p < .001; DS: Chi square = 296,25, p < .001; interaction: Chi square = 2.77 ns.)

4.2   Age

Results from both groups (DS Needed and No DS) were analysed in three age-groups: from 20 to 54 years, from 55–74 years and 75 years or older.

In both groups there are very clear and statistically significant age-group differences: among the youngest respondents (20–54 years) almost all, over 90% are using internet, while in the oldest age-group the internet users are in minority (see Fig. 3). However, in each age-group there are less internet users among those who need disability services than among those who do not need disability services, and all these differences are statistically significant.

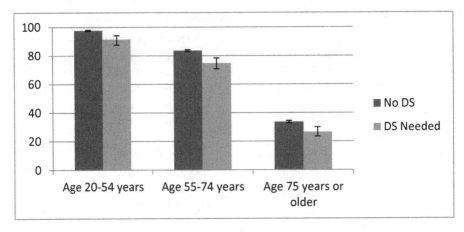

Fig. 3. Comparison of internet usage in groups according to the need for disability services in three age-groups: the percentages of internet users and 99% confidence intervals. (age: Chi square = 5268,65, p < .001; DS: Chi square = 89,27, p < .001; interaction: Chi square = 1.96 ns.)

4.3   Marital Status

Marital status was aggregated to two groups: (i) in a relationship (married or cohabiting) and (ii) no in a relationship (single, divorced, widow). Those who were in a relationship were much more often internet users, and this applies to both groups (see Fig. 4). And again, those who needed disability services used less internet.

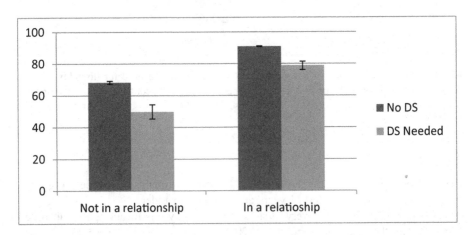

Fig. 4. Comparison of internet usage in groups according to the need for disability services according to marital status: the percentages of internet users and 99% confidence intervals.

4.4   Education

Education level (low, medium and high) was based on the years one had attended to school or studied full-time, and it has been weighted according to different age-groups. In both groups, the proportion of internet users was significantly lower for those who have low educational level than among those with medium or high educational level (see Fig. 5). However, the differences between those, who needed disability services and those who did not, were much more pronounced in each educational level.

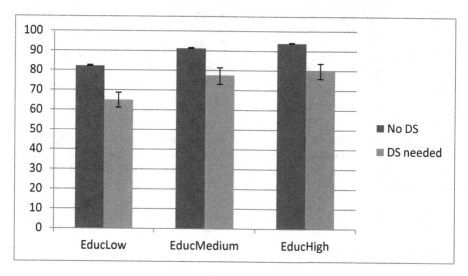

Fig. 5. Comparison of internet usage in groups according to the need for disability services in three education levels: the percentages of internet users and 99% confidence intervals. (education: Chi square = 181,85, p < .001; DS: Chi square = 283,36, p < .001; interaction: Chi square = 3.27 ns.)

4.5   Employment

Among those who are employed (either full-time or part-time), there was no difference between those who needed disability services and those who did not; almost all use internet (Fig. 6). However, among those were not employed, the percentages were much lower in both groups than among employed groups, and also the difference between groups of DS needed and No DS was statistically significant.

4.6   Economic Situation

Economic situation was evaluated by a question "A household may have different sources of income, and more than one of the people living in it may have an income. Considering the total income of your household, how difficult or easy is it to cover your costs?" Answer alternatives varied from "Very difficult" to "Very easy". This variable was reduced to two classes: (i) "difficult" and (ii) "easy". It seems that economic situation did not have much effect on the use of internet (see Fig. 7).

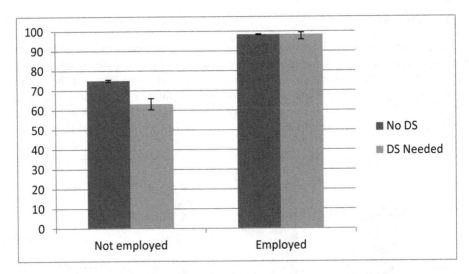

Fig. 6. Comparison of internet usage in groups according to the need for disability services according to employment status: the percentages of internet users and 99% confidence intervals (employment: Chi square = 2195,79, p < .001; DS: Chi square = 86,02, p < .001; interaction: Chi square = 88,89, p < .001)

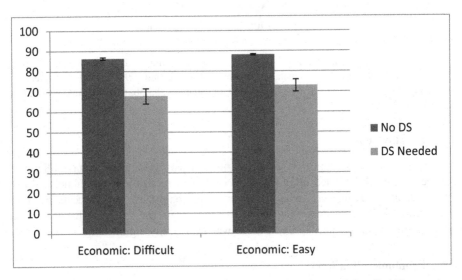

Fig. 7. Comparison of internet usage in groups according to the need for disability services according to economic situation: the percentages of internet users and 99% confidence intervals (economic situation: Chi square = 14,75, p < .001; DS: Chi square = 318,10, p < .001; interaction: Chi square = 3.12 ns.)

5 Discussion

Many studies have highlighted how important internet is for the empowerment and participation of people with disabilities. Internet can also offer valuable information sources and peer support for carers of people with disabilities. Possibilities to benefit from positive impacts of internet appear to be hindered for people who need disability services in Finland, because they have less often internet access at home and use internet less than Finnish people in general. This indicates that there could be a digital disability divide in Finland.

The gap between people with disabilities and people without disabilities can be partly explained by the different age structure. However, the need for disability services is related to the lack of internet access at home and to non-usage of internet in every age group. One possible explanation might be the housing arrangements. Some people with disabilities live in residential housing and might not have personal computer in their disposal.

Based don regression analysis and the Chi-square values, most powerful predictors of the internet usage are age, education level, employment, and marital status (see Table 2). The economic situation, the need of disability services and gender have less predictive power, but do still have statistically significant effect on the internet usage.

Table 2. Results of the regression analysis. Dependent variable: internet usage; independent variables: disability services, age, gender, marital status, education level, employment, economic situation.

Independent variables	Wald Chi-square	$p<$
Disability services	39,10	.001
Age	8774,14	.001
Gender	8,05	.01
Marital status	516,80	.001
Education level	2455,48	.001
Employment	849,44	.001
Economic situation	165,21	.001

This study has following limitations. First, the data was collected between years 2011 and 2015; hence, it might not reflect the current situation in Finland. Secondly, the explanative ability of the survey data is limited because the respondents, who have disabilities, cannot be completely separated from respondents whose family member has disability. This is due to design of the nationwide survey where the data was retrieved. The survey did not include a question about the experienced or diagnosed disability of the respondent. Adding this question for future surveys would improve the possibilities of using them for analysing results from the viewpoint of people with disabilities. In addition, there might be need for making distinction between different disabilities, because digital disability divide could appear between people who have different type of disabilities.

It is also obvious that the designers of the survey have not considered the disability issues. When one compares the different variants of the questionnaire according to age, it can be seen that questions dealing with the need of help are only posed to the eldest respondents; and also the possibility that questionnaire is filled as assisted or by someone else, is only provided for the eldest respondents. It seems that the questionnaire designers have taken into account the needs of ageing citizens, but at the same time totally ignored the existence of the people with disabilities as citizens in Finnish society. Hence, it is understandable that people with disabilities are under represented among the respondents of the survey.

Smart devices are used more and more in everyday life and they can make using internet easier for people with disabilities [11]. However, the impact of smart devices to digital disability divide could not be analysed in this study. The survey did not include any questions about smart devices neither did it make distinction between accessing internet through a computer or through a smart device. There is apparently a need for further research on this topic. Hence, questions related to penetration and use of smart devices would be valuable addition to any survey that aims to follow the development of digital disability divide.

References

1. Watling, S.: Digital exclusion: coming out from behind closed doors. Disabil. Soc. **26**(4), 491–495 (2011)
2. Näslund, R., Gardelli, Å.: 'I know, i can, i will try': youths and adults with intellectual disabilities in Sweden using information and communication technology in their everyday life. Disabil. Soc. **28**(1), 28–40 (2013)
3. Højberg, A.-L., Jeppesen, J.: Examining the effect of networks for students with special educational needs. Scand. J. Disabil. Res. **14**(2), 26–147 (2012)
4. Cruz-Jesus, F., Oliveira, T., Bacao, F.: Digital divide across the European union. Inf. Manag. **49**, 278–291 (2012)
5. Scholz, F., Yalcin, B., Priestley, M.: Internet access for disabled people: understanding socio-relational factors in Europe. Cyberpsychology: J. Psychosoc. Res. Cyberspace **11**(1), 13 p. (2017). https://doi.org/10.5817/CP2017-1-4
6. Çilan, Ç., Bolat, B.A., Coşkun, E.: Analyzing digital divide within and between member and candidate countries of European union. Gov. Inf. Q. **26**, 98–105 (2009)
7. Cruz-Jesus, F., Vicente, M.R., Bacao, F., Oliveira, T.: The education-related digital divide: an analysis for the EU-28. Comput. Hum. Behav. **56**, 72–82 (2016)
8. Brandtzæg, P.B.: Understanding the new digital divide—a typology of Internet users in Europe. Int. J. Hum.-Comput. Stud. **69**, 123–138 (2011)
9. Dobransky, K., Hargittai, E.: The disability divide in internet access and use. Inf. Commun. Soc. **9**(3), 313–334 (2006)
10. Sachdeva, N., Tuikka, A.-T., Kimppa, K.K., Suomi, R.: Digital disability divide in information society: a framework based on a structured literature review. J. Inf. Commun. Ethics Soc. **13**(3/4), 283–298 (2015)
11. Nam, S.-J., Park, E.-Y.: The effects of the smart environment on the information divide experienced by people with disabilities. Disabil. Health J. **10**, 257–263 (2017)

12. Newman, L., Browne-Yung, K., Raghavendra, P., Wood, D., Grace, E.: Applying a critical approach to investigate barriers to digital inclusion and online social networking among young people with disabilities. Inf. Syst. J. **27**, 559–588 (2017)
13. Swedish National Board of Health and Welfare: Still unequal – living conditions for people with functional impairments (2010). http://www.socialstyrelsen.se/publikationer2010/2010-6-21. Accessed 27 Mar 2018
14. Chiner, E., Gómez-Puerta, M., Cardona-Moltó, M.C.: Internet use, risks and online behaviour: the view of internet users with intellectual disabilities and their caregivers. Br. J. Learn. Disabil. **45**, 190–197 (2017)
15. Duplaga, M.: Digital divide among people with disabilities: analysis of data from a nationwide study for determinants of Internet use and activities performed online. PLoS One **16**(6), 1–19 (2017)
16. Ramsten, C., Hammar, L.M., Martin, L., Göransson, K.: ICT and intellectual disability: a survey of organizational support at the municipal level in Sweden. J. Appl. Res. Intellect. Disabil. **30**, 705–713 (2017)
17. National Institute for Health and Welfare (THL). https://thl.fi/fi/tutkimus-ja-asiantuntijatyo/vaestotutkimukset/aikuisten-terveys-hyvinvointi-ja-palvelututkimus-ath/miten-ath-tutkimus-tehdaan. Accessed 13 Apr 2018
18. Kela. Kelan tilastollinen vuosikirja (2012)

Active Digiage? Desirable Futures
for Ageing People

Marina Weck[1(✉)], Tarja Meristö[2], and Nina Helander[3]

[1] Research Unit for Smart Services,
Häme University of Applied Sciences, Hämeenlinna, Finland
Marina.Weck@hamk.fi
[2] FuturesLab CoFi, Laurea University of Applied Sciences,
Nummentie 6, Lohja, Finland
[3] NOVI Research Centre, Tampere University of Technology, Tampere, Finland

Abstract. The changing age structure of population, with its growing number of ageing people, is a worldwide phenomenon among industrialized countries, and Finland is not an exception. This has implications for swiftly rising healthcare and social welfare costs, but also for new type of demand in related services, and thus creates business opportunities for Finnish know-how. Through qualitative semi-structured interviews this research builds understanding on the desires, needs and challenges that the ageing people have in their every-day life and especially in their use of digital technology and different kinds of digital services. This will further provide insight for the service creation for the needs of elderly people in Finland. The results presented in this paper are part of a larger research project, of which this paper represents the pilot study phase.

Keywords: Assistive digital technology · Elderly people · Pilot study

1 Introduction

The changing age structure of population, with its growing number of ageing people, is a worldwide phenomenon among industrialised countries, and Finland is not an exception. This has implications for swiftly rising healthcare and social welfare costs, but also for new type of demand in related services, and thus creates business opportunities for Finnish know-how. Current trend is shifting from a provider-dominated market to a consumer-centric market, where the end customers, the seniors, will control their ageing and quality of life. People want to stay active longer when ageing. The impact of these changes in Finland is already being felt today and is particularly acute at a current time of increased pressure on public budget and growing demands and expectations from people for equal and higher quality services of social welfare and health care. Therefore, the need for a reform emerged, and an overhaul of the structures of the social welfare and health care services system has been going on for several years. The objective is not only to create financially more viable bodies as service organizers, but also to achieve complete horizontal and vertical integration of

© Springer Nature Switzerland AG 2018
H. Li et al. (Eds.): WIS 2018, CCIS 907, pp. 174–183, 2018.
https://doi.org/10.1007/978-3-319-97931-1_14

social welfare and health care services. A priority is also to enable ageing population to remain healthy, active and independent for as long as possible.

Nowadays, digital technologies, particularly health and wellbeing assistive devices and service solutions, are expected to permit ageing people to live independently in their homes longer (see e.g. [1]), to increase essentially their quality of life by compression of morbidity, reducing social isolation and hospitalisations, and hence, to lower health and social care costs. Innovative digital technologies are also expected to bring new opportunities for improving quality of the municipality-based social welfare and health care services and creating socially supportive and age-friendly living environments that enable people to enjoy longer, healthier and more independent lives from an early age up to seniority and being included in the community. Furthermore, adequate utilisation of digital assistive technology for active ageing can also help in achieving objectives of the Finnish social welfare and health care (SOTE) reform, and must be a part of the future municipality-based services delivery system. Advancing integration of digital assistive technology for active ageing into the municipality-based service system requires multiple stakeholders such as government ministries, agencies and communities as well as technology sectors to communicate with each other with the aim of coordinating ongoing activities and creating necessary conditions and consensus on action plans and specifications. To facilitate the communication between multiple stakeholders more empirical knowledge is needed.

Earlier research on new type of services in welfare sector (e.g. [2, 3]) indicates that innovative services have various, many times unforeseen impacts on service system level (e.g. use and costs of services needed) and on individual level (factors related to quality of life). The current research literature lacks the information on innovative technologies' multidimensional (tangible, intangible, financial) impacts on ageing people's lives (in terms of health, well-being, abilities) and on the service system (effects on service needs, use and costs). Moreover, only a small number of empirical investigations have explored the barriers and drivers affecting acceptance and deployment of digital health and wellbeing technologies [4, 5]. According to Niehaves and Plattfaut [1] there are still too little comprehensive consideration and explanation of digital technology acceptance among elderly.

Thus, along with the existing benefits and opportunities, there are also challenges arising: How to ensure that deployed devices of digital assistive technology for active ageing are responsive to the needs, preferences and expectations of individuals and care providers and perceived as trustworthy? How to keep in mind the perspective of people who will be affected by these new technologies and ensure that deployed tools do not fail to provide desirable benefits and services? How to encourage a quicker uptake of new and most advanced tools that respond to needs and preferences of ageing users and care providers throughout the system of social welfare and health care services to ensure larger territorial coverage of a range of the services? How to deal with the large number of different devices and solutions currently existing on the market and high volume of health information these technological tools can generate?

The general aims of the research project are

(i) to increase understanding of perspectives and opportunities for new business models and services utilising digital assistive technologies needed to maximize and sustain aging people's active and independent living at home and

(ii) to generate sufficient evidence that portrays a desirable future for ageing people with regard to digital assistive technologies based on individual and professional users' needs, preferences and practical experiences.

The primary focus lies on the assistive digital technology for active ageing that includes any products such as devices, equipment, instruments and technology and software solutions. The research project attempts to accomplish the following four specific objectives:

- Firstly, to study aging people's needs and preferences for digital assistive technology as well as expectations or conditions affecting their trust, acceptance and usage of innovative technologies that enable them to remain healthier and independent in their own homes for as long as possible.
- Secondly, to identify the core gaps in information among potential users about currently available assistive technology, which respond to ageing people's needs and preferences.
- Thirdly, to study the direct and indirect multidimensional impacts of assistive technology as well as smart living environment on the both individual level, i.e. aging people's health, well-being and ability to live independently at home, and service system level, i.e. service needs and consumption. The discourse of "impact" is not limited only to analysis of desirable outcomes; risks of using digital assistive technology for active ageing will be also addressed.
- And fourthly, to introduce perspectives and opportunities for new businesses and services that will support building the desirable future of aging people as well as proposals for interventions to integrate appropriate tools and solutions of digital assistive technology into the municipality-based service system.

To achieve these objectives the research is divided into two phases: Pilot study and Main study. The purpose of the Pilot study is to build an initial understanding of the research phenomenon and to facilitate the data collection in the Main study. To this end, a Pilot study was conducted with the focus on research questions and design of the appropriate interview guide for the Main study. The results of the Pilot study phase are presented in this paper.

2 Theoretical Framework

Research from the fields of adult development and life span psychology has shown that the aging process is accompanied by a number of physical, cognitive [6], psychological [7] and social [8, 9] changes.

Although, ageing is an individual process, for instance, **physical** functions including various elements such as muscle strength, flexibility, agility, and equilibrium [10] show a declining trend among all people while ageing. Decline in physical health causes challenges for the maintenance of mental health. The concept of mental health can be considered as an umbrella term for psychological and social well-being as well as cognitive functioning. **Psychological** well-being refers to six key-elements such as self-acceptance, positive relations with others, environmental mastery, autonomy, purpose in life, and personal growth. The changes in **cognitive** function that occur in normal human aging involve a decline in the ability to pay attention, working memory, long-term memory, perception, speech, language, decision making, and executive control [11]. While some common age-related stereotypes suggest that older adults are slower at performing many tasks and have poorer memories, the other stereotypes advocate that with age come increased knowledge and wisdom, which can be critical in solving many complex problems of contemporary life [12]. **Social** functions refer to interaction between people occurring in informal and formal contexts [13]. Interaction in informal contexts includes, for example, contacts via phone, email, skype, letters, and meetings with relatives, friends and neighbours. Interaction in formal contexts includes activities such as attending meetings of organisations or clubs, volunteer work, and religious participation. According to some studies, a major reason for a reduction in social participation in old age may be health problems [8, 9].

The purpose of digital health and wellbeing assistive technologies is provide new opportunities for individuals to monitor and support their own health and wellbeing and to create a home environment that is safe and secure to reduce disabilities, falls, fear and stress, to support health.

In the recent years, digital assistive technologies have developed rapidly augmenting the traditional assistive technologies. The term 'digital assistive technology' refers to the use of ICTs for the support of ageing people's everyday tasks and activities [14].

Due to widely accepted beliefs regarding positive relation between these smart technologies and health improvement, quality of life and social welfare and health care services, it is increasingly important that ageing people accept these technologies and make use of them. The level of trust and acceptance as well as motivation to use innovative technologies will rise, when people are convinced that these technologies – useful and responsive to their needs [15, 16] and expectations.

According to the most prominent Technology Acceptance Model (TAM), developed by Davis [17] to understand expectations about information technology, two main variables have an impact on acceptance: perceived usefulness and perceived ease of use. This model has since been widely used, also in the context of digital technology use among elderly people (see e.g. [1]). Another approach represented by the Unified Theory of Acceptance and Use of Technology (UTAUT) [18] suggests that four key constructs such as performance expectancy, effort expectancy, social influence and facilitating conditions are direct determinants of usage intention and behaviour and takes into account sociodemographic and individual factors. Many empirical studies stress the significance of sociodemographic factors such as age, gender, cultural (at the national level) and religious background, family status and individual factors such as education and technological experience for the acceptance level and motivation. However, an important point needs to be taken into account that the sociodemographic background of future ageing people will be certainly different from that of contemporary older adults. [19]

Thus, in order to maximise trust and acceptance of innovative tools of digital assistive technology by ageing people, these tools should be responsive to people's needs, preferences and expectations or conditions supporting trust. The rapid growth of ageing population will likely lead to a wider range of people's needs, preferences and expectations from digital assistive technology and living environments. The importance of understanding what do ageing people actually need for assistance with daily activities when living independently at their own homes and how to respond to these needs is widely acknowledged in the literature (e.g. [20, 21]) and is also highlighted in the recent report of Finnish Ministry of the Environment [22]. Further, it can be assumed that needs, preferences and expectations of ageing people are also related to sociodemographic factors and vary essentially in different living environments and geographical locations.

3 Research Methodology and Data

The general aim of the research is a primary guideline in the choice of research methodology. It has an exploratory character pursuing to observe, interpret and describe the research phenomenon of "desirable future for ageing people with regard to digital assistive technologies". Therefore, a qualitative methodological approach is applied for this research, and face-to-face semi-structured interviews are chosen as a primary method of obtaining sufficiently detailed first-hand data and ensuring co-creation of knowledge between researchers and interviewees.

For interviews in the Pilot study, persona cards were created according to the interviewees' age, sex and living environment (city center, rural area and urban area). Additionally, the following descriptive characteristics were in focus: ability or constraints regarding physical, psychological, cognitive or social dimensions as well as their digital activity, i.e. the ownership and use of digital devices in everyday life. The educational background (academic (A) or non-academic (nA)) was considered as well.

At least one male (M) and one female (F) from each age group with different characteristics and academic background was interviewed. All together 10 pilot semi-structured interviews were conducted to build an understanding about their daily activities, challenges and needs and to create persona descriptions for the further investigations in the Main study. Persona descriptions have been visualised in the form of persona cards, i.e. illustrative persons with story lines of their lives, based on the interviewees' real life experiences (Table 1).

In the Main study, the future needs of ageing customers and society will be clarified through futures research methodology, particularly by using multiple scenario approach, when alternative futures paths in long run will be generated in participatory scenario workshops. Additionally, recommendations based on these scenarios will be made for different persona groups.

Table 1. Persona cards (remark explanation: F = female, M = male, numbers 1–6 = number of interviewed person; nA = non-academic, A = academic)

Age group characteristic	55–64	65–74	75–84	85–>
Living environment				
– Rural area	F2A	M1nA, F5nA	M2A	F1nA
– City center	M3A	F6nA, M4A	F4nA	
– Urban area	F3nA			
Ability/constraints				
– Physical	F3nA	F5nA	M2A, F4nA	F1nA
– Psychological				
– Cognitive			F4nA	
– Social				F1nA
Digital activity				
– Smart phone	F2A, M3A, F3nA	M1nA, F6nA, M4A	M2A	
– Tablet	F2A, M3A, F3nA	F6nA, M4A		
– Laptop	F2A, M3A, F3nA	M1nA, F6nA, M4A	M2A	
– Personal computer		M4A		

4 Results and Implications

The pilot study brought important insight to the main study and its objectives. Aging people's needs and preferences for digital assistive technology seem to be positive, although they are not yet very familiar with the latest devices and applications. Skills and competences to use them are still limited especially in the oldest age group females outside city centers. To get deeper understanding of the impacts on the people's wellbeing and on the new opportunities in business further investigation is needed in the field. Based on literature review [23] it was observed, that elderly people mainly have positive attitude to use electronic services, but many problems were recognized, too. E.g. too small font, unclear symbols or worries about security and safety issues might be reasons for lower use of e-services. Thus, according to Tuohimaa et al. [24] e-health services might have an empowering impact on people's life generally.

Pilot study draws a picture of ten ageing persons, who all have different kinds of needs for services based on their living area and level of activity:

- M2A is an 81 years old male, retired widow with academic background, still working actively in his research area, following the newest information, for instance from science and technology. Thus, he uses smart phone and laptop only for professional and for everyday banking purposes, but not for personal health or wellbeing monitoring, although he has type 2 diabetes.
- M1nA is a 65 years old, retired, married non-academic male person, using mostly smart phone and laptop for musical activities with his band. He is not willing to broaden the use of smart devices, for instance, to social media side or for self-monitoring in terms of wellbeing, because no health problems yet.

- F1nA is an 89 years old lady widow, living alone in her one-family house in the countryside. She is an artist, still painting aquarelles every now and then. She has no interest for smart devices and she has no internet connection or any computer at all in her home. She is active in music and literature, in summertime actively working in her garden with flowers and other plants.
- F2A is a 61 years old female, still active in working life in the research branch, using smart devices actively in her work every day, but also in her semi-professional hobbies in the field of literature, gardening and antiques.
- M3A is a 59 years old man, actively involved in working life in ITC-field. He employs different smart devices daily at work and home. He is very fluent and motivated to use digital technologies in everything what he is doing during working and leisure time.
- F3nA is a 60 years old, married non-academic female, working part-time due to health limitations and physical constraints. She uses smart devices at work, but at home only for some specific everyday needs. In spite of her physical constraints, she is very active person, and gardening, reading and walking are favorite ways of spending free time.
- F4nA is an 82 years old lady widow, living alone in her apartment in the city center. She does not have any smart device and is not willing to learn any of them. She is physically in a very weak condition with slight cognitive constraints, but socially very active. She spends most of her time reading periodical press, watching TV and communicating with her old friends typically on the mobile phone. Due to poor physical health status, she is recipient of different home care services. In particular, she wears a safety button, provided to her by municipal social welfare and health care services.
- F5nA is a 72 years old lady, who is living with her husband in the countryside. She had a stroke in head area four years ago and since that she has been in a wheelchair due to problems in using left side (both hand and foot). Her husband has served as her personal care keeper since that, but they also have a nurse visiting their home three times per day to assist with daily routines. There are these kinds of physical disabilities, but socially she is active and likes to see her family, friends and relatives. However, she doesn't own a smartphone, so the social interaction is limited only to visits. Previously she was active in using computer and finding information through Internet, but after the stroke there has been also signs of slight cognitive disabilities, which seem to have an effect also to her use of computer, that has been decreasing during last couple of years.
- F6nA is a 66 years old lady living in a center of a small town with her husband. She has retired two years ago from her regular job in insurance company. She is physically very active and she doesn't have physical or cognitive disabilities. Socially she is very active, she has few very close friends and she is also actively taking care of her grandchildren living nearby their house. She makes a 5 km long walking round every morning and she also goes to the gym twice a week with her husband. She has a smart phone, which she uses actively. She is also very active in the social media, especially in Facebook. However, even though she has no physical or cognitive disabilities, she is using only those digital technologies that she is very familiar with, and is rather critical to take use any new kind of digital technology.

- M4A is a 68 years old married man, living with her wife in an own house in a center of a small city. He has an academic education and he served for several years in a leading position in a big national company operating in energy sector. He is very technology oriented person, using smart phone, laptop and tablet on every day basis. He has no cognitive or physical disabilities, and he is also rather active socially. With an engineering education background he is enthusiastic to take use of new digital technologies and he actively follows the public discussion around new available technologies.

Based on the interview data and the short narratives of the interviewees, we are able to create two interesting personas from the viewpoint of digital assistive technology and use of services for further investigation:

#1: Active elderly person who is living in the city center near by all different kinds of services

#2: Non-active elderly person with disabilities, living in the rural area far from services

These two personas are rather different when it comes to the use of digital assistive technologies and digital technologies. However, both of these personas are heavy users of different kinds of services, although different types of services, but still they are key customer groups for further investigation and service creation. These two personas will be the focus of the Main study phase of larger research project.

The anticipated findings of the Main study will address both theoretical and practical implications, and in general will provide valuable insights on the desirable future for ageing people with regard to innovative digital technology for active ageing. The findings will support a greater availability of and easier access to digital assistive technology for ageing people and encourage public as well as private social welfare and health care service providers to increase utilisation of the technology in order to deliver more efficient and individually oriented services for ageing people's independent living at home in the future. The findings will also drive innovations in digital assistive technology for active ageing and increase demand for new devices and services.

The aforementioned findings will allow avoiding major risks of protecting outdated status quo, spending public money on something ineffective and protect individuals and communities from financial ruin due to rising costs of social welfare and health care. Ultimately, the findings will facilitate integration of digital assistive technology for active ageing into the municipality-based service system by providing necessary knowledge for communication between multiple stakeholders such as government ministries, agencies and communities as well as technology sectors. This will also serve the cooperation in research and development, replication and co-deployment of digital solutions and products. Thus, the findings will benefit the objectives of the Finnish social welfare and health care (SOTE) reform.

References

1. Niehaves, B., Plattfaut, R.: Internet adoption by the elderly: employing IS technology acceptance theories for understanding the age-related digital divide. Eur. J. Inf. Syst. **23**(6), 708–726 (2014)
2. Ympäristöministeriö: Asunnottomuuden vähentämisen taloudelliset vaikutukset, Ympäristöministeriön raportteja, vol. 7, p. 114 (2011). ISBN 978-952-11-3848-5
3. Sillanpää, V.: Measuring the impacts of welfare service innovations. Int. J. Prod. Perform. Manag. **62**(5), 474–489 (2013)
4. Clark, J.S., McGee-Lennon, M.R.: A stakeholder-centred exploration of the current barriers to the uptake of home care technologies. UK J. Assist. Technol. **5**(1), 12–25 (2011)
5. Heart, T., Kalderon, E.: Older adults: are they ready to adopt health-related ICT? Int. J. Med. Inf. **82**(11), 1–23 (2013)
6. Baltes, P.B., Staudinger, U.M., Lindenberger, U.: Lifespan psychology: theory and application to intellectual functioning. Ann. Rev. Psychol. **50**, 471–507 (1999)
7. Ryff, C.D., Singer, B.H.: Know thyself and become what you are: a eudaimonic approach to psychological well-being. J. Happiness Stud. **9**(1), 13–39 (2008)
8. Bukov, A., Maas, I., Lampert, T.: Social participation in very old age: cross-sectional and longitudinal findings from BASE. Berlin aging study. J. Gerontol. Ser. B: Psychol. Sci. Soc. Sci. **57**(6), 510–517 (2002)
9. Wilkie, R., Blagojevic-Bucknall, M., Belcher, J., Chew-Graham, C., Lacey, R.J., McBeth, J.: Widespread pain and depression are key modifiable risk factors associated social participation in older adults: a prospective cohort study in primary care. Medicine (Baltimore) **95**(31), e4111 (2016). https://doi.org/10.1097/MD.0000000000004111
10. Sugimoto, H., Demura, S., Nagasawa, Y.: Age and gender-related differences in physical functions of the elderly following one-year regular exercise therapy. Health **6**, 792–801 (2014)
11. Glisky, E.L.: Changes in cognitive function in human aging. In: Riddle, D.R. (ed.) Frontiers in Neuroscience. Brain Aging: Models, Methods, and Mechanisms, pp. 3–20. CRC Press, Boca Raton (2007)
12. Park, D.C.: The basic mechanisms accounting for age-related decline in cognitive function. In: Park, D.C., Schwartz, N. (eds.) Cognitive Ageing: A Primer. Psychology Press (2012)
13. Utz, R.L., Carr, D., Nesse, R., Wortman, C.B.: The effect of widowhood on older adults' social participation: an evaluation of activity, disengagement, and continuity theories. Gerontologist **42**(4), 522–533 (2002)
14. Olphert, W., Damodaran, L., Balatsoukas, P., Parkinson, C.: Process requirements for building sustainable digital assistive technology for older people. J. Assist. Technol. **3**(3), 4–13 (2009)
15. Mitzner, T.L., et al.: Older adults talk technology: technology usage and attitudes. Comput. Hum. Behav. **26**(6), 1710–1721 (2010)
16. van Dijk, J.A.G.M.: Digital divide research, achievements and shortcomings. Poetics **34**(4–5), 221–235 (2006)
17. Davis, F.D.: Perceived usefulness, perceived ease of use, and user acceptance of information technology. Manag. Inf. Syst. **13**(3), 319–339 (1989)
18. Verkatesh, V., Morris, M.G., Davis, G.B., Davis, F.D.: User acceptance of information technology: toward a unified view. Manag. Inf. Syst. **27**(3), 425–478 (2003)
19. Flandorfer, P.: Population ageing and socially assistive robots for elderly persons: the importance of sociodemographic factors for user acceptance. Int. J. Popul. Res. **2012**, 13 p. (2012). https://doi.org/10.1155/2012/829835. Article ID 829835

20. Kötteritzsch, A., Weyers, B.: Assistive technologies for older adults in urban areas: a literature review. Cogn. Comput. **8**(2), 299–317 (2016)
21. Mitzner, T.L., Chen, T.L., Kemp, C.C., Rogers, W.A.: Older adults' needs for assistance as a function of living environment. In: Proceedings of the Human Factors and Ergonomic Society, 55th Annual Meeting (2011). http://pwp.gatech.edu/hrl/wp-content/uploads/sites/231/2016/05/hfes2011.pdf
22. Ympäristöministeriö: Älyteknologiaratkaisut ikääntyneiden kotona asumisen tukena. Ympäristöministeriön raportteja, vol. 7 [Smart Technology Solutions Supporting Elderly's Home Life. Support. Reports of Finnish Ministry of the Environment, vol. 7] (2017). https://julkaisut.valtioneuvosto.fi/bitstream/handle/10024/79348/YMra_7_2017.pdf?sequence=1
23. Rosenlund, M., Kinnunen, U.-M.: Ikäihmisten kokemukset terveydenhuollon sähköisten palvelujen käytöstä ja kokemusten hyödyntäminen palvelujen kehittämisessä - kuvaileva kirjallisuuskatsaus [The experience of older people with the use of healthcare electronic services and the utilization of the experience in service development - descriptive literature review]. Finn. J. eHealth eWelfare **10**(2–3), 264–284 (2018)
24. Tuohimaa, H., Ahonen, O., Meristö, T., Rajalahti, E.: E-health solutions as an opportunity for empowering responsibility. Interdisc. Stud. J. ISJ **3**(4), 315–319 (2014)

E-health

Reliability of Health Information in the Media as Defined by Finnish Physicians

Ulla Ahlmén-Laiho[1,2(✉)], Sakari Suominen[3,4], Ulla Järvi[5],
and Risto Tuominen[3,6]

[1] TOTEK Unit, Turku University Hospital, Turku, Finland
humahl@utu.fi
[2] Department of Anaesthesia and Intensive Care,
Faculty of Medicine, Turku University, Turku, Finland
[3] Department of Public Health, Medical Faculty,
University of Turku, Turku, Finland
[4] Department of Public Health, Skövde University, Skövde, Sweden
[5] Tiedetoimittajat Ry, Salo, Finland
[6] Faculty of Health Sciences, University of Namibia, Windhoek, Namibia

Abstract. Mass media is an important forum for the interaction between science and the general public, and media participation has been recognized by the Finnish Medical Association as a duty of physicians. Physicians are an important source of health information for journalists and their perceptions of reliability may influence which medias they are willing to collaborate with. In this study, Finnish physicians were asked to evaluate and define the characteristics of reliability for health information in the media. The survey was filled out by 266 physicians, who estimated that the most reliable mass media sources of health information are scientific publications, medical associations, universities, The Finnish National Institute for Health and Welfare, and other non-profit research centres. The lowest reliability scores were given to online discussion forums, entities representing complementary, and alternative medicine and individual patients. Female physicians and older physicians gave most health information sources higher scores than men or younger respondents. These results highlight a potential conflict between the need to translate scientific language to a form understandable to the general public, and a demand placed by physicians on journalism to be as scientifically accurate and precise as possible. In order to best convey their message to the general public, the professional skills of journalists should be utilised by physicians to overcome this issue.

Keywords: Health journalism · Mass media · Medical journalism
Reliability of health information

1 Introduction

It has been suggested that science achieves its status in society largely through being reported in mass media [1]. In Finland, advances in medical science are one of the most actively followed areas of science [2], and mass media has been proven to be an important source of health information to Finnish patients [3]. The country has been

© Springer Nature Switzerland AG 2018
H. Li et al. (Eds.): WIS 2018, CCIS 907, pp. 187–199, 2018.
https://doi.org/10.1007/978-3-319-97931-1_15

ranked in the top three of the Freedom of Speech index [4], and media self-regulation in Finland has been lauded as comparably healthy and effective [5, 6], which all makes Finland an interesting subject in the study of the interactions between mass media and the medical community. Science communication aimed at the general public has three important collaborating bodies: scientists, journalists and the audience [7]. The medical profession enjoys the same sort of given trust in society as does traditional mass media [8], and this trust is a vital part of social cohesion and order [9]. Finnish health journalists, as well as their colleagues in other countries, have been shown to identify as representatives of medical science, as opposed to other views on health and medicine [10, 11]. This is beneficial to physicians in the sense that health information reported in the media can have an impact on the patient-doctor relationship, the forming of practices and guidelines in healthcare [12, 13] and possibly also political decision-making regarding healthcare [14]. According to previous studies, purposeful educational media campaigns dealing with health have at least some effect [15–17], and the media is frequently assumed to be capable of exerting a strong influence on the public's opinion concerning health and illness.

Healthcare professionals often view the field of health communication from a utilitarian viewpoint – as a means for educating and changing opinions [18]. This ideology of often one-directional conveying of ideas has been criticised as an entity that strengthens the positional power of certain professions in the society such as physicians [18], and the information selected by scientists to be offered to the media has been shown to shape health reporting [19, 20]. In recent years, research dealing with health journalism has shifted from merely attempting to convey scientific facts to defining how health, the human body and illness are defined and discussed in the society [18]. According to a prior Finnish study, the biomedical model appears to be dominant, as compared to other views on these matters [21]. Physicians benefit, to some extent, from this setting [22, 23], which journalists also recognise [24, 25]. There exists a general demand of accuracy when it comes to health journalism [26, 27] and healthcare professionals have publicly criticized health journalists' ability to convey accurate, objective information [19, 28].

Physicians are an important data source for journalists when reporting on health, medicine and illness [25, 29]. A Finnish study has shown that physicians do not complain to Finland's self-regulatory media body, The Council for Mass Media in Finland, more often than other professionals [30]. Some profession-specific issues, however, may affect the physicians' interaction with journalists and mass media such as the demands of medical confidentiality [30]. According to a Finnish study, health journalists consider the perceived reliability of the source of information a determining factor in whether a physician might be willing to collaborate with said media sources [10].

In epidemiological research, the reliability of information is defined as the repeatability of results using the same data [31]. A related term is validity, which seeks to evaluate how accurately the chosen data describes the phenomenon being studied. A great deal of scientific research is carried out not only in order to gain knowledge, but also with the aim of improving the reliability of prior results and thus increasing the independence and objectivity of science [32]. In fields of applied science, such as clinical medicine, reliable information is a cornerstone of patient safety and evidence-based treatment, but the scientific ethos is also a part of the status of medicine in society.

The reliability of the internet as a source of medical information has been evaluated by individual physicians [33–35], but recent studies on physicians' perceptions of the source reliability of health information are not available. A study done in Finland in the 1990s showed that a third of Finnish physicians felt that media health reporting was reliable, and a fifth felt it distorted facts; 44% felt that health reporting was ideologically biased and only 13% felt it was neutral [36]. In the same study, physicians rendered highest reliability scores to health-centred magazines and relative good scores to radio and television whereas general magazines and newspapers were ranked next-best. Lowest scores were given to tabloids [36]. Finnish physician respondents in the earlier study mentioned expressed that health reporting in the media is important and that they would have wanted to see more of it [36]. In that prior study, physicians were critical towards their own profession: 41% felt that the medical profession had not a good track record in conveying medical information to the general public [36].

The field of media has greatly changed after that earlier study was published [3] but more recent data regarding the views of physicians is not available. The association between physicians' perception of the reliability of health information media sources and their willingness to collaborate with journalists has, to the best of the authors' knowledge, not been examined before.

2   Purpose and Methods of This Study

The aim of the study was to explore physicians' perceived reliability of different health information sources in the media, and to evaluate their willingness to participate in a journalistic process.

Depending on the data the study utilised a combined qualitative-quantitative approach. The use of quantitative methodology follows the tradition of media research within mainstream social sciences [18, 37], whereas the interpretation and content analysis of the freeform answers takes into account the current research paradigms of health journalism in cultural sciences [18, 37].

Nearly all (94%) of Finnish physicians are members of the Finnish Medical Association [38]. A demographically representative sample of 1198 potential participants was drawn, with appropriate consent of the holder of the registry, from the membership registry of the Finnish Medical Association. An electronic cross-sectional survey was carried out by a commercial electronic research instrument (Webropol). The recipients were offered two months of time for responding, and non-responders were automatically reminded maximally three times via e-mail. Reasons for non-responsiveness were not studied, although the research group was contacted by a few non-responders who reported that they did not feel their expertise was sufficient to allow them to reply or that they were too busy. The electronic questionnaire was returned by 266 respondents (22%), a number corresponding with the participation rates of the Finnish Medical Association's prior surveys regarding Finnish physicians.

The first part of the survey established the participants' background demographics regarding age, medical specialty, stage of specialisation, employment sector, and their level of involvement in medical research. Although the recipients were asked to select their precise year of birth, for analysis they were combined into three age groups (born before 1965, born within the period of 1965 to 1984, born after the year 1984). This classification was based on the common stages of a Finnish physician's career: the youngest age bracket would likely be non-specialised or in specialty training, the group in the middle would already have a more stabilised career after probably having finished specialty training, and the oldest age bracket would comprise of those in a senior career position and of those already retired. The level of academic involvement was inquired by the following options: has never participated in research/has participated in research before/is preparing a doctoral dissertation/holds a PhD/is a holder of the Title of Docent/is a holder of the title of Professor. For analysis, the respondents were grouped into those holding at least a PhD and others. Docents and professors grouped together were also compared to those holding a PhD but no higher title, and to those in the PhD process or having no current or prior academic involvement.

The respondents were asked to evaluate twenty different media sources of health information on a nine-point Likert scale, in which one was equal to highly unreliable and nine to highly reliable. The participants were then asked to list characteristics of a source that they considered particularly reliable and characteristics of sources the considered particularly unreliable. The number of descriptive terms was not limited for these two questions, and closed alternatives were not offered. The frequencies of different characteristics mentioned were counted and categorised by the researchers, combining synonyms. More detailed statistical analysis of these descriptions was not carried out since categorising them contained a risk of subjectivity by the interpreting researcher. However, to ensure the validity of the categorisation and the calculation of items mentioned, the Webropol system's own word cloud function was utilised to ensure that the results gleaned by an automatic word recognition tool were sufficiently similar to the frequencies calculated by the researcher.

SPSS was used for the statistical analysis of the numerical data. The Chi-square test was used to evaluate the differences between proportions and Student's t-test was used to evaluate the differences between two mean values. Evaluation of more than two mean values was based on One-Way Analysis of Variance (ANOVA). The general sum index of reliability was computed by adding up all the numerical values the respondent assigned to all examined media sources. The frequency distribution of the sum index was close to normal, so a multiple linear regression model could be fitted to study the effects of selected background factors on the overall reliance to mass media, while having the effects of other studied factors simultaneously controlled.

3   Results

3.1   Respondent Demographics

Women comprised 64.3% of respondents. The age distribution was as follows: born between 1945–1954 12.0%; born between 1955–1964 28.6%; born between 1965–1974 22.2%; born between 1975–1984 27.8%, and born after this 9.4%. Out of all respondents, 59.8% had finished specialist training and 24.8% were in the process of doing so. The great majority (80.1%) of respondents worked in public healthcare;

26.3% were employed in the private sector. Two thirds (76.3%) of the physicians surveyed spend more than half of their working hours doing clinical patient work.

The age, employment sector and gender distributions of the respondents were similar to those of Finnish physicians in general [39].

3.2 Survey Results

The highest reliability scores were assigned to scientific publications, followed by medical associations, universities, The Finnish National Institute for Health and Welfare and other non-profit research centres, The Ministry of Health and Social Services, and the administrative bodies of the Finnish public healthcare system. The lowest reliability scores were given to online discussion forums, entities representing complementary and alternative medicine (CAM) and individual patients. Female physicians gave most surveyed information sources higher scores than men (Table 1).

Table 1. The reliability of sources of health information in the media as evaluated by Finnish physicians *(P values are only given for statistically significant differences. CAM = complementary and alternate medicine)*

Information source	All respondents	Women	Men	p
Domestic scientific publications	8.10	8.13	8.05	
International scientific publications	7.84	7.8	7.92	
Specialty-centred and other physician associations	7.83	7.9	7.72	
University or other research unit	7.77	7.85	7.64	
The Finnish Institute for Health and Welfare	7.73	7.88	7.44	<0.01
The Finnish Medical Association and equivalents	7.58	7.71	7.35	<0.05
The Ministry of Health And Social Services	7.47	7.67	7.12	<0.001
The administration of Finnish public healthcare	7.22	7.29	7.10	
Individuals researchers and research groups	6.70	6.77	6.57	
Individual physicians from the public sector	6.11	6.18	5.98	
Patient organisations	5.91	6.12	5.53	<0.01
Pharmaceutical companies	5.52	5.63	5.32	
Health-centred magazines	5.27	5.26	5.31	
Individual physicians from the private sector	5.17	5.26	5.02	
News agencies	4.98	5.08	4.80	
Newspapers	4.67	4.62	4.77	

(continued)

Table 1. (*continued*)

Information source	All respondents	Women	Men	p
TV and radio	4.59	4.65	4.50	
Individual patients	3.26	3.26	3.26	
Entities and individuals representing CAM	2.46	2.63	2.16	<0.05
Online discussion forums	1.89	1.92	1.85	

Respondents who had a PhD or who were holders of the title of Docent or Professor gave foreign scientific publications slightly but not significantly ($p > 0.05$) higher reliability scores (8.07) than those without scientific experience (7.76). Physicians who had gone through clinical specialty training trusted the administrative bodies of public healthcare ($p < 0.01$) and patient advocate organisations ($p < 0.05$) less (7.06 and 5.72) than those who had not undergone specialty training (7.46 and 6.18).

Those respondents who spent more than half of their working hours in clinical work trusted medical associations ($p < 0.05$) and medical specialty associations ($p < 0.01$) (7.67 and 7.95) more than others (7.3 and 7.95 respectively).

Respondents born before the year 1965 trusted information from pharmaceutical companies (5.82; $p < 0.05$) more than the two younger age brackets. Those born in the period 1965–1984 gave a reliability score of 5.37; those born after 1984 gave a score of 4.96. In a linear regression model, when the effects of other background factors were simultaneously controlled, older participants and women expressed higher overall reliability than younger or male respondents.

The most significant determinants of reliability were adherence to scientific principles, impartiality, peer review, expertise and quality factors commonly associated with published research. Half of female respondents mentioned scientific principles while a quarter of male participants did so. Men were more likely to mention broadness of viewpoint but otherwise there were little differences between genders (Table 2).

Table 2. Characteristics of reliable sources of health information mentioned at least once by physicians (*CAM = complementary and alternate medicine*)

Characteristic	All (n = 266)	% of women (n = 171)	% of men (n = 95)
Scientific, representing medical science, evidence-based	112	52.0	25.3
Objectivity, impartiality, neutrality, no commercial interests	57	19.3	25.3
(Widely) peer-reviewed	44	15.2	18.9
Expertise	41	16.4	13.7
Repeatable study of high quality being quoted, sample size big enough	26	12.3	5.3

(*continued*)

Table 2. (*continued*)

Characteristic	All (n = 266)	% of women (n = 171)	% of men (n = 95)
A university or some other publicly funded, governmental or otherwise well-known entity behind the information	19	7.6	6.3
Information sources are named and the associated references listed appropriately	18	5.8	8.4
Source has medical training, highly educated, professional training in healthcare	18	7.0	6.3
Extended clinical or other experience from the field	16	4.7	8.4
A wide perspective, good background research done, integrative, sees the big picture	17	8.2	13.7
The publication is known to be prestigious, scientific and critical	15	5.8	5.3
Is not based on only one source, one person's opinion or one case	10	4.7	2.1
Openness, honesty, self-critical, sources evaluated critically	10	2.3	6.3
A large research consortium or conclave of experts is behind the data	8	4.7	0.0
The author is esteemed, well-known	6	0.6	5.3
Someone whose job makes them responsible for what they say about health	4	0.6	3.2
The content is not emotionally coloured	3	1.2	1.1
The physician surveyed has personal experience of a source being reliable before	3	1.2	1.1
Non-judgmental, no agenda	3	0.6	2.1
Controlled, supervised reporting	2	0.6	1.1
No anonymity	2	0.6	1.1

Characteristics of unreliability that were most frequently listed by respondents included subjectivity, attempting to further one's commercial or ideological interests, appealing to the audience's emotions, making unscientific claims, and being associated with complementary and alternative medicine. Women were more inclined to list emotional content as a characteristic of unreliability (Table 3).

Table 3. Characteristics of unreliable sources of health information mentioned at least once by physicians *(CAM = complementary and alternate medicine)*

Characteristic	All (n = 266)	% of women (n = 171)	% of men (n = 95)
Singular case, one person's opinion, subjectivity	102	44.4	27.4
Attempt to further financial or other personal interests, having an agenda	77	22.2	41.1
Tone appeals to emotions, content based on emotions	39	17.5	9.5
Information of unscientific nature	35	14.0	11.6
CAM, being based on belief instead of science	28	9.4	12.6
Lack of expertise, lacking background research, lack of training	28	8.2	14.7
Sensationalism, attention-seeking, flashy and unfounded headlines	27	11.7	7.4
Source material scarce or missing or unreliable	24	11.1	5.3
Fanaticism, having a background ideology, prejudice	21	4.1	14.7
Lack of criticism, especially towards data sources	12	2.9	7.4
Represents an anonymous opinion or online forums where anyone can say whatever they want	11	4.7	3.2
Faulty viewpoint, false generalisations, speculation	11	5.3	2.1
Hearsay and rumours, second-hand information	10	2.3	6.3
Representing one ideological organisation	8	2.9	3.2
Narrow viewpoint, does not see the big picture	7	4.1	0.0
Simplistic, one-sided	5	0.6	4.2
Physician is under the personal impression that a certain source is unreliable	3	1.8	0.0
Certain medias are unreliable categorically, such as tabloids	3	1.2	1.1
Paranoia and conspiracy theories	2	0.0	2.1
Empty promises, miracle drug, game-changing	2	1.2	0.0
Creating conflicts, making the opposite side look bad	2	0.6	1.1

4 Discussion

According to a Finnish study repeated at a few years' intervals [2], the general public trusts science more than it trusts the media, through which the general public gets most of its health information. Physicians' opinions may well affect the consumption of health journalism by their patients; a source a physician has recommended may well be the first or only one a patient turns to, and perceived reliability may well determine which sources are recommended by the physician. However, the publications estimated by the respondents of the present study to be most reliable by those surveyed may be difficult for laypersons to comprehend, which might also affect whether their contents will be utilised by the general public.

According to the results of this present study, Finnish physicians expect a scientific viewpoint from health sources they consider reliable. This may be at odds with a demand for a more pluralistic view of health and illness [23] and health journalism has been accused of not being sufficiently critical of the medical establishment [24, 40].

Media researchers have suggested before that, in demanding journalists to have a lot of substance expertise, physicians may not be seeing their own expert roles clearly [41]. Not all scientists see popularisation of science and communicating with the general public as a part of their work, but at least many Finnish social scientists have been shown by Pitkänen and Niemi [42] to do so. All in all, the views of physicians as compared to Finnish health journalists when it comes to reliable health reporting are in many respects quite similar [10], and these specialised journalists may have reasonable influence on how health reporting is carried out.

It isn't always easy for a journalist to discern who actually is an expert in a certain subject matter, especially if they appear to hold significant academic credentials. When the media questions someone's expertise the situation may inadvertently end up strengthening the expert's perceived value [43]. Physicians demanding a high level of medical expertise from the media and demanding that journalistic products to only reflect science may cause some challenges in collaboration particularly journalists who have not specialised in these issues, since the precise and specific language of the natural sciences does not lend itself well to effective popularisation of medicine. This dilemma has been acknowledged before, although prior to the present study, no data has been available to support the idea.

In order to reach a compromise between scientific accuracy and understandable content, the expertise of both journalists and the scientific community is needed. This has been acknowledged by the Finnish Journalist Association and the Finnish Medical Association, who have together formulated guidelines for reporting on medical issues [44]. These guidelines remind journalists that they are obligated to seek the truth, and that physicians again have a duty to participate in public discussion through the media. This creates a fruitful ground for collaboration.

Especially in the light of the recent rise of more pluralistic views of health in media, the patient's viewpoint is an element which a journalist may want to make use of as a means to offer a point of relatability for the audience. From the physicians' point of view in this survey, such material presented in the media may be problematic in its subjectivity since it is not based on research data. The participants of this study described unreliable sources with terms such as subjectivity, non-scientific thinking and being based on individual opinions – all characteristics befitting interviews of individual patients. According to a prior study that surveyed the opinions of Finnish health journalists [10], media professionals saw such material as much less problematic than the physicians in the present study.

Those participants who did a substantial amount of clinical work were more confident of the reliability of medical associations as information sources. This may be due to them being more familiar with those professional organisations than researchers are. As compared to an earlier study where Finnish health journalists were asked to rate the reliability of the same data sources, they assessed these organisations to be less reliable than the respondents of this present study did [10]. This may be due to the fact that these associations, unlike some of their European counterparts, are also labour unions and thus can be seen as having a goal to further the economic and other interests of their members instead of underlining solely their scientific role.

Scientific publications do not represent the only health information source utilized by physicians [45]; mass media serves not only laypersons but also physicians as a source of health information, as do internet sources which are not produced by mass media outlets. According to Roshan et al. [46], online sources can give patients and physicians false, imprecise and conflicted information. Emond et al. [47] have suggested that uncertainty about the reliability of information may be a key reason for medical professionals of not instructing patients to seek health information in the media. Due to a lack of medical training, patients have a limited ability to estimate the reliability of available medical information [48], and even a third of the general public in Finland estimates that they cannot gauge the reliability of health information available online [3]. This creates a pressure for professionals to participate in evaluating and improving the quality of health reporting.

Commercial entities also have an effect on where media gets its health information. In a study involving 37 countries [49], medical journalists described the pharmaceutical industry as a very active provider of information. The fact that older respondents in the present study were less critical towards these companies can be explained by historical reasons: negative attitudes towards collaboration and financial connections between physicians and pharmaceutical companies have not been frowned-upon for long, and the regulation of these relationships is also a phenomenon borne during the last few decades. The reliability estimate given by the respondents in this present study was similar to the results of an earlier study [10] in which Finnish health journalists were surveyed. It is possible that the familiarity of physicians with pharmaceutical companies may have increased their perceived reliability. Even though younger respondents were more sceptical to the reliability of such information, they still gave higher reliability scores to pharmaceutical companies than they did to news agencies or newspapers. Considering that commercial or other personal interests were listed by the physicians as characteristics of unreliability in media, the relatively short history of negative attitudes towards a close relationship between physicians and pharmaceutical companies may well explain this finding.

The compliance percentage may affect the reliability of the results. However, the percentage of replies out of those who were selected as part of the initial pool of respondents is similar to that of an earlier study dealing with social scientists and the media [42], and the demographics of respondents in this present study were verified to match the demographics of Finnish physicians' in general [39, 50]. Since nearly all Finnish physicians are members of the Finnish Medical Association, drawing the sample from its member register can be expected of not having significantly distorted sample demographics. Reasons for non-compliance were not studied, and it is possible that those who did reply may represent a subgroup more interested or experienced in the health journalism than those who did not respond.

As part of the scientific community, physicians may have increasing need for media collaboration in the future. During the 2010s universities and other research facilities have begun expending more sources on outward communication, PR and even so-called marketing of science [51]. Interaction with the rest of society has sometimes even been declared as a major task for universities [1, 52], a significant part of obtaining research funding [1, 53], and some have even suggested communication with the rest of society to be part of the scientific community's process of justifying its funding [7].

All in all, the surveyed Finnish physicians consider science to be the foundation of reliable health reporting and are somewhat suspicious of more subjective and pluralistic approaches that aim for relatability to rouse the interest of the general public. Journalists may be rather good at acknowledging the limits of their knowledge [54]; physicians may not be as willing to lean on the expertise of journalists on formulating their messages into a form that is understandable and enticing to the general public. By educating both journalists and physicians about each other's viewpoints and challenges in their fields it may be possible to enhance collaboration between these groups. Research, such as this present study that explores the differences and similarities between these professions, may assist in avoiding problems and setting mutual goals for high-quality reporting on health in the media. The similarities between the views of the physicians surveyed here to results from a prior study regarding social scientists [42] may mean that the challenges of science communication are universal across scientific disciplines. This could then mean that potential solutions found between the media and one group of science representatives could be utilised by other groups as well. Achieving a more thorough image of the encounters between journalism and medical science will require further research with a broader approach, for which the results of this present study can offer some starting points.

References

1. Väliverronen, E.: Tiede ja ympäristöongelmat julkisuudessa. Tampereen yliopisto: Tiedotusopin laitos, pp. 16, 36–37, 40, 43 (1994)
2. Tieteen tiedotus ry: Tiedebarometri 2016 (2016). http://www.tieteentiedotus.fi/files/Tiedebarometri_2016.pdf. Accessed 21 Mar 2018
3. Ek, S., Niemelä, R.: Onko internetistä tullut suomalaisten tärkein terveystiedon lähde? Informaatiotutkimus 29(4) (2010)
4. Reporters Without Borders Press Freedom Index (2018). https://rsf.org/en/ranking. Accessed 21 Mar 2018
5. Fielden, L.: Regulating the Press – A Comparative Study of International Press Councils. Reuters Institute (2012)
6. Kirchner, L.: Self-regulation done right. How Scandinavia's press councils keep the media accountable. Columbia Journal. Rev. News Front (2012). http://www.cjr.org/the_news_frontier/self-regulation_done_right.php?page=all. Accessed 21 Mar 2018
7. Miettinen, N.: Popularisoinnin polttopisteessä: lääketieteen yleistajuistaminen mediassa kielellisenä, viestinnällisenä ja yhteiskunnallisena toimintana. Thesis. Jyväskylän yliopiston kielten laitos (2016)
8. Matikainen, J.: Sosiaalisen ja perinteisen median rajalla. Viestinnän tutkimuskeskus CRC, Viestinnän laitoksen tutkimusraportteja 3/2009, p. 75. Helsingin yliopisto (2009)
9. Kohring, M., Matthes, J.: Trust in news media. Development and validation of multidimensional scale. Commun. Res. 34(2), 231–252 (2007)

10. Ahlmén-Laiho, U., Suominen, S., Tuominen, R., Järvi, U.: Finnish health journalists' perceptions of collaborating with medical professionals. Commun. Comput. Inf. Sci. 450, 1–15 (2014)

11. Finer, D., Tomson, G., Björkman, N.-M.: Ally, advocate, analyst, agenda-setter? Positions and perspectives of Swedish medical journalists. Patient Educ. Couns. 30(1), 71–81 (1997)

12. Soumerai, S.B., Dennis, R.-D., Kahn, J.S.: Effects of professional and media warnings about the association between aspirin use in children and Reye's syndrome. Milbank Q. 70(1), 155–182 (1992)

13. Maclure, M., Dolmuth, C.R., Naumann, T., et al.: Influences of educational interventions and adverse news about calcium-channel blockers on first-line prescribing of antihypertensive drugs to elderly people in British Columbia. Lancet 1997(352), 943–948 (1998)

14. Kunelius, R., Renvall, M.: Terveydenhuolto: julkisuus, politiikka ja kansalaiset. In: Torkkola, S. (ed.) Terveysviestintä. Helsinki, Tammi (2002)

15. Bala, M., Strzeszynski, L., Cahill, K.: Mass media interventions for smoking cessation in adults. Cochrane Database Syst. Rev. (1), CD004704 (2008)

16. Robinson, M.N., Tansil, K.A., Elder, R.W., et al.: Mass media health communication campaigns combined with health-related product distribution: a community guide systematic review. Am. J. Prev. Med. 47(3), 360–371 (2014)

17. Wakefield, M.A., Loken, B., Hornik, R.C.: Use of mass media campaigns to change health behaviour. Lancet 376(9748), 1261–1271 (2010)

18. Torkkola, S.: Sairas juttu. Tutkimus terveysjournalismin teoriasta ja sanomalehden sairaalasta. Tampereen yliopisto (2008)

19. Ruuskanen, J., Jalanko, H.: Lääketiede joukkoviestimissä. Duodecim 113(14), 1407 (1997)

20. Corbett, J.B., Mori, M.: Medicine, media, and celebrities: news coverage of breast cancer, 1960–1995. Journal. Mass Commun. Q. 76(2), 229–249 (1999)

21. Kärki, R.: Lääketiede julkisuudessa. Prometheus vai Frankenstein. Tampere, Vastapaino (1998)

22. Zola, I.: Medicine as an institution of social control. Sociol. Rev. 20(4), 487–504 (1972)

23. Illich, I.: Limits to Medicine. Medical Nemesis: The Expropriation of Health. Marion Boyars, Lontoo (1995)

24. Järvi, U.: Toimittaja katsoo potilasta – uhri vai sankari. Toimittajat haluaisivat juttuihinsa nykyistä useammin potilaan näkökulman. Suomen Lääkärilehti, 311–317 (2002)

25. Järvi, U.: Potilas ja media. Potilaan rooli terveysjournalismin eri lajityypeissä. Unpublished thesis, Jyväskylän yliopisto, Viestintätieteiden laitos (2003)

26. Nelkin, D.: Medicine and media. An uneasy relationship: the tensions between medicine and the media. Lancet 347(8), 1600–1603 (1996)

27. Kangaspunta, S., Huusko, M.: Mahdollisuuksien avaruus. In: Terveyden ja hyvinvoinnin yhteisötelevisio -tutkimusprojektin väliraportti, pp. 42–43. Tampereen yliopisto, Tampere (2001)

28. Poikolainen, K.: Viestintä vaarantaa terveytesi. Duodecim 105(22), 1790–1795 (1989)

29. Väliverronen, E.: Lääketiede mediassa. Duodecim 121, 1394–1399 (2005)

30. Ahlmén-Laiho, U., Suominen, S., Järvi, U., Tuominen, R.: Complaints made to the council for mass media in Finland concerning the personal and professional lives of doctors. In: Eriksson-Backa, K., Luoma, A., Krook, E. (eds.) WIS 2012. CCIS, vol. 313, pp. 91–103. Springer, Heidelberg (2012). https://doi.org/10.1007/978-3-642-32850-3_9

31. Hopkins, W.: Measures of reliability in sports medicine and science. Sports Med. 30(1), 1–15 (2000)

32. Patja, K.: Seurausta kannattaa epäillä syystäkin. Suom Lääkärilehti 1–2, 26–27 (2015)

33. Keogh, C.J., McHugh, S.M., Moloney, M.C., et al.: Assessing the quality of online information for patients with carotid disease. Int. J. Surg. 12(3), 205–208 (2014)

34. Alba-Ruiz, R., Bermudex-Tamayo, C., Pernett, J.J., et al.: Adapting the content of cancer web sites to the information needs of patients: reliability and readability. Telemed. e-Health 19(12), 956–966 (2013)

35. Goslin, R.A., Elhassan, H.A.: Evaluating internet health resources in ear, nose, and throat surgery. Laryngoscope 123(7), 1626–1631 (2013)

36. Puska, P., Wiio, O.: Lääkärit ja terveyttä koskeva joukkoviestintä. Suom Lääkäril 48, 2569 (1993)

37. Järvi, U.: Median terveyden lähteillä: miten sairaus ja terveys rakentuvat 2000-luvun mediassa. Thesis. Jyväskylän yliopiston viestintätieteiden laitos (2011)

38. Suomen Lääkäriliitto: Lääkärimäärä kasvaa (2017). https://www.laakariliitto.fi/uutiset/ajankohtaista/laakarimaara-kasvaa/. Accessed 21 Mar 2018

39. Suomen Lääkäriliitto: Lääkäriliiton vuositilasto 2015 (2016). Saatavilla: http://www.laakariliitto.fi/site/assets/files/1268/vuositilastot_2015_fi.pdf. Accessed 21 Mar 2018

40. Lupton, D., McLean, J.: Representing doctors: discourse and images in the Australian press. Soc. Sci. Med. 46(8), 947–958 (1998)

41. Leikola, A.: Tiede, viesti, toimittaja. Kirjassa Rydman, J. (toim.), Puhutaanko oikeista asioista: tiedevalistuksen tila Suomessa s. 65–71. Helsinki, Tieteellisen seurain valtuuskunta (1994)

42. Pitkänen, V., Niemi, M.K.: Hallitsematon ja houkutteleva media. Yhteiskuntatieteilijöiden näkemyksiä julkisesta asiantuntijuudesta. Yhteiskuntapolitiikka 81(2016): 1 (2016)

43. Billings, L.: The case of the deviant doctor and journalists on defense: a study of science, rhetoric and boundary-work in the media. In: Conference Papers - International Communication Association, 2005 Annual Meeting, New York, NY, pp. 1–12 (2005)

44. Suomen Lääkäriliitto and Suomen Journalistiliitto: Lääkärien ja toimittajien yhteinen tiedotussuositus (2013). https://www.laakariliitto.fi/site/assets/files/2708/tiedotussuositus_140108.pdf. Accessed 21 Mar 2018

45. Egle, J., Smeenge D., Kassem K., Mittal V.: The internet school of medicine: use of electronic resources by medical trainees and the reliability of those resources. J. Surg. Educ. (72), 316–320 (2015)

46. Roshan, A., Agarwal, S., England, R.J.A.: Role of information available over the Internet: what are the parents of children undergoing tonsillectomy likely to find? Ann. Roy. Coll. Surg. Engl. 90(7), 601–605 (2008)

47. Emond, Y., de Groot, J., Wetzels, W., van Osch, L.: Internet guidance in oncology practice: determinants of health professionals' Internet referral behavior. Psycho-Oncology 22(1), 74–82 (2013)

48. Chen, X.I., Siu, L.L.: Impact of the media and the Internet on oncology: survey of cancer patients and oncologists in Canada. J. Clin. Oncol. 19(23), 4291–4297 (2001)

49. Larsson, A., Oxman, A.D., Carling, C., Herrin, J.: Medical messages in the media – barriers and solutions to improving medical journalism. Health Expect. 6, 323–331 (2003)

50. Parmanne, P., Vänskä, J., et al.: Lääkärimäärä kasvaa eläköitymisaallosta huolimatta. Suom Lääkärilehti 24, vsk 69, 1811–1812 (2014)

51. Väliverronen, E.: Tiedeviestintä ja asiantuntijuus – tutkijoiden muuttuva suhde julkisuuteen. Yhteiskuntapolitiikka 80(2), 221–232 (2015)

52. Strellman, U., Vaattovaara, J.: Esipuhe. In: Strellman, U., Vaattovaara, J. (ed.) Tieteen yleistajuistaminen, pp. 9 –13. Helsinki, Gaudeamus (2013)

53. Kiikeri, M., Ylikoski, P.: Tiede tutkimuskohteena. Filosofinen johdatus tieteentutkimukseen, p. 191. Helsinki, Gaudeamus (2004)

54. Järvi, U., Vuorenkoski, L., Vainikainen, T.: Toimittaja taiteilee lääkeviestinnän ristiaallokossa. Kysely lääketieteen toimittajien näkemyksistä lääketieteen tuottajista ja tiedon luotettavuudesta. Tiedotustutkimus 2005, 4–5 (2005)

Preferred Biosignals to Predict Migraine Attack

Hanna-Leena Huttunen[⊠] and Raija Halonen

University of Oulu, P.O. Box 4500, 90014 Oulu, Finland
{hanna-leena.huttunen,raija.halonen}@oulu.fi

Abstract. Migraine is classified to two classes, with aura and without aura, and migraine seizures last usually several hours. The goal of this study was to identify the most important symptoms of migraine to be monitored by wearable sensors to predict the migraine attack. The purpose of wearable sensors is to guide patients to take the migraine medication in time, and to support their own care. Self-measurement is a growing trend worldwide and sensor technology has been used for several years in activity wristbands, smartphones, rings, mobile phones, and mobile applications. The study was conducted as an operational study, randomised for those who had been diagnosed with migraine by a doctor. The study was divided into two parts, at first a questionnaire was sent to 17 people in social media. On the basis of the questionnaire, a qualitative interview was conducted for 12 persons with migraine. Responses to the questionnaire were compared to the results of the interview, and the answers to the research questions were sought. Migraine patients considered important that device reports quality of sleep, pulse, blood pressure, stress levels, sleep apnea, and energy consumption.

Keywords: Migraine · Prodromal symptoms · Wearable sensors
Health promotion · Self-measurement

1 Introduction

The purpose of this study was to analyse which biosignals migraine patients would like to measure to help them in managing their migraine. With an intelligent device, the emergence of migraine can be predicted, and patients can be assisted in their own care monitoring. Furthermore, wearable sensors make self-monitoring more efficient and users more aware of their own health (see [1]).

Wearable sensors collect information from users and provide feedback in real time using health applications. Self-measurement technology is about individuals measuring biological, physical, behavioural or environmental information. For several years, self-measurement has been a rising global trend utilised for activity wristbands, smartphones, rings, mobile phones and mobile applications [2, 3].

The aim of the study was to find out the most important biosignals from the view point of patients with migraine that the intelligent device should measure to predict the emergence of migraine attack. In addition, the study investigated the willingness of users to use an electronic migraine diary to support their own care. The main research question was:

Which are the six most important biosignals a device should measure to predict the incoming migraine attack?

The survey was answered through questionnaires and qualitative interviews. The questionnaires were answered by 17 persons with a migraine diagnosis.

The results of this study show that migraine patients are able to propose the six biosignals that a wearable sensor should measure to detect a migraine attack. With this study, we can define a device that will help migraine patients to detect pre-symptoms and assist them in monitoring their own care and take a medicine in time. Additionally, migraine patients provided researchers with valuable information on the emergence of migraine attacks to develop future devices for migraine treatment.

2 Related Work

Migraine can be divided to two classes, with aura and without aura. In migraine with aura, the pain is preceded by visual disturbances, numbness, muscle weakness and difficulty in speech. Migraine without migraine usually begins without the aura symptoms. From neurological diseases, migraine is the most common wide-ranging gene-regulated illness [4]. Migraine is one of the most expensive diagnosis for European health care as 10 to 15% of population suffer from it. Migraine has been associated with other illnesses such as stroke, depression, allergy, and blood pressure. At the European level, migraine costs 111 billion EUR per year [5, 6]. Because of hormonal changes, women suffer from migraine more than men [7]. Migraine is divided into four stages: pre-symptoms, migraine aura, headache, and post-symptoms. Migraine attacks last for 4–72 h and change rapidly. Common migraine pre-symptoms include fatigue, yawning, increased appetite, hunger for sweet, irritability, and feeling cold. The pre-symptoms of migraine with aura lasts for 5–60 min, and may include also lightening eyes, smelling sensation, visual field defects, sound sensitivity, and facial acuity. At the end of the aura phase, a pulsating headache begins, and also nausea and vomiting are common [8]. Migraine can be treated with two types of medication: preventive daily medication and acute medication after detecting pre-symptoms. The efficacy of medicines depends on which phase of the migraine attack the medication is taken. The best response to treatment with acute medication occurs when the drug is taken before the headache begins [9].

Digitalisation is part of future healthcare; the demands of self-care are growing in the world and more effective solutions needs to be developed [10]. Information and communication technology (ICT) can be used to take the health history of the entire patient into consideration at various stages of treatment. New technology and genetic information enables to design an individual care flow and to prevent the emergence of diseases. Patients can use sensor technology to measure and monitor their own health. Studies show that monitoring of one's own care results better results than using traditional therapy without aid from technology [7, 11]. Evolving technology offers new ways to observe and enhance health and physical fitness [2, 3]. Applications can collect information about user activity and wellbeing using psychical activity trackers, bluetooth-containing heart rate monitors and other sensors [3]. Sensors used for self-measurement have become smaller and can be better used with mobile technologies [12]. In the United States, about 60% of adults monitor weight, diet, or fitness, and 33% monitor blood pressure, blood sugar, headaches and sleep [13]. However, only one in five utilises digital technology to follow these variables, the rest are using older technologies such as pen and paper [14]. Due to the potential of wearable devices, data-gathering internet services and the storage of large data volumes, interest in self-measurement and data analysis has increased [15]. Analysing body and mind functions is no longer exclusive to science, medical researchers and technology specialists, but smart phones make it possible to monitor and store daily life for almost everyone [16].

There are several different devices available on the market, and the interest of the devices to be sold in promoting individuals' own health has received a lot of attention as the new generation of portable devices emerges [17, 18]. Wearable devices are designed to measure, for example, pulse, daily rest, quality of sleep, activity, stress and mood. Feedback allows users to understand and modify their activities and behaviours and thereby promote their own health [19]. The structure of wearable devices is generally small and light, and can be attached to, for example, a wrist or incorporated into shoes, clothing or sporting equipment [20]. Measuring human biosignals from the wrist turned out to be useful in predicting the emergence of diseases. Biosignals provide useful information on physiological changes such as changes in skin temperature, pulse and sleep. The market has advanced sensors that can be used to measure migraine pre-symptoms [21, 22]. A study of migraine patients revealed their willingness to use sensors to detect pre-symptoms in order to take medication in time. Most of them would like the device to be located in a wrist part of a watch so that migraine alert is easily recognisable [23].

Mobile devices, monitors and applications enable healthcare development, as they can be combined with a variety of sensors to collect and evaluate physiological data from the human body. Sensor networks work together via a wireless network. They allow to achieve a wide variety of opportunities to track and understand large-scale, real-life phenomena [7, 24]. Mobile devices are used in healthcare and wireless data transfer facilitates efficient data processing [30]. Sensor information is necessary to evaluate the patient's condition, determine the correct diagnosis, and to make treatment decisions and follow-up plans [11].

Increased self-consciousness helps to focus on certain behaviour and can improve well-being [25]. Earlier studies about migraine patients' willingness to wear sensors to detect migraine pre-symptoms and their pre-symptoms revealed that 88.8% of the respondents wanted a device to detect an upcoming migraine attack. The study also showed that most of the participants wanted the device to be located on the wrist, either in the watch, bracelet, or skin patch [23]. Sleep quality is associated with migraine birth and sleep disorder is a major trigger of migraine, also raising the body's stress hormone [26]. A study of wearable sensor to detect migraine attacks by using the Empatica E4 wristband showed that migraine attacks start at night and migraine patients wake up to headaches. The study also showed that the emergence of migraine attacks is unique and can be detected by sensors [1].

3   Research Methods

The study focused on migraine patients by means of qualitative research aimed at understanding a small group in the real world. The main method was qualitative interview, one of the most important tools when collecting qualitative data (see [27]). The study was explorative in nature as very little knowledge was available about the use of body sensors to detect migraines or their pre-symptoms (see [28, 29]).

3.1   Data Collection

The target group of the study was a random group of migraine sufferers. Collection of the data was carried out in three phases (see Fig. 1). In the first phase, people were asked to participate in research through social media. Migraine diagnosis was a criterion for participating. Twenty-two people with migraine came forward and a migraine questionnaire form in October 2016 in cooperation with the migraine Association. There were 17 responses to the questionnaire, which resulted in a qualitative interview for 12 participants. An e-mail survey and a qualitative interview were conducted in the fall of 2017. Five persons were not interviewed because they did not live in the area. The questions for the interview were compiled on the basis of a literature review. After evaluating the question quality, an invitation letter was sent to the informants.

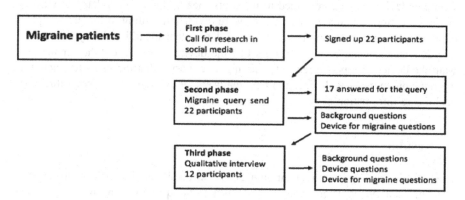

Fig. 1. Qualitative research data collection steps

The email inquiry was open to respondents for two weeks and it was responded only once per person. All questionnaires were correctly filled, so no rejection was made. The questionnaires were analysed and based on analysis the qualitative interview questions were defined. The interviews were conducted with a semi-structured questionnaire with open questions. The study concluded open questions to allow the widest possible picture of the pre-symptoms of migraine and their identification. The interviews were conducted at Oulu during one week, and they lasted about one hour. The interviews were arranged to be pleasant and peaceful to make the setting as natural as possible.

3.2   Analysis of Data

The analysis of the questionnaire was divided into two phases. In the first phase, a migraine questionnaire was categorised into two main categories, background information and device issues. The questions of the interview were divided into three main categories, background information, intelligent devices and migraine sensitive sensors. The results of the survey were analysed with Excel tool and cross-table was made. The interview material was read several times to get a full picture and responses were recorded and tabulated. Similarities were sought from the material, and it was organised into categories and named in accordance with the content. The categories were summarised and combined according to the survey and the interview. The background information was classified according to age, sex, hobby, profession, migraine type, pre-symptoms, medication, count of migraine attacks, trigger of migraine attack, time when migraine attacks occur and if relatives suffer from migraine. The data were analysed for typical symptoms associated with migraine and were classified according to the pre-symptoms and the main symptoms.

Questions about the device were classified according to the users' interest, what kind of smart technology users are familiar with, whether the users have wearable devices at home, where the users use wearable devices, what kind of experiences the users have with wearable devices, what motivates the users to wear wearable device, what problems the users have encountered when using wearable devices, and if wearable devices have contributed to the users' health. Questions related to wearable device detecting migraine pre-symptoms were divided according to the pre-symptoms of migraine, whether the users would use a device that identifies the symptoms of a migraine attack, what would the users like the device to measure, whether the users want the device to report directly to the migraine diary, what the users feel about the migraine pre-symptoms device, and how the users feel if the device reports directly to health care information systems.

4   Results

The material was collected in autumn 2017 via email inquiry and by means of a qualitative interview. There were 17 responses to the questionnaire, but only 12 participants participated in a qualitative interview.

4.1   Personal Background Questions

The first phase of the survey was answered by 16 women and one man. Twelve respondents were selected to qualitative interview and all interviewees were women and their age distribution was from 9 to 58 years. Most of them were in the age group of 30–49 years.

Most respondents suffered from migraine with aura, but respondents also had migraine without aura, and one respondent had both. For example Emma, 41 yrs, suffering from migraine with aura described: *"Behind the right eye starts a strange feeling, which gradually spreads and intensifies to ache. This is accompanied by sensitivity to odour and light, nausea (no vomiting), intermittent numbness of the head, or weakening of thought activity. Duration usually 72 h, usually starting in the morning."*

Ann, 34 yrs, suffering from migraine without aura informed: *"I feel pulsation in the left eye for multiple days or forehead range. Sometimes also nausea."* Jenny, 45 yrs, suffers from migraine both with and without aura and reported about her migraine attacks: *"It begins with a powerful headache that medication does not help, but the symptoms worsens. Then there is over sensitivity (tone, light, smells). Nausea, muscle pain, and eye pain."*

One respondent had no information on migraine form because the migraine had been diagnosed only recently. Sally, 9 yrs, was not sure if she suffered migraine with aura or not and explained: *"First comes stomach pain, fatigue and paleness. After that hard headache. If the medicine is not taken at the right time, I will start to vomit."*

Ten respondents were employees, one was unemployed, and one was a schoolchild. All respondents at work worked with computer. All respondents had physical exercise as a hobby.

One questions was to solve if the respondents' relatives had migraine. The respondents had close relatives with diagnosed migraine, and a few respondents had also children with migraine diagnose. Nine mothers and seven sisters suffered from migraine. Four children, two fathers, two brothers and two grandmothers also suffered from migraine. The results proposed that migraine is more common in female relatives. The purpose of the interviews was to find out the typical migraine attacks of the respondents and describe their migraine patterns.

For most respondents, stress, bright lights, excessive clothing, excessive sleeping, blood sugar variations, strong smells, stiffness of the muscles, too heavy exercise, eating chocolate and fatty foods, or menstruation triggered a migraine attack.

The majority of respondents (13) had at least two migraine attacks per month. Two respondents suffered more than five attacks per month, and two respondents suffered 3–4 migraine attacks per month. 14 migraine patients identified migraine symptoms. The most common of them were feeling cold, graving, muscle pain, difficulty finding words and visual disturbances. Three respondents could not classify their pre-symptoms.

4.2   Device Questions

The questions about the device were to determine if the migraine patients used intelligent technology in their everyday life to promote their own health. In the interview, the respondents raised four intelligent devices, but all respondents did not identify smart phones, smartphones, tablets, sports watches and computers as intelligent technologies, so all respondents could not present these four possibilities for the interviewer.

Eleven respondents used a smartphone but one of the respondents couldn't recognise it as smart device. Four respondents recognised that the tablet and computer were intelligent devices that they used in everyday life. Four of the respondents used smartwatch every day in their work, collecting data during sports performance, monitoring their own progress and monitoring sleep quality. The interviewers wanted to know why the respondents had not obtained wearable devices to measure their own health. Most of the respondents mentioned that there is no need to acquire a smart device or have not bothered to acquire it. One of the respondents didn't know why he should have a smart device in his own life.

The interviews sought answers to the questions of which of the identified six (6) most important biosignals the device should measure to predict a migraine attack (see Fig. 2). Another question was about pressing a button to synchronise the information with the migraine diary, whether the device should be available through the healthcare provider, and if information should be synced directly to the health care information system.

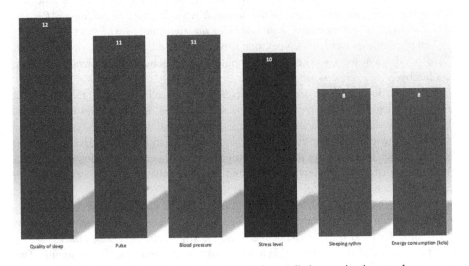

Fig. 2. The six most important biosignals for predicting a migraine attack

Figure 2 lists the desired biosignals revealed by the interviews. Figure 2 shows that all respondents wanted the device to measure sleep of quality (12), next preferred were pulse (11), blood pressure (11), stress level (10), and sleep rhythm and energy consumption were preferred by eight respondents. These six features were raised important for the device to measure to predict the incoming migraine attack.

All 17 respondents who responded to the questionnaire were willing to take the migraine report to the migraine diary. In the interviews, the same question was repeated and all twelve were willing to pass the information to the migraine diary. One respondent said she fills the migraine diary manually and finds it very laborious. The "reset" button would help migraine patients to be able to monitor the frequency of migraine attacks. One respondent explained: *"Yes I could press the button. With the migraine diary we could see e.g. the density of migraine attack and think what was triggering the attack."* Another told: *"The migraine diary would help my life if I could anticipate the attacks and take my medicine in time before the situation gets worse."* From the responses, it emerged that the device should be fast and easy to use to maintain interest in the device.

One interviewee described his migraine diary and told how migraine attack had occurred during sports, when the muscles have been tense and when he had been ill. Another reported: *"Ten years ago my migraine got chronic and I don't want to get into such situation anymore."* An anticipating device and migraine diary together help in forecasting pain attacks. One of the patients revealed: *"I'm really afraid of the pain attacks as they take all my ability to act. As a one-parent, one should always be competent to act."* The respondents considered it important that the migraine diary is available in a mobile application that can be consulted by a physician/nurse if necessary. They also considered that if they press the acknowledge button, the information goes to the health care information system and is available to the nursing staff and can be visited when needed. One patient confirmed: *"All that improves my healthcare I will do. In future, I'd like to know the statistics of how often my migraine knocks and if the attack was prevented by the medicine."*

15 respondents considered it important that the device should be available from a health centre, occupational health care, neurologist or other healthcare provider. 12 respondents were willing to buy the device by them self.

5 Discussion

The aim of the study was to find out if migraine patients would like to monitor their biosignals to reveal pre-symptoms like light sensitive eyes, sound, sensitivity of the smell, facial defect, lack of field of vision, blinking lights in the eyes, or combinations of such symptoms. This study strengthens earlier studies that migraine is a genetic-regulated illness and it is inherited from generation to generation. Because of hormonal changes, women suffer from migraine more than men and migraine sickness is located in the 25–44 age group [1, 4, 23]. In this study most of the respondents were 30–49 years old, and they had been diagnosed with migraine over the years. Respondents' close relatives, such as mothers and daughters, had also been diagnosed with migraine. Of the respondents' mothers, nine had had migraines, seven of daughters had migraines, four children had migraines, and migraine had been diagnosed with two grandmothers. Respondents had migraine with aura and without aura and one of the respondents had no information on the type of migraine. All respondents at work did work with computer. Each respondent had some degree of exercise as a hobby.

Migraine symptoms occur in the majority of patients and symptoms often occur a day before the actual migraine attack. The most common pre-symptoms were fatigue, yawning, increased appetite, hunger for sweet, irritability and feeling cold [23]. Half of the participants suffered from migraine with aura and they were more likely to detect the oncoming migraine attacks and to medicate themselves in time. Patients with migraine without aura, headaches began unexpectedly but they still suffered from pre-symptoms, which they could not interpreted as oncoming migraine. Previous study has demonstrated that sleep quality is associated with migraine birth and sleeping disorder is a major migraine trigger and also raises the body's stress hormone [26]. In this study most of the respondents had migraine attack during the night.

Measuring human biosignals on the wrist is proved useful in predicting the emergence of diseases [23]. The six most important biosignals were sleep quality, pulse, blood pressure, stress levels, sleep rhythm, and energy consumption. Biosignals provide useful information on physiological changes that improve the availability of treatment.

There are various mobile devices on the market, including applications that enable healthcare development, as they can be combined with a variety of sensors to evaluate collected data [12, 24]. The study shows that migraine patients are willing to support their self care with mobile application, which will automatically record the migraine diary information. The "reset" button would help migraine patients be able to monitor the number and frequency of migraine attacks. Data gathering allows migraine patients to avoid a migraine attack by reacting faster. Feedback allows the user to understand and modify their activities, behaviours and thus promote their own health [19].

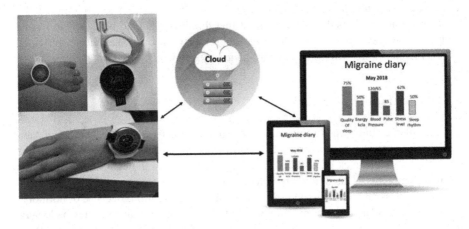

Fig. 3. Architecture for wearables

6 Conclusions

To conclude, it looks that in the future, more and more health promotion services will become electronic when technology develops at a speed. Technology can help migraine patient in everyday life when pre-symptoms of migraine are easier to identify and treatment can be started faster. Technology helps migraine patients to stay at work for longer, to have less sick leave, and to know their own health care themselves. The sensors used for self-measurement are small and can be used with wearable devices and mobile technology [12]. Earlier research [23] shows that migraine patients want to use a smartwatch or intelligent bracelet that can measure the pre-symptoms of a migraine attack. The current study proposed that migraine patients considered it important that the device measures the quality of sleep, pulse, blood pressure, stress levels, sleep rhythm, and energy consumption. All of the respondents were willing to use a device that reads and syncs the information about migraine attack to migraine diary by a confirm button.

Measuring human biosignals from the wrist is recognised to be useful in predicting emergence of diseases [1] and biosignals provide useful information on physiological changes which can be used to improve the availability of treatment [7, 11]. The current study listed sleep quality, pulse, blood pressure, stress levels and sleep rhythms as well as energy consumption as the six most important biosignals of a device to measure.

The current study proposes that people are willing to use sensor-based wearables that are connected with other systems such as diaries and interaction with other actors. Figure 3 depicts an architectural view for such a system.

As a conclusion, self-measurement is rising worldwide and migraine patients are willing to use smart devices to support their own care. Measuring the pre-symptoms of patients with migraine can promote well-being and illness management.

There are only few studies in the measurement of the pre-symptoms of migraine so far. As studies differ it is difficult to find out how effective a device detecting these six biosignals would be. Further studies are needed to assess the benefits and cost implications of supporting sensors in support and control of migraine in the long term.

References

1. Koskimäki, H., Mönttinen, H., Siirtola, P., Huttunen, H.L., Halonen, R., Röning, J.: Early detection of migraine attacks based on wearable sensors: experiences of data collection using Empatica E4. In: Proceedings of the 2017 ACM International Joint Conference on Pervasive and Ubiquitous Computing and Proceedings of the 2017 ACM International Symposium on Wearable Computers, pp. 506–511. ACM, September 2017
2. Na, H.S., Choi, Y.S., Park, T.S.: Mobile robot for personal exercise training in ubiquitous healthcare environment. In: Proceedings of the 2nd International Conference on Interaction Sciences: Information Technology, Culture and Human, pp. 742–744. ACM, November 2009
3. Klasnja, P., Pratt, W.: Managing health with mobile technology. Interactions 21(1), 66–69 (2014). ISSN 1072-5520
4. Pietrobon, D., Striessnig, J.: Neurobiology of migraine. Nat. Rev. Neurosci. 4(5), 386–398 (2003)
5. Kaattari, A., Tiirinki, H., Paasivaara, L., Nordstrom, T., Taanila, A.: Major user of primary health care services in Northern Finland birth cohort. Soc. Medicat. Mag. 52(3), 199–200 (2015)
6. Kallela, M.: What's new in migraine pathophysiology and genetics. Duodecim 121(6), 665–674 (2005)
7. Chan, M., Campo, E., Estève, D., Fourniols, J.Y.: Smart homes-current features and future perspectives. Maturitas 64(2), 90–97 (2009)
8. Linde, M., et al.: The cost of headache disorders in Europe: the Euro-Light project. Eur. J. Neurol. 19(5), 703–711 (2012)
9. Burstein, R., Collins, B., Jakubowski, M.: Defeating migraine pain with triptans: a race against the development of cutaneous allodynia. Ann. Neurol. 55(1), 19–26 (2004)
10. Olesen, J., Gustavsson, A., Svensson, M., Wittchen, H.U., Jönsson, B.: The economic cost of brain disorders in Europe. Eur. J. Neurol. 19(1), 155–162 (2012)
11. Ko, J., Lu, C., Srivastava, M.B., Stankovic, J.A., Terzis, A., Welsh, M.: Wireless sensor networks for healthcare. Proc. IEEE 98(11), 1947–1960 (2010)

12. Choe, E., Lee, N., Lee, B., Pratt, W., Kientz, J.: Understanding quantified-selfers' practices in collecting and exploring personal data. In: Proceedings of the 32nd Annual ACM Conference on Human Factors in Computing Systems (CHI 2014), pp. 1143–1152 (2014)
13. Swan, M.: The quantified self: fundamental disruption in big data science and biological discovery. Big Data 1(2), 85–99 (2013)
14. Lupton, D.: The diverse domains of quantified selves: self-tracking modes and dataveillance. Econ. Soc. 25(1), 101–1229 (2016)
15. Rettberg, J.W.: Seeing Ourselves Through Technology: How We Use Selfies, Blogs and Wearable Devices to See and Shape Ourselves. Palgrave Macmillan, London (2014)
16. Pantzar, M., Ruckenstein, M.: The heart of everyday analytics: emotional, material and practical extensions in self-tracking market. Consum. Mark. Cult. 18(1), 92–109 (2014)
17. Fritz, T., Huang, E.M., Murphy, G.C., Zimmermann, T.: Persuasive technology in the real world: a study of long-term use of activity sensing devices for fitness. In: Proceedings of the SIGCHI Conference on Human Factors in Computing Systems, pp. 487–496 (2014)
18. Yang, H., Yu, J., Zo, H., Choi, M.: User acceptance of wearable devices: an extended perspective of perceived value. Telemat. Inform. 33(2), 256–269 (2016)
19. Crawford, K., Lingel, J., Karppi, T.: Our metrics, ourselves: a hundred years of self-tracking from the weight scale to the wrist wearable device. Eur. J. Cult. Stud. 18(4–5), 479–496 (2015)
20. Parviainen, J.: Quantified bodies in the checking loop: analyzing the choreographies of biomonitoring and generating big data. Hum. Technol. 12(1), 56–73 (2016)
21. Pagán, J., et al.: Robust and accurate modeling approaches for migraine per-patient prediction from ambulatory data. Sensors 15(7), 15419–15442 (2015)
22. Pagán, J., Risco-Martín, J.L., Moya, J.M., Ayala, J.L.: Grammatical evolutionary techniques for prompt migraine prediction. In: Proceedings of the Genetic and Evolutionary Computation Conference, pp. 973–980. ACM, July 2016
23. Huttunen, H.L., Halonen, R., Koskimäki, H.: Exploring use of wearable sensors to identify early symptoms of migraine attack. In: Proceedings of the 2017 ACM International Joint Conference on Pervasive and Ubiquitous Computing and Proceedings of the 2017 ACM International Symposium on Wearable Computers, pp. 500–505. ACM, September 2017
24. Krishnamachari, B.: Networking Wireless Sensors. Cambridge University Press, Cambridge (2005)
25. Bentley, F., et al.: Health mashups: presenting statistical patterns between wellbeing data and context in natural language to promote behavior change. ACM Trans. Comput. Hum. Interact. 20(5), 27 (2013). Article 30. https://doi.org/10.1145/2503823
26. Mönttinen, H., Koskimäki, H., Siirtola, P., Röning, J.: Electrodermal activity asymmetry in sleep - a case study for migraine detection. In: Eskola, H., Väisänen, O., Viik, J., Hyttinen, J. (eds.) EMBEC & NBC 2017, vol. 65, pp. 835–838. Springer, Singapore (2017). https://doi.org/10.1007/978-981-10-5122-7_209
27. Myers, M.D., Newman, M.: The qualitative interview in IS research: examining the craft. Inf. Organ. 17(1), 2–26 (2007)
28. Gable, G.G.: Integrating case study and survey research methods: an example in information systems. Eur. J. Inf. Syst. 3(2), 112–126 (1994)
29. Baskerville, R.L.: Investigating information systems with action research. Commun. AIS 2 (3es), 4 (1999)
30. Thiyagaraja, S., Dantu, R.: Finger blood flow monitoring using smart phones. In: Proceedings of the 8th International Conference on Body Area Networks, BodyNets 2013, pp. 237–239, ICST, Brussels, Belgium (2013). ISBN 978-1-936968-89-3

Interpreting Behaviour and Emotions for People with Deafblindness

Riitta Lahtinen[1] and Stina Ojala[2](✉) (iD)

[1] ISE Research Group, University of Helsinki, Helsinki, Finland
[2] Department of Future Technologies, University of Turku, Turku, Finland
stina.ojala@utu.fi

Abstract. This case study investigates interpreting emotions and behaviour for the deafblind. Here we give examples on the different methods used for enhancing emotions based on sign language, speech-to-text and other types of interpreting. The group in question consists of individuals with a hearing impairment (the deaf and hard-of-hearing groups), individuals with a dual-sensory impairment and individuals with a deafblindness. The study investigates the interpreting process as a means to increase a person's social inclusion and well-being. The examples given in the article consist of different types of interprets received by the individuals within a film watching event. A further note is made on venue layout and individual needs with regards to interpreting needs and preferences.

Keywords: Behaviour · Interpreting · Deafblindness · Social inclusion

1 Introduction

This research investigates relaying emotional content within interpreting process especially with regards to interpreting for people with deafblindness or a dual-sensory impairment. This process includes three main categories: linguistic interpreting, guiding and environmental description. Emotional content can be included in each of these parts: one can verbalise emotions within linguistic interpreting, environmental description benefits from so-called emotional haptices (emotional response hand [1]), and guiding may include walking in time with music.

Even though nowadays it is possible to use on-demand film databases, going to the cinema is still popular. There are more than the film that goes into cinema-going experience. One goes to the cinema with a friend, there is an audience, one might buy sweets etc. to be enjoyed during the film. All of these parts form the holistic cinema-going experience. One can also better focus on the film and doesn't have the same disturbances as at home. The possibility to watch a film on a DVD made it possible to get this experience accessible to the people with deafblindness or dual-sensory impairment.

Finnish legislation allows a person with deafblindness, a dual-sensory or a hearing impairment to receive interpreting services, which are paid by the Finnish social security institute (Kela). The users of interpreting services have individual interpreting profiles, which include the communication and interpreting methods and other

H. Li et al. (Eds.): WIS 2018, CCIS 907, pp. 211–220, 2018.
https://doi.org/10.1007/978-3-319-97931-1_17

individual needs with regards to interpreting, such as necessary technical aids. Interpreting methods may include spoken language, sign language, sign supported speech, speech-to-text or methods relaying information through touch, such as tactile sign language, haptices or other tactile-based methods.

Interpreting for an individual may involve a working pair. The interpreters may use different interpreting methods simultaneously according to the individual's wishes and needs. The working pair might include one using tactile sign language for linguistic information and the other using haptices for situational awareness. Another individual might wish for speech-to-text interpreting for linguistic information and haptic methods for situational interpreting. A working pair might consist of a speech-to-text and a signing interpreter working together. The individual needs may wary from one situation to another.

The need for different interpreting methods varies. One needs to change the direction of gaze between two information sources when following a film and speech-to-text interpreting. This strains the functional vision of the person with a visual impairment as one needs to accommodate between a near and a far target in succession. This process is called accommodation of eyes [2, 3].

The emotional content in the films are expressed for example with intonation and vocal quality changes and/or with music. The perception and processing of vocal quality changes requires the ability to process the subtle nuances in the quality of voice. These qualities are highly varied and individual, and the disambiguation needs practice [4]. This ability is impaired in a hearing impairment. The musical qualities are also difficult to decipher with hearing aids or cochlear implants due to their limitations [5]. These musical textures are also culturally-bound and highly dynamic. Often there are both music and speech used simultaneously in the films, and this increases the challenges for deciphering the auditory environment [6; 206–207]. For the above reasons, the interpreting is very important for relaying the emotional content in the film, that is, to support the individuals' functional hearing and sight.

1.1   Audiovisual Translation

An audiovisual interpreter verbalises the scene or picture, that is s/he tells what s/he sees [7]. Audiovisual interpreter concentrates on translating between visual and auditive channels only. Audiovisual describer on the other hand relays the scene holistically and includes also auditive information in the interpretation if working with people with deafblindness. The interpretation of the scene in the film when interpreting for a person with a dual-sensory impairment relies strongly on the visual processing of the interpreter. The people with a visual impairment can enjoy the visual story-telling of the film via audio description when the interpreter verbalises what s/he sees. Within the interpreting the process tells about how one perceives the space and how the soundscape creates the visual space. One can also mimic the changes between static and dynamic story-telling by systematic choices in verbal story-telling to depict the changes in the percepts of the character in the film. The translation studies also acknowledge the intermodal translation processes, which bring the film accessible to the people with a visual and/or hearing impairment.

1.2   Sign Language Interpretation in the Cinema

Contrary to working with spoken languages, sign language interpreting includes both linguistic and non-linguistic interpretation. The non-linguistic interpretation includes environmental description. The co-operation with the cinemas usually is smooth, so that one can negotiate to be able to see the preview and get the manuscript of the film to be able to prepare. The most demanding part of the task is to produce the interpretation not facing the screen in the cinema, because it is very difficult to disambiguate the characters based on auditory disambiguation only. This difficulty is based on the fact that all of us use our vision to help speech perception when there are more than one sound source present [6].

The iconicity of sign languages, that is, the sign may indicate certain characters of the referent, for example the aspect or manner of movement, can be used in making the message as concise as possible to save time. The basic sign for walking changes shape when the person is limping or running fast. In spoken English the word changes, but in a signed language the basic sign is modified accordingly. This adds an extra layer to the interpretation – to find the most descriptive signs for a specific situation. Also gestures from the film may be incorporated into the interpret. This is highlighted when interpreting for a person with deafblindness as the visual elements in the film should be incorporated into the signed interpret.

It might be that the interpreter has to treat the information quite independently from the source to elicit a similar emotional response to the interpret. For example the funny elements might be quite different from one language to another. The so-called cultural interpretation might be highly adequate but not necessarily equivalent to the source. When interpreting a film, the relaying of emotions is more important than being equivalent. Translation is not just translating words and sentences but expressing meanings in the other language. The main goal of interpreting for the deafblind is to relay the feel and emotional content of the film by condensing the message and still maintaining the correct product. Interpreting and relaying of emotions and facial expression are an integral part of interpreting.

In order to produce a coherent end product in interpreting, one has to be able to combine different interpreting methods and change them when in need flexibly and creatively to accommodate the changing situations, both on screen and with the film-goer's hearing and sight status. There might also be a drastic change to the interpreting so that in the beginning it might be possible to follow the signing first in free space then move to a visual frame but towards the end of the film there might be a need for hands-on signing.

1.3   Speech-to-Text Interpreting in the Cinema

Speech-to-text is an intralingual interpreting method. It includes conveying speech in a visual form, that is text. Within the process the text needs to be modified in real time and to be readable for the reader with regards to the functional properties of the vision [8].

Sometimes one is able to get the manuscript of the play beforehand, and that makes it easier to accomplish the preliminary edit. The edit requires work as one must make text readable and concise. If the material is on the computer, one can advance on the text on time with the film. It is very important to time the text correctly so that one doesn't give away the plot during the interpreting process (including operas, [9]).

When using speech-to-text interpreting the client cannot follow both interpret and the screen simultaneously and this inability is more severe with people with dual-sensory impairment. In that situation the person might follow speech-to-text screen only. In that scenario the interpret product has to be able to denote the dialogue shifts on screen. Also there might be a need to refer to the visual story-telling on screen. That is called environmental description within interpreting. If music is used to convey emotions, the interpreter should be able to convey the same emotions with text-based options. Virkkunen states, that whenever music has a strong role in the story, subtitles become less important. That is the main difference between subtitling for hearing people and speech-to-text interpreting for the people with hearing or dual-sensory impairment. Because of the rhythm and timing of the film, the description on film consists condensed description [10; 22]. It might only include one single word and thus, there is a need for thorough choice of the word. There is one single descriptive word within the material of this study /quietly vaimeasti/.

The interpreting methods adapt to the hearing and vision status of the client. The voice quality indicates emotions, but it might also result in decreasing intelligibility for the hearing-impaired listener [11]. The intelligibility is further decreased for the dual-sensory impaired person, because then the audiovisual elements of speech are not available either [12]. The behavioural description of characters in the film is incorporated in the hands-on and tactile forms of interpreting, while linguistic content governs speech-to-text and visual forms of interpreting.

1.4   Situational Awareness

Before the film starts, the interpreter and the client have to agree on what types of description are to be used. The methods include e.g. drawing on the body, and object handling. There might be different senses involved, such as olfactory and taste, as well as using haptics. The objects here might have included boxing gloves where you could have smelled leather, possibly sweat and you could have tried them on or at least explored them haptically as the storyline of the film is about a Finnish boxer.

The events at the Finnish Deafblind Association usually start with environmental description time (usually 15 min). The information within includes e.g. information on attendance, including seating order. There might also be information relevant to the event, such as this time it includes information about the film - era, places, characters, style of clothing etc. Some of this information can also be repeated after the film, as that is the chance to clarify anything that the person has missed during the film.

In the UK there are events arranged by VocalEyes. The events include the possibility to feel the theatre play scene and clothing of the actors as well as possibility to interview them. There is also an annual "Feel the Force" - science fiction event for the visually impaired. The name depicts the possibility to use one's sense of touch to gather information on film sets and clothes the characters wear.

The prior knowledge of number as well as hearing and visual status of the participants is important in order to book a suitable venue. This information also includes the number of interpreters and the need of them to have the screen on their field of vision. The special requirements include the need for seating arrangements in such a way that everyone will be able to follow the film using their functional hearing and vision supported by various types of interpreting methods.

A prior notice of the film event was published in the Finnish Deafblind Association magazine called Tuntosarvi. There were 7 participants in the film event. Six of them had dual-sensory impairment and one was hearing and sighted. The organiser of the event (author RL) organised the environmental description for the event. The venue was the Frans Leijon meeting room of the Finnish Deafblind Association. The room has adaptive lighting and a built-in induction loop.

2 Materials and Methods

The Happiest Day in the Life of Olli Mäki is a 2016 Finnish drama film. It tells the story of a Finnish boxer Olli Mäki and it is based on true events. He was the first Finn to have a fight at the Olympic Stadium in Helsinki in 1962. The film is feature-length black-and-white film (96 min). The 10 s scene used as the material of this study is at time stamp 72.11. The scene used because there was no dialogue, abundance of facial expression, emotions, actions and movement.

The material of the pilot study consists of a black-and-white film depicting 1960's. This is accomplished using different aspects in the film including the clothes, hair styles, traffic and furniture. Also the black-an-white element of the film forms a part of the feel. This is an important fact to relay in interpreting, so that the participant doesn't expect colours as it might be that s/he has problems in colour vision.

The interpretation received by the participants is spontaneous and real-time. The visual and hearing conditions are adapted to be best possible in order to making the experience as convenient and fun as possible for the participants. The lighting conditions have to be of good quality. The use of functional vision can be obtained when the venue has adaptive lighting system. That allows the participants to find the most suitable place for their visual status. People differ in the lighting conditions they need. There is a main lighting with adaptation possibility as well as a suppletive light above the table. When watching the film there is a need for some lighting so the signing and the facial expressions of the interpreters can be followed. In the beginning of the event all the light were on, but when the film started the lights were dimmed somewhat. This is similar to the behaviour of lighting in the cinema.

The venue map has the induction loop pattern depicted as a dotted line (Fig. 1). The figure depicts the seating order of the participants. The size of the venue is 5×7 m. The oval table in the middle of the room is 3.5×1.1 m. There is a 32" tv in the corner. The numbers relate to the participants (Fig. 1; Tables 1 and 2). The filled grey squares depict the participants and the number indicates their position in the communication list. The triangles with black edges denote interpreters and the numbers within indicate the participant following the interpreter. The circle denotes the organiser of the event (author RL). The figure also indicates the places of the table and the tv as they were not mobile. There was a free seating order, so everyone was able to choose their place according to their needs (need to see the tv screen, use of one or two interpreters, etc.).

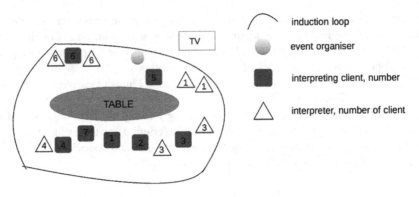

Fig. 1. Venue map

Table 1. Participants' communication and interpreting methods used

Participant	Interpreter(s)	Independent percept	Interpreting	Main source	Communication
1. Deaf, sighted	2 FSL interpreters	Emotion content	Linguistic content	Film	Sign language
2. Deaf, visual impairment	2 FSL interpreters	Strong emotions	Emotional and linguistic content	Interpret	Sign language
3. Deafened, visual impairment	2 speech-to-text interpreters, hybrid with SSF	No	Emotional and linguistic content	Interpret	Finnish
4. Blind, hearing impairment	1 interpreter with touch-based information	Auditive information from film	Emotional content	Film	Finnish
5. Visual and hearing impairment	No	Emotional and linguistic content	No	Film	Finnish
6. Deafblind	2 FSL interpreters	No	Linguistic and emotional content	Interpret	FSL hands-on and haptices

The chairs in the room were movable and some of them did not have armrests. This is an important feature with regards to tactile methods of interpreting to be as ergonomic and easy to produce and perceive as possible. The movability of the chairs is an integral part of the seating plan, as here interpreting is an integral part of the experience

Table 2. Information received from the film

Information	Users, communication numbers	Content
Visual	1, 2, 5, 7	Close-up of Olli meeting Eelis Eelis smiles and pats Olli's cheeks with both hands Eelis grabs Olli and hugs him Their heads are close to each other Olli puts on his morning gown The audience surrounds them
Auditive	4, 5	Great (male voice, quiet, not clear) (claps, murmur) Great (male voice quietly) (murmur)
Speech-to-text	3	Close-up of smiling Eelis, then Eelis hugs Olli firmly: Well done, well done, Olli! Olli puts on his morning gown while flashlights from cameras flash. Raija walks in
Subtitling	4, 5	Gosh, Olli! Well done Gosh. (Quietly)
Hands-on movement	6	Eelis depicted by one and Olli by the other hand. Speed of meet in hand movements. The intensity and duration of the hug depicts the joy of the meeting. The depiction also includes who greets whom. The interpreter uses the hands, arms and the upper back within the interpretation. It might also be possible to accomplish the interpret of the boxing match standing position where the hands represent the boxers
Audio description		A close up of a smiling, dark-haired, 30 year old man, Eelis' face. He looks at the shorter, blond, 26-year-old Olli, comes closer to him and pats his cheeks eagerly, takes him into his arms and hugs him while patting Olli's shoulder with his other hand. Olli looks down and seems to be content. Olli puts on his morning gown

of watching a film. The soft seats in a cinema might be comfortable, but they become clumsy when one attempts to produce or perceive touch-based methods of interpreting when one cannot position yourself optimally for the interpreting.

The optimal hearing conditions were obtained with the mobile induction loop, which was installed around the seating area. All the participants were seated inside the loop, because the loop only transfers the signals within. There was a separate microphone to pick up the sound from the tv. Tv audio output was not available for the direct connection for the induction loop. During the discussion the speakers took turns to speak, and there was only one voice source at a time. The organiser gave floor to speakers one by one. All of the participants used the telecoil capacity of their hearing aids and cochlear implants [5].

There are special requirements for the timing and information processing with regards to watching the film with a group of people with dual-sensory impairment. To receive interpreting via several different sensory channels simultaneously takes a lot of energy so pauses are very important for the participants. Furthermore, there are requirements to the timing of the event as a whole, as there are special requirements for the preparation of timing of the film and information flow. The group decided to have one 15 min break during the film. This was based on the information that to be receiving interpreting with tactile and touch-based methods for 1.5 h continually is very strenuous for the participant. Furthermore, the break also allows a silent period for the participants who are listening to the film via different assistive listening devices.

The description track was read by a female voice in the film. A female voice is usually perceived as being soft and emphatic, but with a hearing loss, the higher formants (resonance areas) of a female voice might decrease the discrimination ability of the speech [13]. This difficulty is increased by the severity of the hearing impairment. However, the type of the hearing impairment affects the variation - if the hearing impairment affects lower frequencies the female voice is more intelligible whereas if the hearing impairment affects higher frequencies the male voice is more intelligible respectively.

2.1   Participants' Communication and Interpreting Methods

People with a dual-sensory impairment, deafblindness or hearing and visual impairment all have their individual communication methods. Some may use sign language, such as Finnish Sign Language (FSL), some so-called Sign Supported Finnish (SSF), which is a visual communication method based on spoken Finnish language and some use spoken Finnish, either in spoken or written format. The individuals differ in their perception and production of language, as some individuals might speak themselves but receive information back in e.g. written format or by using SSF. The communication table is organised by the primary sensory impairment, the communication and interpretation methods used (1–8, Fig. 1 squares for participants and triangles respectively for the interpreters). All of the interpreters had been specialised in interpreting for the deafblind incl. environmental description. The film was visually perceived in various degrees by participants 1, 2, and 5 and induction loop was used by 4 and 5 (Table 1).

2.2   Received Information from the Film

The participants were using different interpreting methods in connection to the film experience. The following list provides information on what types of information they perceived from the film both independently and via different types of interpreting methods (Table 2).

3   Conclusions

After watching the film there was a discussion on the usability and accessibility of audio description track for each participant. The audio description as a concept was new for all of the participants. The participants who used hearing aids and cochlear implants thought that the speaking rate and the overlap of music and speech was difficult to follow. This is similar to the group discussion where there are many voices simultaneously. This is the first difficulty in a hearing impairment [6]. The comments from cochlear implant users were similar, but the special comment from this group was relating to the volume ratio between music, speech and audio description. The simultaneous audio description and other sounds made word discrimination difficult. The speaking rate was also a challenge for this group. Overall, the hearing impaired group noticed that listening for continuous auditive signal was very strenuous as many comments included the fact that towards the end the film was more difficult to follow. The audio description was described as being simple and neutral, but in some scenes the audio description felt to be more successful and relaying also the more subtle feelings. The boxing scene was particularly successful with regards to tactile and other types of interpreting [14]. The physical strenuosity of tactile forms of interpreting resulted in aches and pains in the hands of the receiver. This was avoided somewhat by having a break in film.

The difficulties with regards to audio description included volume ratios, speaking rate and the qualities of the female voice. This raises a question whether the audio description track is accessible for the hearing impaired users. On the other hand, the practice in listening the voice resulted in the audio description being easier to listen to towards the middle of the film before the tiredness takes over. Furthermore, audio description track can be beneficial to the interpreters as it tells about non-audible events on screen. The variety of methods in interpreting for the deafblind gives an option to vary between different methods to diminish the workload. This is especially true for the methods using the sense of touch.

This type of film screening events bring the cinema-going scene more accessible for the deafblind and dual-sensory impaired people. It is easier to plan one's visit when you have prior knowledge of the venue, the assistive devices available and that there is some interpreting services available. Even though some of the cinemas have a telecoil loop, it might not be in use or the staff does not know how to use it. Also, in a regular cinema one might have difficulties in finding one's seat and it is not possible to know if it is suitable before the film begins.

If there was an additional menu on the DVD with the character voice samples, it would help the people with visual impairment to connect the characters from the very beginning of the film. Also, there might be an option for clothing description. This would approximate the events where people with visual impairment have the possibility to interview the actors and feel their clothes in theatres (cf. VocalEyes events). The holistic film experience might also include certain objects to be felt and explored in connection to the film.

References

1. Lahtinen, R.: Haptices and haptemes: a case study of developmental process in touch-based communication of acquired deafblind people. Academic dissertation, University of Helsinki (2008)
2. Goldberg, M.: Control of gaze. In: Kandel, E.R., Schwartz, J.H., Jessell, T.M. (eds.) Principles of Neural Science, 4th edn. McGraw-Hill, New York (2000)
3. LEA-test for visual impairments. http://www.lea-test.fi. Accessed 8 June 2018
4. Waaramaa, T.: Emotions in voice. Acoustic and perceptual analysis of voice quality in the vocal expression of emotions. Academic dissertation, University of Tampere (2009)
5. Limb, C.J., Roy, A.T.: Technological, biological, and acoustical constraints to music perception in cochlear implant users. Hear. Res. **308**, 13–26 (2014)
6. Aulanko, R., Jauhiainen, T.: Puheen kuuleminen ja havaitseminen. In: Aaltonen, O., Aulanko, R., Iivonen, A., Klippi, A., Vainio, M. (eds.) Puhuva ihminen: Puhetieteiden perusteet, pp. 205–219. Otava, Keuruu (2009)
7. Hirvonen, M.: Multimodal representation and intermodal similarity cues of space in the audio description of film. Academic dissertation, University of Helsinki (2014)
8. Laurén, S.: Kielen sisäinen tulkkaus. In: Käden käänteessä. Viittomakielen kääntämisen ja tulkkauksen teoriaa sekä käytäntöä. Diakonia-ammattikorkeakoulun julkaisuja XX, pp. 199–226 (2006)
9. Virkkunen, R.: Tekstitys oopperassa. Juvenes-Print, Tampere (2001)
10. Lahtinen, R., Palmer, R., Lahtinen, M.: Environmental Description. A1 Management UK, London (2010)
11. Ojala, S., Lahtinen, R., Palmer, R., Äärelä, A.: Enhancing emotions through touch – haptices as a special case. Linguistic Lettica. Latviešu Valodas Institūta Žurnals, pp. 34–49 (2016). ISSN 1407-1932. http://www.lulavi.lv/media/upload/tiny/files/LL24_sakums%20saturs.pdf
12. Andersen, T.S., Tiippana, K., Lampinen, J., Sams, M.: Modeling of audiovisual speech perception in noise. In: ASVP (2001)
13. Ojala, S., Raimo, I.: Akustiikkaa ja artikulaatiota eli miltä puhe näyttää. In: Aaltonen, O., Aulanko, R., Iivonen, A., Klippi, A., Vainio, M. (eds.) Puhuva ihminen: Puhetieteiden perusteet, pp. 174–182. Otava, Keuruu (2009)
14. Mesch, J.: Tactile Sign Language: Turn Taking and Question in Signed Conversations of Deaf-blind People. Gallaudet University Press, Washington (2001)

Need for eHealth Ethics

Minna M. Rantanen[⊠], Juhani Naskali[iD], and Jani Koskinen[iD]

Turku School of Economics, University of Turku, Turku, Finland
{minna.m.rantanen, juhani.naskali, jasiko}@utu.fi

Abstract. The healthcare is an area where ethics has justifiably gained a central position, and this fact has acted as a safeguard for people and society. However, the increasing use of information technology has brought forth new kind of situations that the traditional medical ethics approach has not faced before. There is need for a new approach of eHealth ethics that covers the needs for modern healthcare to ensure that the ethicality will be ensured today and future likewise. We argue that a fruitful approach for this is the synthesis of traditional medical ethics and IS-ethics. In this article we look the four principles of medical ethics together with IS-ethics approaches by Moor and Brey to see what kind of values should be protected and what are the needs for justified use of information technology in healthcare.

Keywords: eHealth · Ethics · Values · New approach

1 Introduction

Information systems are an inseparable part of modern healthcare. Electronic medical records, electronic health records and other electronic information systems have changed the way that healthcare functions and is moderated. Despite the major impact of information technology (IT) on the healthcare this relationships seems to be poorly understood [1–3]. Since healthcare strongly relies on technology, the potential risks with technology are also potential risks for successful healthcare [4, 5].

Technology causes change in the social system to which is implemented and this change can be unpredictable as well. When an information system is changed or implemented it will change the organisation as well [6–9]. Technological products, such as information systems, influence their social context by either through affordances or through constrains, enabling or discouraging certain behaviour or use [10]. Thus, the way that the information system is designed also plays an important role in this unpredictable interaction. As information systems are always designed by human beings that are trying to fulfil certain goals, information systems are never value free [11–13].

Values are abstract ideals of what is important in life, that people strive to realise in the real world and thus, often act upon their values. [10, 14] Thus, values that are held in importance while making decisions about information systems affect the inbuilt values of a system. For instance, if efficiency of the system is a value that is held by the people developing the information system, the value of efficiency is probably going to be build in that system. However, this value might not be valued by other people that

H. Li et al. (Eds.): WIS 2018, CCIS 907, pp. 221–232, 2018.
https://doi.org/10.1007/978-3-319-97931-1_18

are going to be using or are otherwise in interaction with the system. Thus, we should aim to find the values that are beneficial to all human beings affected by the information system that is designed. However, we have to be able to justify why specific values are preferred instead of others and then the ethics comes forward.

The field of IT-ethics has attempted to find the ethically justified way to make systems for the people [10]. However, we argue that there is a special need for eHealth ethics, since modern healthcare is in many ways different from the traditional organisation. First, healthcare has strong background in ethics [15, 16]. Second, healthcare is depended on the healthcare information systems and in case of malfunction the negative consequences can be irreversible [17]. Third, current development trend brings individuals closer to practitioners with eHealth solutions and makes the modern healthcare even more complex socio-technical system [18].

Thus, in this paper we consider some aspects of eHealth ethics and represent some values that could be a part of its basis. Since ethics without action is not going to make a change, we also consider how eHealth ethics could be applied in practice when developing and assessing health related information systems. The aim of this paper is to spark a discussion about the need and content eHealth ethics. Thus, we do not argue that our description of eHealth ethics or its application is the only way of making ethically justified health related information systems, but rather present it as one proposal for a more ethical approach on eHealth.

In the next section we describe the background of eHealth and explain why eHealth ethics as a new way of viewing healthcare information systems is required. In the Sect. 3 we discuss different kinds of applied ethics that are in relation to eHealth ethics and describe what eHealth ethics is. In the Sect. 4 we consider ways that could be used to apply eHealth ethics in practice. Finally, we conclude in Sect. 5.

2 Background

As a topic eHealth is widely discussed in conferences, in the literature, and in the media. Despite the frequent use of the term there is no consensus about the definition of eHealth. Many definitions have been proposed and used to describe broad range of technology in various different settings. [19–21]

According to Shaw et al. [21] the most popular definition with most citations is Eysenbach's [22] high-level definition of eHealth:

> "e-health is an emerging field in the intersection of medical informatics, public health and business, referring to health services and information delivered or enhanced through the Internet and related technologies. In a broader sense, the term characterises not only a technical development, but also a state-of-mind, a way of thinking, an attitude, and a commitment for networked, global thinking, to improve health care locally, regionally, and worldwide by using information and communication technology".

Despite that this definition is more like an idea of eHealth than clear definition, it fits our purposes well. However, we can no-longer state that the field of eHealth is emerging. Also we use the term healthcare informatics to describe the intersection of medical informatics, public health and business. Thus, our definition for eHealth in this paper is *"eHealth is a sub-field of healthcare informatics, referring to health services and information delivered or enhanced trough the Internet and related technologies"*.

Healthcare informatics can also be described as an interdisciplinary field in the cross-roads of information systems and healthcare. Information systems science as a field has its roots in the managerial aspects of the computer assisted organisations even there are also other paradigms, such as the Scandinavian participatory approach [23]. Thus, the paradigms of the field have been shifting towards wider consideration of the nature of an information system, that acknowledges also the social aspects in relation to the technical ISs [24]. This shift can be seen also in the field of health informatics, as example there is an increasing interest towards customer-centric information systems such as personal health records [25–27].

Also the field of healthcare is going through a paradigm shift from sickness centricity towards more preventive healthcare [28]. Simultaneously, the expert driven nature of healthcare is shifting, as the customers of healthcare are more interested in health issues and due to technological changes more capable of getting more information, thus breaking the long standing information monopoly of the healthcare professionals [29]. Thus, healthcare informatics are amid of the paradigm turmoil.

Technology has played a major role in the paradigm shifts of healthcare as White [30] noted a decade ago. Now healthcare systems globally are facing the problem of ageing population and thus, are in pressure to become more efficient [18, 28]. Once again technology is playing an important role in this change. However, the change is no longer happening only within the healthcare institutions but also in the customer side. Technologies which endorse patient engagement and self-care are gaining more and more popularity, and changing the healthcare systems. [18]

It is apparent that these changes will change the nature of healthcare drastically. Healthcare is no longer all about practitioners healing sick patients, but rather a complex cooperation between professionals and people with the help of technology. Due to this tectonic shift, we can no longer view healthcare information systems solely from the perspective of healthcare. We have to take into account also the individuals who are taking care of their selves with technological systems connected to healthcare. Thus, new ways of viewing healthcare information systems are needed.

Healthcare and medicine have a long history that is interrelated with ethics for millennia. Ethical values have guided the practitioners as well as the development of the field in general [15, 16]. We still need to understand the ethical aspects and consequences in relation to healthcare and technology. Thus, ethics should be embraced as a basis for the modern eHealth now and in the future.

However, due to the evolving and complex state of the healthcare we can no longer rely merely on the ethical basis of the healthcare. We also need to consider ethical values of the individuals that are becoming more active actors in the complex sociotechnical system of modern healthcare. Besides understanding the values of practitioner and individuals, we also need to understand values that are incorporated in healthcare information systems (HISs), since information systems are never value free [11–13].

A good example of a value that is built in information technology is the value of efficiency that often seems to be the goal of the healthcare development. Efficiency is based on the speed of computers likewise its advanced freedom from limitation of space and location. Efficiency itself is not a bad value—from utilitarian point it is also ethical as it enables the production of more good—but if it is the core value we may have situation where anything inefficient is seen as bad which obviously is not true. Also, if efficiency is seen as the most important value, surpassing all others, such as quality of care and compassion, it will inevitably create problems. Therefore, without noticing these kind of embedded values and ethical issues following those values underneath the outcome can be unpredictable and in many cases undesirable.

We should clearly question efficiency as a core value of healthcare and medicine based on this short analysis. But which values could be considered to be the basis of modern healthcare and thus, also as a value base for technology used in it? To analyse this, we need to understand ethics of both healthcare and technology. To make a real change, we also need a way to pass this understanding to the developers and stakeholders of HISs. For these purposes we propose a new form of applied ethics that we have here named as eHealth ethics, which combines healthcare ethics and computer ethics.

3   eHealth Ethics

3.1   Healthcare Ethics

As stated earlier healthcare, medicine, and ethics have a long history [15, 16]. Likewise, from the beginning of nursing, the ethical nature of the work of the profession has been emphasized [15]. Ethical codes define the duties of nurses, give guidelines for ethical actions, express the virtues of nurses and provide nurses with core values and standards [31]. Thus, it is obvious that ethics cannot be overridden by efficiency.

Thus, ethical reflexity towards the work process has a major role in the field of healthcare and is – or at least should be – the standard position in the field [16]. Thus, as ethics is an inseparable part of healthcare and when developing or implementing a HIS, we should understand the underlying values that have manifested through ethical principles (here the four principles of medical ethics) in action.

Thus, is this current situation we can turn towards the four principles of medical ethics which have been the basis of medical ethics: respect for autonomy, beneficence, non-maleficence, and justice [32–34]. Information systems developed for the healthcare should thus fulfil these principles to incorporate the values of healthcare.

Autonomy
Principle of autonomy is aimed at securing the rights of individual to be treated without forced paternalistic manners. Leino-Kilpi [35] stated that there are four points for autonomy of patient.

First, human rights and values has to be respected [35]. We need to understand the value of people as themselves. This is very Kantian approach—people should always seen as ends in themselves, not merely as means [36]. Thus, when designing an information system, one should respect the people that are affected by the system.

Secondly, patient needs information about health services and they need to have access to their own information [35]. The current trend is to give patients access to their health information [37]. This right for patients to their own information from ethical perspective is also underlined by Koskinen [38]. However, the information in many cases is not easy to understand by layman and there is obvious need for improving how the information system are developed. Those should also serve the needs of patients if we want to achieve autonomy of patients instead of supporting paternalistic structures with information systems.

Thirdly, informed consent is needed for a patient to be autonomous [35]. If a patient cannot give consent that is based on their own judgement, they do not have autonomy. Informed consent can be fulfilled only if the information needs of patients are fulfilled. Even if there are systems that support giving and making consents—like Omakanta in Finland—it does not be enough if there is no information available to make decisions, yet alone informed ones.

Fourthly, the privacy and confidentiality must be respected [35]. If there are risks of losing privacy, patients possibility to be open and have trustworthy relationship with healthcare (professionals) is endangered. Thus, the security issues in HISs should be taken seriously if we want to secure the trust towards healthcare.

Beneficence and Non-maleficence

Beneficence and non-maleficence are principles which have to be analysed together in healthcare as there are many cases where some harm must be done to achieve the created good. In practise, there should always be substantial beneficence for patient to be ethically justified practise [39]. For HISs this means that they may not cause harm but always be beneficial. There is clear advantages of using HIS that works well increased effectiveness, more information for medical decision making etc.

The problem is, that in many cases the promises that are put in HIS, are not met. There have been even life-endangering situations that information systems has been caused in healthcare [40, 41]. Thus, there exist and ethical demand to ensure that new HISs create more beneficence for patients than previous system. This should be taken care when designing and implementing new systems.

Justice

Justice – it is not easy to say what kind of healthcare would be just. Campbell et al. [39] announce that for treating people without consideration of their worth, the need should probably be the basis for delivering care. It is obvious that there usually are needs in excess of the resources of healthcare and we need to find solution to use resources ethically. Equal and fair treatment of people when they are in need of help justifies the existence of healthcare. People should have access to care which they need and which healthcare can arrange with allocation of its limited resources [42].

We need to use information technology to improve our healthcare but such way that we are not violating the other principles. Technology—likewise efficiency—has instrumental value in healthcare but not intrinsic and thus it must serve the good for society not be the main goal.

The four principles have received some criticism but they are still used in practise and research despite of limitations they have [43, 44]. Thus, these principles should be considered as a simplification of the codes of ethics – as a necessary but not as a sufficient condition to be taken care in context of HISs too.

3.2   Computer Ethics

Computer ethics (also known as IS ethics) is a branch of ethics concerning the unique ethical issues that wouldn't exist without computers (or other information technology) [45]. One of the breakthrough articles was written by Moor in 1985 [46], and after that researchers have continued to examine modern ethical dilemmas from this unique perspective. Just as Environmental Ethics has emerged as a field of ethics relating to the moral relationship between humans and the environment, Computer Ethics concerns the moral questions of what *should* and *shouldn't* be done in situations that involve IS [47].

While the uniqueness of Computer Ethics has been a source of some debate and its legitimacy as a unique field has been challenged [48], there are many examples of unique cases where it is difficult or impossible to use everyday analogues to situations concerning information technology. While simply involving a computer is not enough for an ethical issue to be considered computer ethics, some cases are unique enough to warrant a special category of examination. In such instances, it is imperative to clear up all related concepts. For example, copying a file is not analogous to borrowing or reproducing or stealing a physical object, but a distinct act of its own. As such, the morality of copying files in different situations is nearly impossible to analyze without incorporating the technological perspective of Computer Ethics [10, 46, 47, 49].

This type of new acts and situations often create what Moor calls policy vacuums, which computer ethicists attempt to fill [47]. A policy vacuum is created by fast technological development that makes it hard or even impossible to adjust laws and policies fast enough to fit the current situation. Examples of such vacuums exist, for example, in regards to cyborgs, nanotechnology and AI [50–52]. Here we attempt to, at least partially, bridge such a gap in eHealth.

3.3   eHealth Ethics as a Framework

As technological development has made and will continue to change how our healthcare will evolve, we need to be able to combine the ethical knowledge from the fields of healthcare and technology. There has been proposal that the four principles of medical ethics could serve as common language between the medical and IS professionals [13].

However, it seems that ethical guidelines or codes—such as the four principles—of healthcare are not used or widely known by developers of HIS's even though IS field has developed the ethical codes of their own [53]. If ethical principles for healthcare and medicine are not followed/understood in the development or procurement of HIS the outcome hardly is fulfilling the demands of those principles. The developed system necessarily creates ethical consequences to the whole healthcare system as it dynamically changes the whole system instead of being mere isolated static technological implementation [6–9, 54].

When designing systems for healthcare the ethics of the medical profession, values of patients and society must be reflected in the system; if they are not, the system does not (or at least may not) answer to the needs of the field, and thus we get systems which do not answer to the needs of the healthcare or society. Of course there may be need for rethinking and revising those ethical principles but there is need to have something to base on today and we leave the revision of those principles out of scope of this paper.

Why these ethical principles are seen as important for IS professionals that develop systems? Why it is not enough that healthcare as buyer of HIS makes sure that systems are in line with values and regulation in the healthcare? Koskinen et al. [13] stated that these principles could be common ethical ground for both healthcare professional and developers of information systems. The common ethical language would help the developers to understand values that must respected in healthcare. Likewise, the need for healthcare professionals to see how technology is affecting organisation would be more easily to be shown, when risks could be stated with language that shows the ethical consequences. Thus, there is need for strong participatory approach in eHealth ethics.

However, we see that before we have possibility to participatory actions we need for more detailed view for the ethics of eHealth, that should be focused by researchers. We claim that even the four principles may be a good, simplified tool for practitioners, the more detailed codes should be also looked to meet the needs of varied ethical issues that emerges with technology.

Our aim is to develop the synthesis of IS-ethics (based on Moor [46] and Brey [10]). There is lot of other IS-ethical theories and directions but in this paper we look only the those above mentioned ones. Moor can be seen as one of founders in IS-ethics approach (called computer ethics by Moor) who did make the problems of computerisation visible. Thus, we chose to use it as it points the relevance of IS focus in ethics.

If Moor is one of the founders of IS-ethics, Brey is an advocate of more modern research and is focusing on wider aspects of technology in level of society and what are the fundamentals that technology should supported in good society. These together with the four principles are basis of our first draft for eHealth ethics that should be evaluated by public discourse and real life problems faced in healthcare. Thus our approach is somewhat similar—but not same—as RRI (responsible research and innovation) that is seen to be more fruitful than mere philosophical-theoretical approach by offering the more practical way of looking ethical issues concerning ISs [55].

It must be noted that even Stahl et al. [55] see that although RRI has its advantages there is still need for computer ethics as such. We see that our approach is the between of those views by relying heavily on ethical theories but looking towards the participatory approach at the same time.

4   eHealth Ethics in Practice

Moor [46] shows we need to consider the ethical consequences of information technology and see that legislation cannot be seen as sufficient safeguard. A complementing regulative approach for legislation is soft law that includes professional guidelines and codes of ethics.

Soft law means varied, rule of law kinds of norms that do not fulfil the characteristic of the legislation as soft laws are crated different way than laws are. Government authority may formulate those to support specific legislation and its application. Soft laws can be also created by co-operation of governmental official and private actors to work as norms that should be followed. Likewise specific branches of industry or professional groups may enforce norms that they should comply with (example standards of accounting) [56]. Soft laws (here ethical codes) are important as they guide toward actions that are in line with values of society.

The four principles are an example of soft law, in a sense that they guide the work of medical professionals. However, medical professionals and organisations are bound to follow also other ethical codes and standards when treating people [57, 58]. If the public intent is to keep the healthcare systems ethically justified, it is mandatory to extend this thinking also to the development of HISs in more extended rate than it appears to be currently. Thus, the eHealth ethics—not seen only as medical ethics—as a field should cover not only the healthcare professionals, but also the developers of HISs and the public authorities behind the resolutions on behalf of the society.

However, this has not been the situation in the previous and current way in procurement, development and implementation of HIS [59–61]. The HISs are tools for achieving improved health and quality of life for citizens and as with any other healthcare tools, it must function in the maximum quality achievable within reasonable limits. If—and when—these systems are created without the aid of ethical analysis and guidelines, the whole purpose of the dependant field, i.e. healthcare, is compromised.

The four principles of medical ethics is a promising ethical basis for HIS development because of its universal and yet case-by-case adaptable nature. They are theoretically simple, generalisable, well established in the field of healthcare and when more deeply inspected, yet still cover quite well the needs of HISs as well as healthcare as a field. As every philosophical theory, it does not solve all possible problems; rather its strength is that it can be used as a common ethical basis to be used for both healthcare and HIS development.

Hence, different professionals can derive and sharpen their own, more specific ethical codes and rules and still have a common ethical basis for discussions and analysis of actions. To summarise, the usage of the four principles in context of technology does not remove all the problems, but it allows different participants to use a common language in development of modern healthcare. Used in this way it would be a major improvement compared to current procurement, development and implementation of HISs.

However, we need more research and analysis about he values that the eHealth ethics is based on. Although the four principles provide a good basis from the perspective of healthcare, also more general values should be examined to guarantee the respect of patients and citizens. Also due to fast development of technology and policy vacuums that it easily creates, we are not suggesting that eHealth ethics should be a static but rather an always evolving framework that has inbuilt the participatory approach. Thus, in future we hope to develop this framework further by considering a wider spectrum of values than the four principles of medical ethics form perspective of Healthcare side and also other IS-ethical theories should be evaluated and pondered for creating sustainable and ethically justified soft laws and codes in context of eHealth.

5   Conclusions

This paper has three main contributions. First, it views the change of the eHealth from perspective practitioners and individuals that are taking more active role in the healthcare with help of the fast developing technology. Although, individual paradigm changes have been noted before, there is very little consideration on how we can manage this change as a whole. Second, this paper introduces eHealth ethics - a possible way of managing this change by developing ethically justified healthcare information systems. Third, the contribution is not limited to a theoretical framework, but this paper also introduces codes as possible practical implementation to eHealth ethics.

However, as noted before, this paper is just a first draft and introduction of eHealth ethics in hopefully long and fruitful discussion about the topic. Thus, further analysis is needed and welcomed. Also, participatory approach should be brought to this discourse of ethical issues in healthcare to ensure that the core values of whole society could be founded and implemented as code of eHealth ethics. Otherwise there is risk that we come up with codes that are not internalised by society. We as researchers can offer new ideas and view for wider discussion and this is the point of this paper; offer one proposal for ethical guidelines for modern healthcare to be evaluated by open discourse —first by researchers but hopefully by larger audience too if our idea seen promising one.

References

1. Nguyen, L., Bellucci, E., Nguyen, L.T.: Electronic health records implementation: an evaluation of information system impact and contingency factors. Int. J. Med. Inform. 83 (11), 779–796 (2014). https://doi.org/10.1016/j.ijmedinf.2014.06.011. http://www.sciencedirect.com/science/article/pii/S1386505614001233
2. Murray, E., et al.: Why is it difficult to implement e-health initiatives? A qualitative study. Implement. Sci. 6(1), 6 (2011). https://doi.org/10.1186/1748-59086-6
3. Ammenwerth, E., et al.: Impact of CPOE on mortality rates-contradictory findings, important messages. Methods Inf. Med. 45, 586–594 (2006)
4. Meeks, D.W., Smith, M.W., Taylor, L., Sittig, D.F., Scott, J.M., Singh, H.: An analysis of electronic health record-related patient safety concerns. J. Am. Med. Inform. Assoc. 21(6), 1053–1059 (2014). https://doi.org/10.1136/amiajnl-2013-002578
5. Larsen, E., Fong, A., Wernz, C., Ratwani, R.M.: Implications of electronic health record down time: an analysis of patient safety event reports. J. Am. Med. Inform. Assoc. ocx057 (2017). https://doi.org/10.1093/jamia/ocx057
6. Lyytinen, K., Hirschheim, R.: Information systems as rational discourse: an application of Habermas's theory of communicative action. Scand. J. Manag. 4(1), 19–30 (1988). http://dx.doi.org/10.1016/0956-5221(88)90013-9. http://www.sciencedirect.com/science/article/pii/0956522188900139
7. Lyytinen, K., Newman, M.: Explaining information systems change: a punctuated sociotechnical change model. Eur. J. Inf. Syst. 17(6), 589–613 (2008). https://doi.org/10.1057/ejis.2008.50
8. Luna-Reyes, L.F., Zhang, J., Gil-García, J.R., Cresswell, A.M.: Information systems development as emergent socio-technical change: a practice approach. Eur. J. Inf. Syst. 14 (1), 93–105 (2005)
9. Mumford, E.: The story of socio-technical design: reflections on its successes, failures and potential. Inf. Syst. J. 16(4), 317–342 (2006)
10. Brey, P.: The strategic role of technology in a good society. Technol. Soc. 52, 39–45 (2018)
11. Nissenbaum, H.: How computer systems embody values. Computer 34(3), 118–119 (2001)

12. Tavani, H.T.: Ethics & Technology: Ethical Issues in an Age of Information and Communication Technology, 2nd edn. Wiley, Hoboken (2007)
13. Koskinen, J.S., Heimo, O.I., Kimppa, K.K.: A viewpoint for more ethical approach in healthcare information system development and procurement: the four principles. In: Eriksson-Backa, K., Luoma, A., Krook, E. (eds.) WIS 2012. CCIS, vol. 313, pp. 1–9. Springer, Heidelberg (2012). https://doi.org/10.1007/978-3-642-32850-3_1
14. Friedman, B., Kahn, P.H., Borning, A., Huldtgren, A.: Value sensitive design and information systems. In: Doorn, N., Schuurbiers, D., van de Poel, I., Gorman, M. (eds.) Early Engagement and New Technologies: Opening Up the Laboratory, vol. 16, pp. 55–95. Springer, Dordrecht (2013). https://doi.org/10.1007/978-94-007-7844-3_4
15. Kangasniemi, M., Pakkanen, P., Korhonen, A.: Professional ethics in nursing: an integrative review. J. Adv. Nurs. 71(8), 1744–1757 (2015). https://doi.org/10.1111/jan.12619
16. Laukkanen, L., Suhonen, R., Leino-Kilpi, H.: Solving work-related ethical problems: the activities of nurse managers. Nurs. Ethics 23(8), 838–850 (2016)
17. Rantanen, M., Heimo, O.I.: Problem in patient information system acquirement in Finland: translation and terminology. In: Kimppa, K., Whitehouse, D., Kuusela, T., Phahlamohlaka, J. (eds.) HCC 2014. IAICT, vol. 431, pp. 362–375. Springer, Heidelberg (2014). https://doi.org/10.1007/978-3-662-44208-1_29
18. Fiaidhi, J., Kuziemsky, C., Mohammed, S., Weber, J., Topaloglou, T.: Emerging it trends in healthcare and well-being. IT Prof. 18(3), 9–13 (2016). https://doi.org/10.1109/MITP.2016.45
19. Oh, H., Rizo, C., Enkin, M., Jadad, A.: What is ehealth (3): a systematic review of published definitions. J. Med. Internet Res. 7(1), e1 (2005). https://doi.org/10.2196/jmir.7.1.e1
20. Showell, C., Nøhr, C.: How Should We Define eHealth, and Does the Definition Matter? pp. 881–884. IOS Press, Amsterdam (2012). https://doi.org/10.3233/978-1-61499-101-4-881
21. Shaw, T., McGregor, D., Brunner, M., Keep, M., Janssen, A., Barnet, S.: What is ehealth(6)? Development of a conceptual model for ehealth: qualitative study with key informants. J. Med. Internet Res. 19(10), e324 (2017). https://doi.org/10.2196/jmir.8106. http://www.jmir.org/2017/10/e324/
22. Eysenbach, G.: What is ehealth? J. Med. Internet Res. 3(2), e20 (2001). https://doi.org/10.2196/jmir.3.2.e20
23. Muller, M.J., Kuhn, S.: Participatory design. Commun. ACM 36(6), 24–28 (1993). http://doi.acm.org/10.1145/153571.255960
24. Hirschheim, R., Klein, H.K.: A glorious and not-so-short history of the information systems field. J. Assoc. Inf. Syst. 13, 188–235 (2012)
25. Lahtiranta, J., Koskinen, J.S.S., Knaapi-Junnila, S., Nurminen, M.: Sensemaking in the personal health space. Inf. Technol. People 28(4), 790–805 (2015)
26. Cabitza, F., Simone, C., Michelis, G.D.: User-driven prioritization of features for a prospective interpersonal health record: perceptions from the Italian context. Comput. Biol. Med. 59, 202–210 (2015). https://doi.org/10.1016/j.compbiomed.2014.03.009. http://www.sciencedirect.com/science/article/pii/S0010482514000729
27. Lee, G., Joong, Y.P., Soo-Yong, S., Jong, S.H., Hyeon, J.R., Jae, H.L., Bates, D.W.: Which users should be the focus of mobile personal health records? Analysis of user characteristics influencing usage of a tethered mobile personal health record. Telemed. e-Health 22, 419–428 (2016)
28. Demiris, G.: New era for the consumer health informatics research agenda. Health Syst. 1(1), 13–16 (2012). https://doi.org/10.1057/hs.2012.7
29. Piras, E.M., Zanutto, A.: "One day it will be you who tells us doctors what to do!". Exploring the "personal" of PHR in paediatric diabetes management. Inf. Technol People 27(4), 421–439 (2014). https://doi.org/10.1108/ITP-02-2013-0030

30. White, R.E.: Health information technology will shift the medical care paradigm. J. Gener. Intern. Med. **23**(4), 495–499 (2008)

31. Numminen, O., Van Der Arend, A., Leino-Kilpi, H.: Nurses' codes of ethics in practice and education: a review of the literature. Scand. J. Caring Sci. **23**(2), 380–394 (2009)

32. Gillon, R.: Medical ethics: four principles plus attention to scope. BMJ. Br. Med. J. **309** (6948), 184 (1994)

33. Beauchamp, T.L.: Methods and principles in biomedical ethics. J. Med. Ethics **29**(5), 269–274 (2003)

34. Lee, L.M.: A bridge back to the future: public health ethics, bioethics, and environmental ethics. Am. J. Bioethics **17**(9), 5–12 (2017)

35. Leino-Kilpi, H.: Patient's Autonomy, Privacy and Informed Consent, vol. 40. IOS Press, Amsterdam (2000)

36. Kant, I.: The Metaphysics of Morals. Cambridge University Press, Cambridge (2017)

37. Essen, A., et al.: Patient access to electronic health records: differences across ten countries. Health Policy Technol. **7**, 44–56 (2018)

38. Koskinen, J.: Datenherrschaft–an ethically justified solution to the problem of ownership of patient information. Ph.D. thesis, University of Turku, Finland (2016)

39. Campbell, A.V., Jones, D.G., Gillett, G.: Medical Ethics, 4th edn. Oxford University Press, Melbourne (2005)

40. Dobson, J.: Understanding failure: the London ambulance service disaster. In: Dewsbury, G., Dobson, J. (eds.) Responsibility and Dependable Systems. Springer, London (2007). https://doi.org/10.1007/978-1-84628-626-1_7

41. Kaipio, J., et al.: Usability problems do not heal by themselves: national survey on physicians' experiences with EHRS in Finland. Int. J. Med. Inform. **97**, 266–281 (2017). https://doi.org/10.1016/j.ijmedinf.2016.10.010. http://www.sciencedirect.com/science/article/pii/S1386505616302258

42. Denier, Y.: On personal responsibility and the human right to healthcare. Camb. Q. Healthc. Ethics **14**(2), 224–234 (2005)

43. Page, K.: The four principles: can they be measured and do they predict ethical decisionmaking? BMC Med. Ethics **13**(1), 10 (2012)

44. Christen, M., Ineichen, C., Tanner, C.: How "moral" are the principles of biomedical ethics? – a cross-domain evaluation of the common morality hypothesis. BMC Med. Ethics **15**(1), 47 (2014). https://doi.org/10.1186/1472-6939-15-47

45. Maner, W.: Unique ethical problems in information technology. Sci. Eng. Ethics **2**(2), 137–154 (1996)

46. Moor, J.H.: What is computer ethics? Metaphilosophy **16**(4), 266–275 (1985)

47. Weckert, J.: Computer Ethics. Routledge, Abingdon (2017)

48. Tavani, H.T.: The uniqueness debate in computer ethics: what exactly is at issue, and why does it matter? Ethics Inf. Technol. **4**(1), 37–54 (2002). https://doi.org/10.1023/A:1015283808882

49. Bynum, T.: Computer and information ethics. In: Zalta, E.N. (ed.) The Stanford Encyclopedia of Philosophy, Winter 2016 edn. Metaphysics Research Lab, Stanford University, Stanford (2016)

50. Moor, J., Weckert, J.: Nanoethics: assessing the nanoscale from an ethical point of view. In: Discovering the Nanoscale, pp. 301–310 (2004)

51. Moor, J.H.: Should we let computers get under our skin? In: The Impact of the Internet on Our Moral Lives, pp. 121–137 (2005)

52. Bostrom, N., Yudkowsky, E.: The ethics of artificial intelligence. In: The Cambridge Handbook of Artificial Intelligence, pp. 316–334 (2014)

53. Gotterbarn, D., Bruckman, A., Flick, C., Miller, K., Wolf, M.J.: ACM code of ethics: a guide for positive action. Commun. ACM **61**(1), 121–128 (2017). https://doi.org/10.1145/3173016

54. Heimo, O.I., Kimppa, K.K., Nurminen, M.I.: Ethics and the inseparability postulate. In: ETHIComp 2014, Pierre & Marie Curie University, Paris, France, 25th–27th July 2014 (2014)

55. Stahl, B.C., Eden, G., Jirotka, M., Coeckelbergh, M.: From computer ethics to responsible research and innovation in ICT: the transition of reference discourses informing ethics-related research in information systems. Inf. Manag. **51**(6), 810–818 (2014). https://doi.org/10.1016/j.im.2014.01.001. http://www.sciencedirect.com/science/article/pii/S037872061400007X

56. Tala, J.: Lakien laadinta ja vaikutukset. Edita (2005)

57. World Medical Association: Declaration of Helsinki – ethical principles for medical research involving human subjects (2013). https://www.wma.net/policies-post/wma-declaration-ofhelsinki-ethical-principles-for-medical-research-involving-human-subjects/

58. The United Nations Educational, Scientific and Cultural Organization: Universal Declaration on Bioethics and Human Rights (2005)

59. Vayena, E., Salathe, M., Madoff, L.C., Brownstein, J.S.: Ethical challenges of big data in public health. PLOS Comput. Biol. **11**(2), 1–7 (2015). https://doi.org/10.1371/journal.pcbi.1003904

60. Deutsch, E., Duftschmid, G., Dorda, W.: Critical areas of national electronic health record programs—is our focus correct? Int. J. Med. Inform. **79**(3), 211–222 (2010)

61. Heeks, R.: Health information systems: failure, success and improvisation. Int. J. Med. Inform. **75**(2), 125–137 (2006)

Combating Health Inequalities Using IT: The Case of Games for Controlling Diabetes and Obesity in Chicago's South Side

N. Wickramasinghe$^{(\boxtimes)}$

Epworth HealthCare and Deakin University, Melbourne, Australia
Nilmini.work@gmail.com

Abstract. Diabetes and obesity are serious chronic diseases that are increasing at alarming escalating rates globally; however lower socio-economic groups of populations are over represented and current attempts to stem such increases have not proved to be successful. This paper proffers the potential of serious games that invoke social influence dynamics and are developed around culturally and socially relevant contexts as a way to address this disturbing and growing problem. This paper begins with a brief review of how serious games can be used as an effective learning and communication medium as well as outlining the benefits of social influence before applying the constructs to an Urban Health (Chicago) context. The paper demonstrates how, in this context, games can be used as a pedagogical tool to foster superior learning and understanding. Playing games or using other simulation-oriented applications can offer a visual portrayal of situations, from which this population can garner understanding and applicability to clinical constructs and knowledge.

Keywords: Diabetes · Obesity · Serious games · Health inequality
Urban health · Gaming

1 Introduction

Games, particularly digital games such as console-based videogames and computer games, have recently become recognized as providing rich and effective learning contexts for participants/players [1–4]. Known as "serious games", they are generally accepted to be games used for training, advertising, simulation, or education [5] that are designed to run either on personal computers (PCs) or video game consoles (e.g. Xbox or PlayStation 2). There are a growing number of video and computer games whose primary purpose is something other than to entertain [6].

A major player in the field of serious games is The Woodrow Wilson International Center for Scholars (a public-private partnership) whose goal is to assist in the development of a new series of policy education, exploration, and management tools which utilize contemporary computer game designs, technologies, and development skills [7]. As part of this goal the *Serious Games Initiative* plays a greater role in helping to organize and accelerate the adoption of computer games for a variety of challenges facing the world today [7].

© Springer Nature Switzerland AG 2018
H. Li et al. (Eds.): WIS 2018, CCIS 907, pp. 233–241, 2018.
https://doi.org/10.1007/978-3-319-97931-1_19

1.1   Serious Games for Healthcare

The efficacy of serious games for a number of clinical and healthcare applications has been identified [8, 9] as there are numerous opportunities for using them in informing, educating and training patients, medical students and medical professionals in ways that ensure not only a more efficient but also a more enjoyable way of learning. In the healthcare environment, there is scope to:

(a) explore the link between knowledge and behaviour - an effective serious game can provide a useful environment for communicating specific knowledge, challenging skills and showing outcomes;
(b) develop cooperative games which can enable players to increase communication inside and outside the game about self-care, and their feelings about their condition and understanding (for example, educating children about the dangers of smoking);
(c) design games to encourage better health behaviour and not just better health knowledge.

2   American Healthcare

For the better part of the 20th century, and now into the 21st, the United States has rightfully claimed the best medical care system in the world [10]. Looking at the miraculous cures, incredible surgical feats, control of infectious disease, and other aspects of American medicine, it is difficult to dispute the claim. But there is another story when one looks at the health of the nation's urban poor [10]. The health care system in the United States seems to hardly touch many of the most vulnerable individuals and communities [11]. Additionally, when medical care is delivered, it is often inadequate to meet the complex health, social, economic, educational, and environmental needs of inner-city urban residents [10].

The paradox of the modern American medical system is that, although it has an unparalleled capacity to treat and repair (particularly with regard to trauma and infectious disease), it is often ill-prepared to prevent illness, especially within the complex context of the urban environment. Although this contradiction has implications for the entire American population, its impact is greatest for those with the fewest resources, including the urban poor [11]. For inner-city residents who often live close to large academic health centers, the paradox is all the more acute. Even though the "best care in the world" may literally be right next door, poor urban residents experience some of the worst health conditions, live in some of the least-healthy environments, and have some of the worst health indices of any population group in the nation - in some instances comparable to those found in developing nations.

2.1   The Challenges of Urban Health

The South Side of Chicago has a population of approximately 752,496 of which over 93% are African American [12]. Many of these residents suffer from not only poverty, but also poor health. In fact, despite its proximity to a prestigious academic institution (University of Chicago), the community has experienced startlingly high rates of many preventable diseases and deaths [12]. By the late 1990s, Chicago's health department statistics indicated that the neighbourhoods in the south side had the highest age- and sex-adjusted rates of morbidity and mortality from cardiovascular and cerebrovascular disease in the entire city [12]. Residents also suffer disproportionate incidences of diabetes, cancer, some pulmonary diseases, HIV-related illnesses, and substance abuse [12].

Adequately addressing these health challenges has been further complicated by long-standing attitudes of mistrust between the University and the local community. Many in the community believed that the University was only interested in the community as a place to conduct research, and that it continued to build and increase its size at the expense of the community. On the other hand, many at the university have been perplexed and resentful because they felt the community did not recognize the institution's commitment to programs and employment or the personal contributions of the University's faculty and staff in providing health care for the community.

3   Social Influence

Social networks consist of a finite set of actors or people and the relationships between them [13]. Most commonly, those relationships are categorized into strong and weak ties [14]. According to Granovetter [15] strong ties are intimate bonds between family members or close friends that are maintained regularly and permanently. Tending to be concentrated in particular groups, strong ties are of informal nature and occur between network members with a shared social identity. In contrast, weak ties emerge as non-intimate bonds between acquaintances. Maintained infrequently and inconsistently, weak ties may be formal contacts and are more likely to link members of different small groups [16]. Weak ties tend to generate informational support whereas informal and strong ties are associated with the provision of emotional support [16].

Christakis and Fowler [17] conducted a 32 year longitudinal study regarding the spread of obesity in a large offline social network. Their results show, that the susceptibility of a person to become obese increases when close members in the social network become obese [17]. Thus, the chance of becoming obese is positively correlated with the closeness and strength of the relationship. Though the design and findings of their study have been criticized, e.g., in [18], a number of papers supports their line of argument. Talking about epidemic diseases in social networks, [19] distinguishes between communicable diseases transmitted through e.g., bacteria and viruses, such as influenza and HIV, and non-communicable diseases, e.g., cancer and diabetes, that can – by definition – not be transmitted. However, he acknowledges the diffusion of ideas and behaviours, as well as contagious trends and habits, provides a powerful substitute for physical mechanisms to spread diseases and results in a so-called "social infection". Thus, the risk factors for non-communicable diseases, such as overweight and obesity, can be spread across social networks. In addition, the relationship between social influence, network structures and obesity was also identified as an important factor in obesity [21].

Online social networks are applications that allow users to build a semi-public or public profile within a bounded system, to create explicit linkages to other users and to communicate by sharing information or sending messages between each other [20]. Organized around people, online social networks are structured as egocentric networks within which the individual is at the centre of their personal network [21]. Online social networks exhibit a high similarity to offline social relationships, as they offer similar functionalities as unmediated spaces [22]. They display people's (extended) offline social network and are primarily used to maintain and reinforce existing offline relationships [23]. Online social networks can be of a general nature or address a special or niche subject. For instance, online health communities allow people to seek information, communicate with others with the same or similar problems, to share health guidance and compare treatment and medication strategies [24]. Maloney-Krichmar and Preece [25] investigated an online health community for two and a half years and found that this community provided emotional support between its members. The accessibility from everywhere at any time, anonymity of the medium as well as the access to greater expertise are regarded as the main benefits of this online health community [25]. Having studied an online health social network for six months, Ma et al. [26] found that users' weight changes correlate positively with the number of their friends and their friends' weight-change performance. The study revealed that the online influence and its propagation distance appear to be greater than in real-world social networks [26].

Individual behaviours and lifestyle choices shaped by the offline and online social environment are driving - if not significantly impacting - the global obesity epidemic [27]. Individual behaviours, in particular health-related behaviours such as physical activity, diet, sleep, smoking, alcohol consumption as well as adherence to medical treatments and help-seeking behaviour [28], appear to be of significance in this context. Hence, investigating the relationship between online social networks and health-related behaviours, including dietary and physical activity patterns, forms the focus of this research.

To better understand this relationship, we ground our study on multiple disciplines including sociology, information systems, network research and social network analysis [29]. Based on evidence of studies focusing on the relationship between offline social networks and health-related behaviours, we propose that online social networks influence an individual's health-related behaviour and subsequently his or her health and thus we design an online-social network application to test this.

3.1   The Role of Information and Communication Technologies (ICTs)

The causes of obesity and diabetes are multifaceted and result from a confluence of several factors. Individual medical conditions may determine a person's susceptibility to gain weight but cannot explain the dramatic increase in the number of obese and diabetic people worldwide [30]. Changes in individual behaviours leading to an increased intake of high-caloric foods and a decrease of physical activity are suggested to be a key contributor to the global obesity epidemic [27]. Moreover, social networks have been identified as one of the most important dimensions of people's social environment that may enable or constrain the adoption of many behaviours, including health-promoting behaviours [31].

Previous studies have focused on the spread of obesity within traditional (offline) social networks [17, 32]. As ideas, behaviours and trends are passed on within people's social environment, a person-to-person spread of obesity within social networks has been suggested [17].

Lately, the dramatic growth of electronic (online) social networks has resulted in a blurring of the boundaries between the real and virtual world [33]. Online social networks have become part of many people's everyday life and are – just as "real world contacts" – suggested to influence the diffusion and adoption of health-related behaviours [26]. Given that online social networks are becoming more important in people's daily lives, this paper designs the Health 2.0 Facebook application Calorie Cruncher, which aims to support the investigation of the relationship between online social networks and health-related behaviour in the context of obesity and diabetes.

Thus, it would appear logically at least that games that were appropriately designed to be culturally and socially appropriate and relevant should be able to invoke social influence dynamics to enable better health behaviours to ensue. This is the thesis of the research stream proffered in the paper.

4   The Efficacy of Serious Games for Reducing Health Disparities

The motivation for using serious games to combat health inequalities can be explained by goal-setting theory. From Tetlock and Kim [34], we learn how individuals are motivated by goals, and the achievement of these same goals. Goals should be both accessible and attainable [35] and, in order to direct ourselves, we set ourselves goals that are:

- clear (not vague) and understandable
- challenging (to assure stimulation and avoid boredom)
- achievable (to minimize the chance of failure).

The selection of learning objects [36] and objectives therein should be selected so that they can be incorporated in the learner's goal-setting system (i.e., via a game encapsulating a "serious" message). Any work or effort required to achieve the game's objectives should be designed so that a student perceives it as being achievable. Learning object-driven instructional activities should be clear and easy to conceptualize, but also challenging enough to maintain intellectual engagement [36]. Goal-setting (via games) that integrates a patient's personal healthcare goals as well as helping attain his/her goals towards understanding can lead to "multi-pronged motivation" [36].

Role playing games can be used to meet self-actualization needs (following Abraham Maslow's *Hierarchy of Needs*); such needs revolve around the intrinsic growth of what is already in an organism (in this case, "bringing out" what is already within a person). A health-oriented serious game could be considered as a complex learning object; such a game could be extremely effective in scenarios (i.e. in East

Baltimore) which involve a "social impact" or social problem. The pedagogy behind this game (in terms of learning objectives) would include enabling patients (learners) to practice decision-making skills, problem analysis, and cause-and-effect relationships. We agree with the fact that more detailed research is required in order to determine the relationship between various objects and learners' motivation, self-concept, self-efficacy, and overall performance [36].

5   Design Science Research Methodology

In order to appropriately design the proposed serious games a design science research methodology (DSRM) combined with a user-centred design focus and coupled with co-creation aspects will be employed.

The design science research methodology process model has been used with great success by Peffers et al. [37]. The model is consistent with the principles and guidelines of design science research established in previous research studies such as Hevner et al. [38]. Table 1 explains the application of the DSRM to the Facebook application Calorie Cruncher developed in this paper. While Fig. 1 provides initial deign templates of the application.

Table 1. Design Science Research Methodology (DSRM)

DSRM activities	Activity description	Application in this study
Problem identification and motivation	Identify and describe the importance of the problem	Data collection for the measurement of the influence of friends on the individual's body weight, design implications for the application
Definition of objectives for the application	Define the artefact that accomplishes the objectives	Design of an application that provides access to the users' network of friends and that gathers data on the users' health-related behaviours
Design and development	Identify the requirement for the solution and create the artefact	Design of the application based on qualitative interviews
Demonstration	Use artefact to solve problem	Proof of concept of the application
Evaluation	Iterate back to the design of the artefact	Identification of areas to improve the application
Communication	Publish and communicate the results	Conference publications and road shows to communicate and discuss the results in order to develop this project further

Adapted from Peffers et al. [37]

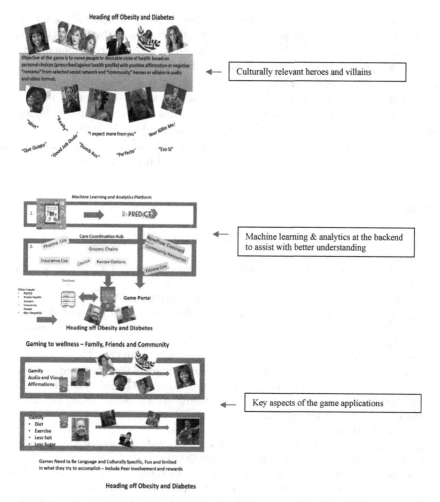

Fig. 1. Screen shots of templates of the game with culturally appropriate images and socially relevant language for the urban health environment South side Chicago (provided by ARIASIS)

6 Discussion and Conclusions

The Information Age has necessitated several changes in the way organizations operate; success for organizations is now inextricably linked to fostering and nurturing their intellectual assets. The south side of Chicago health inequality example provided in this paper, coupled with the fast-paced environment of the Information Age, means that new learning techniques and pedagogies are also required to facilitate the learning experience and ensure superior, effective and efficient learning and transfer of knowledge ensues. To address this need we believe that the use of serious games to demonstrate clinical concepts is an important initiative.

The stakeholder implications of this study are important, especially for patients (end users) who are better prepared to understand clinical concepts which they have never experienced in a scenario which is both entertaining and educational (serious games). This paper has served to demonstrate the potential efficacy of using serious games in the urban health environment. In so doing it has described some of the educational and fun characteristics of serious games and how this can be transferred into a clinical setting. It is the position of this paper that these arguments are important and should be considered and that the adoption of such initiatives in the Urban Health environment will assist in combatting inherent health inequalities and serve to stem the growing rats of diabetes and obesity in this segment of the population.

References

1. Gee, J.P.: What Video Games Have to Teach Us About Learning and Literacy. Palgrave Macmillan, New York (2003)
2. Klein, J.H.: The abstraction of reality for games and simulations. J. Oper. Res. Soc. **36**(8), 671–678 (1985)
3. Prensky, M.: Digital Game-Based Learning. McGraw-Hill, New York (2001)
4. Stapleton, A.J., Taylor, P.C.: Physics and playstation too: learning physics with computer games. In: Australian Institute of Physics 15th Biennial Congress, Darling Harbour, NSW, 8–11 July 2002
5. Herz, J.C.: 50,000,000 star warriors can't be wrong. Wired (10) (2002)
6. Jenkins, H.: Game design as narrative architecture. In: Wardrip-Fruin, N., Harrigan, P. (eds.) First Person: New Media as Story, Performance, Game. MIT Press, Cambridge (2004). http://mediaartscultures.eu/jspui/bitstream/10002/616/1/FP-ch4.pdf. Accessed Feb 2018
7. The Woodrow Wilson International Center for Scholars (2006). http://www.wilsoncenter.org. Accessed 8 Oct 2006
8. Howell, K.: Games for health conference 2004: issues, trends, and needs unique to games for health. Cyberpsychology Behav. **8**(2), 103–109 (2005)
9. Lowood, H.: Game studies now, history of science then. Games Cult. **1**(1), 78–82 (2006)
10. Hero, J.O., Blendon, R.J., Zaslavsky, A.M., Campbell, A.L.: Understanding what makes Americans dissatisfied with their health care system: an international comparison. Health Aff. **35**(3), 502–509 (2016)
11. Pearlstein, S.: Free market philosophy doesn't always work for health care. Washington Post, 8 June 2005
12. Cain, L.P.: Annexation. In: The Electronic Encyclopedia of Chicago. Chicago Historical Society (2005). Accessed 8 Sept 2016
13. Wasserman, S., Faust, K.: Social Network Analysis: Methods and Applications. Cambridge University Press, Cambridge (1994)
14. Kneidinger, B.: Facebook und Co. VS Verlag für Sozialwissenschaften, Wiesbaden (2010). https://doi.org/10.1007/978-3-531-92455-7
15. Granovetter, M.S.: The strength of weak ties. Am. J. Soc. **78**(6), 1360–1380 (1973)
16. Rostila, M.: A resource-based theory of social capital for health research: can it help us bridge the individual and collective facets of the concept? Soc. Theory Health **9**(2), 109–129 (2011)
17. Christakis, N.A., Fowler, J.H.: The spread of obesity in a large social network over 32 years. N. Engl. J. Med. **357**(4), 370–379 (2007)

18. Cohen-Cole, E., Fletcher, J.M.: Is obesity contagious? Social networks vs. environmental factors in the obesity epidemic. J. Health Econ. **27**(5), 1382–1387 (2008)
19. Gershenson, C.: Epidemiology and social networks. Sociol. Methods **22**(1), 199–200 (2011)
20. Hammond, R.A.: Social influence and obesity. Curr. Opin. Endocrinol. Diab. Obes. **17**(5), 467–471 (2010)
21. Kaplan, A.M., Haenlein, M.: Users of the world, unite! The challenges and opportunities of social media. Bus. Horiz. **53**(1), 59–68 (2010)
22. Arnaboldi, V., Passarella, A., Tesconi, M., Gazze, D.: Towards a characterization of egocentric networks in online social networks. In: Proceedings of the Sixth International Workshop on Mobile and Networking Technologies for Social Applications, Crete (2011)
23. Boyd, D.M., Ellison, N.: Social network sites: definition, history, and scholarship. J. Comput.-Med. Commun. **13**(1), 210–230 (2007)
24. Hwang, K.O., et al.: Social support in an internet weight loss community. Int. J. Med. Inform. **79**(1), 5–13 (2010)
25. Maloney-Krichmar, D., Preece, J.: A multilevel analysis of sociability, usability, and community dynamics in an online health community. ACM Trans. Comput.-Hum. Interact. **12**(2), 1–32 (2005)
26. Ma, X., Chen, G., Xiao, J.: Analysis of an online health social network. In: IHI 2010, pp. 297–306 (2010)
27. WHO: Obesity and overweight (2011). http://www.who.int/mediacentre/factsheets/fs311/en/index.html. Accessed 11 July 2011
28. Hyyppä, M.T.: Healthy Ties. Springer, Dordrecht (2010). https://doi.org/10.1007/978-90-481-9606-7
29. Steiny, D.F.: Networks and persuasive messages. Commun. Assoc. Inform. Syst. **24**(1), 473–484 (2009)
30. WHO: Obesity: preventing and managing the global epidemic. Report of a WHO consultation. WHO Technical report Series 894, Geneva (2000)
31. McNeill, F.: A desistance paradigm for offender management. Criminol. Crim. Justice **6**(1), 39–62 (2006)
32. Fowler, J.H., Christakis, N.A.: Dynamic spread of happiness in a large social network: longitudinal analysis over 20 years in the Framingham Heart Study. BMJ **337**, a2338 (2008). https://doi.org/10.1136/bmj.a2338
33. BVDW: https://www.bvdw.org/presseserver/bvdw_socialmedia_kompass_2010/100818_bvdw_socialmedia_kompass_2010_final.pdf
34. Tetlock, P.E., Kim, J.: Accountability and judgment in a personality prediction task. J. Pers. Soc. Psychol. Attitudes Soc. Cogn. **52**, 700–709 (1987)
35. Nash, S.S.: Learning objects, learning object repositories, and learning theory: preliminary best practices for online courses. Interdiscip. J. Knowl. Learn. Objects **1**, 217–228 (2005)
36. Nash, S.S.: Social impact "Serious Games" and online courses (2005). http://www.xplanazine.com/archives/2005/06/social_impact_a.php. Accessed 5 Sept 2005
37. Peffers, K., Tuunanen, T., Rothenberger, M.A., Chatterjee, S.: A design science research methodology for information systems research. J. Manag. Inform. Syst. **24**(3), 45–77 (2007)
38. Hevner, A.R., et al. (2004). http://aisel.aisnet.org/misq/vol28/iss1/6/

Author Index

Printed in the United States
By Bookmasters